MW01701867

AMERICAN ACADEMY™
OF OPHTHALMOLOGY

1

Update on General Medicine

Last major revision 2015–2016

2016–2017

BCSC

Basic and Clinical Science Course™

Protecting Sight. Empowering Lives.™

Published after collaborative review with the European Board of Ophthalmology subcommittee

The American Academy of Ophthalmology is accredited by the Accreditation Council for Continuing Medical Education to provide continuing medical education for physicians.

The American Academy of Ophthalmology designates this enduring material for a maximum of 10 *AMA PRA Category 1 Credits*™. Physicians should claim only the credit commensurate with the extent of their participation in the activity.

CME expiration date: June 1, 2018. *AMA PRA Category 1 Credits*™ may be claimed only once between June 1, 2015, and the expiration date.

BCSC® volumes are designed to increase the physician's ophthalmic knowledge through study and review. Users of this activity are encouraged to read the text and then answer the study questions provided at the back of the book.

To claim *AMA PRA Category 1 Credits*™ upon completion of this activity, learners must demonstrate appropriate knowledge and participation in the activity by taking the posttest for Section 1 and achieving a score of 80% or higher. For further details, please see the instructions for requesting CME credit at the back of the book.

The Academy provides this material for educational purposes only. It is not intended to represent the only or best method or procedure in every case, nor to replace a physician's own judgment or give specific advice for case management. Including all indications, contraindications, side effects, and alternative agents for each drug or treatment is beyond the scope of this material. All information and recommendations should be verified, prior to use, with current information included in the manufacturers' package inserts or other independent sources, and considered in light of the patient's condition and history. Reference to certain drugs, instruments, and other products in this course is made for illustrative purposes only and is not intended to constitute an endorsement of such. Some material may include information on applications that are not considered community standard, that reflect indications not included in approved FDA labeling, or that are approved for use only in restricted research settings. **The FDA has stated that it is the responsibility of the physician to determine the FDA status of each drug or device he or she wishes to use, and to use them with appropriate, informed patient consent in compliance with applicable law.** The Academy specifically disclaims any and all liability for injury or other damages of any kind, from negligence or otherwise, for any and all claims that may arise from the use of any recommendations or other information contained herein.

Cover image: From BCSC Section 10, *Glaucoma.* Typical gonioscopic appearance of angle recession. *Courtesy of Steven T. Simmons, MD.*

FSC www.fsc.org MIX Paper from responsible sources FSC® C103061

Printed in the United States of America

Basic and Clinical Science Course

Louis B. Cantor, MD, Indianapolis, Indiana, *Senior Secretary for Clinical Education*
Christopher J. Rapuano, MD, Philadelphia, Pennsylvania, *Secretary for Ophthalmic Knowledge*
George A. Cioffi, MD, New York, New York, *BCSC Course Chair*

Section 1

Faculty

Herbert J. Ingraham, MD, *Chair,* Danville, Pennsylvania
A. Luisa Di Lorenzo, MD, Troy, Michigan
Maria Jancevski, MD, Birmingham, Michigan
Jaclyn L. Kovach, MD, Naples, Florida
Maria A. Woodward, MD, Ann Arbor, Michigan
A. Jan Berlin, MD, *Consultant,* Portland, Maine
Steven L. Mansberger, MD, MPH, *Consultant,* Portland, Oregon

The Academy wishes to acknowledge the following committees for review of this edition:

Vision Rehabilitation Committee: John D. Shepherd, MD, Omaha, Nebraska

Practicing Ophthalmologists Advisory Committee for Education: Steven J. Grosser, MD, *Primary Reviewer,* Golden Valley, Minnesota; James M. Mitchell, MD, *Primary Reviewer,* Edina, Minnesota; Edward K. Isbey III, MD, *Chair,* Asheville, North Carolina; Alice Bashinsky, MD, Asheville, North Carolina; David J. Browning, MD, PhD, Charlotte, North Carolina; Robert G. Fante, MD, Denver, Colorado; Bradley Fouraker, MD, Tampa, Florida; Dasa Gangadhar, MD, Wichita, Kansas; James A. Savage, MD, Memphis, Tennessee

EBO

European Board of Ophthalmology: Bahram Bodaghi, MD, PhD, *EBO Chair,* Paris, France; Christina N. Grupcheva, MD, PhD, FEBO, *EBO Liaison,* Varna, Bulgaria; Sébastien Abad, MD, PhD, Paris, France; Boris Bienvenu, MD, PhD, Caen, France; Sylvain Choquet, MD, Paris, France; Michel Drancourt, MD, PhD, Marseille, France; Thomas Hanslik, MD, PhD, Brest, France; Pierre Hausfater, MD, PhD, Paris, France; Gerard Helft, MD, PhD, Paris, France; Ina Kötter, MD, PhD, Hamburg, Germany; Frédérique Kuttenn, MD, Paris, France; Anne Leger, MD, Paris, France; David Saadoun, MD, PhD, Paris, France; Damien Sène, MD, PhD, Paris, France; Pascal Sève, MD, PhD, Lyon, France; Hélène Vallet, MD, Paris, France

Financial Disclosures

Academy staff members who contributed to the development of this product state that within the past 12 months, they have had no financial interest in or other relationship with any entity discussed in this course that produces, markets, resells, or distributes ophthalmic health care goods or services consumed by or used in patients, or with any competing commercial product or service.

The authors and reviewers state that within the past 12 months, they have had the following financial relationships:*

Dr Bienvenu: Crossject (C, L), CSL Behring (C), Genzyme (C), Octapharma (C), Sanofi (C)

Dr Bodaghi: Abbott Medical Optics (C), Allergan (C, S), Bausch + Lomb Surgical (C), Novartis Pharmaceuticals (S), Santen (C), Xoma (C)

Dr Browning: Aerpio (S), Alimera Sciences (C), Diabetic Retinopathy Clinical Research (S), Genentech (S), Novartis Pharmaceuticals (S), Pfizer (S), Regeneron Pharmaceuticals (S)

Dr Choquet: Celgene (L), Janssen (L), Roche France (C)

Dr Fante: Ophthalmic Mutual Insurance Company (C)

Dr Fouraker: Addition Technology (C), Alcon Laboratories (C), Keravision (C), Ophthalmic Mutual Insurance Company (C)

Dr Grosser: Ivantis (O)

Dr Grupcheva: Johnson & Johnson (L), Laboratoires Théa (L)

Dr Helft: Abbott (L), AstraZeneca (L), Bayer (L), Boehringer Ingelheim (C, L)

Dr Isbey: Alcon Laboratories (S), Allscripts (C), Bausch + Lomb (S), Medflow (C)

Dr Jancevski: Aldeyra Therapeutics (C)

Dr Kötter: AbbVie (L), Actelion (L), Bristol-Myers Squibb (L), Chugai (L), Novartis (S), Pfizer (L), Roche (S), UCB (L)

Dr Mansberger: Alcon Laboratories (C), Allergan (C, S), Envisia Therapeutics (C), Mobius (S), National Eye Institute (S), Santen (C)

Dr Savage: Allergan (L)

Dr Sève: Actelion (C), GSK (L), Pfizer (L), Sobi (L)

Dr Woodward: National Eye Institute (S)

*C = consultant fees, paid advisory boards, or fees for attending a meeting; L = lecture fees (honoraria), travel fees, or reimbursements when speaking at the invitation of a commercial sponsor; O = equity ownership/stock options of publicly or privately traded firms (excluding mutual funds) with manufacturers of commercial ophthalmic products or commercial ophthalmic services; P = patents and/or royalties that might be viewed as creating a potential conflict of interest; S = grant support for the past year (all sources) and all sources used for a specific talk or manuscript with no time limitation

The other authors and reviewers state that within the past 12 months, they have had no financial interest in or other relationship with any entity discussed in this course that produces, markets, resells, or distributes ophthalmic health care goods or services consumed by or used in patients, or with any competing commercial product or service.

Recent Past Faculty

James P. Bolling, MD
Anne Louise Coleman, MD, PhD
Eric P. Purdy, MD
Gwen Sterns, MD
Jonathan Walker, MD

In addition, the Academy gratefully acknowledges the contributions of numerous past faculty and advisory committee members who have played an important role in the development of previous editions of the Basic and Clinical Science Course.

American Academy of Ophthalmology Staff

Dale E. Fajardo, *Vice President, Education*
Beth Wilson, *Director, Continuing Professional Development*
Ann McGuire, *Acquisitions and Development Manager*
Stephanie Tanaka, *Publications Manager*
D. Jean Ray, *Production Manager*
Beth Collins, *Medical Editor*
Naomi Ruiz, *Editorial Assistant*

American Academy of Ophthalmology
655 Beach Street
Box 7424
San Francisco, CA 94120-7424

Contents

General Introduction

The Basic and Clinical Science Course (BCSC) is designed to meet the needs of residents and practitioners for a comprehensive yet concise curriculum of the field of ophthalmology. The BCSC has developed from its original brief outline format, which relied heavily on outside readings, to a more convenient and educationally useful self-contained text. The Academy updates and revises the course annually, with the goals of integrating the basic science and clinical practice of ophthalmology and of keeping ophthalmologists current with new developments in the various subspecialties.

The BCSC incorporates the effort and expertise of more than 80 ophthalmologists, organized into 13 Section faculties, working with Academy editorial staff. In addition, the course continues to benefit from many lasting contributions made by the faculties of previous editions. Members of the Academy's Practicing Ophthalmologists Advisory Committee for Education, Committee on Aging, and Vision Rehabilitation Committee review every volume before major revisions. Members of the European Board of Ophthalmology, organized into Section faculties, also review each volume before major revisions, focusing primarily on differences between American and European ophthalmology practice.

Organization of the Course

The Basic and Clinical Science Course comprises 13 volumes, incorporating fundamental ophthalmic knowledge, subspecialty areas, and special topics:

1 Update on General Medicine
2 Fundamentals and Principles of Ophthalmology
3 Clinical Optics
4 Ophthalmic Pathology and Intraocular Tumors
5 Neuro-Ophthalmology
6 Pediatric Ophthalmology and Strabismus
7 Orbit, Eyelids, and Lacrimal System
8 External Disease and Cornea
9 Intraocular Inflammation and Uveitis
10 Glaucoma
11 Lens and Cataract
12 Retina and Vitreous
13 Refractive Surgery

In addition, a comprehensive Master Index allows the reader to easily locate subjects throughout the entire series.

References

Readers who wish to explore specific topics in greater detail may consult the references cited within each chapter and listed in the Basic Texts section at the back of the book.

These references are intended to be selective rather than exhaustive, chosen by the BCSC faculty as being important, current, and readily available to residents and practitioners.

Study Questions and CME Credit

Each volume of the BCSC is designed as an independent study activity for ophthalmology residents and practitioners. The learning objectives for this volume are given on page 1. The text, illustrations, and references provide the information necessary to achieve the objectives; the study questions allow readers to test their understanding of the material and their mastery of the objectives. Physicians who wish to claim CME credit for this educational activity may do so online by following the instructions at the end of the book.

Conclusion

The Basic and Clinical Science Course has expanded greatly over the years, with the addition of much new text and numerous illustrations. Recent editions have sought to place a greater emphasis on clinical applicability while maintaining a solid foundation in basic science. As with any educational program, it reflects the experience of its authors. As its faculties change and as medicine progresses, new viewpoints are always emerging on controversial subjects and techniques. Not all alternate approaches can be included in this series; as with any educational endeavor, the learner should seek additional sources, including such carefully balanced opinions as the Academy's Preferred Practice Patterns.

The BCSC faculty and staff are continually striving to improve the educational usefulness of the course; you, the reader, can contribute to this ongoing process. If you have any suggestions or questions about the series, please do not hesitate to contact the faculty or the editors.

The authors, editors, and reviewers hope that your study of the BCSC will be of lasting value and that each Section will serve as a practical resource for quality patient care.

Objectives

Upon completion of BCSC Section 1, *Update on General Medicine,* the reader should be able to

- describe the various factors to consider in critically reviewing clinical research
- explain the importance of the randomized, controlled clinical study in evaluating the effects of new treatments
- describe the classification, pathophysiology, and presentation of diabetes mellitus, as well as the diagnostic criteria for this disease
- describe the various therapeutic approaches for diabetes mellitus, including new insulins and oral agents
- classify the levels of hypertension by blood pressure measurements
- list the major classes of antihypertensive medications and some of their characteristics and adverse effects
- discuss the indications for dietary and pharmacologic treatment of hypercholesterolemia
- describe the various diagnostic procedures used in the evaluation of patients with coronary artery disease
- state the current treatment options for ischemic heart disease, heart failure, and cardiac arrhythmias
- list the common causes of stroke in patients encountered by ophthalmologists
- distinguish between obstructive and restrictive, reversible and irreversible, pulmonary diseases, and give examples of each type
- discuss the major behavioral disorders and possible therapeutic modalities for these conditions (including the ocular adverse effects of psychoactive medications)

- list some of the factors associated with a patient's adherence or nonadherence to medical regimens
- explain the rationale for and value of screening programs for various systemic diseases
- discuss the major disease processes affecting most of the adult population, and briefly explain how preventive measures may reduce the morbidity and mortality that these diseases cause
- list the most prevalent types of cancer for men and for women together with the appropriate screening methods for detecting them
- describe current concepts about the etiologies of most malignancies
- describe traditional as well as more novel approaches to the treatment of various types of cancer
- describe the ophthalmic manifestations of the major systemic diseases covered in this volume
- list the most common human pathogens and their manifestations
- discuss the epidemiology, clinical features, and treatment of human immunodeficiency virus infection
- list the newer antiviral, antifungal, and antibacterial agents and their benefits and adverse effects
- describe the early manifestations and treatment of malignant hyperthermia
- describe the current American Heart Association guidelines for performing cardiopulmonary resuscitation

CHAPTER 1

Using Statistics in Clinical Practice

Ophthalmologists use clinical research to establish best practices for patient care. Clinical research can be complex, requiring an interdisciplinary group of clinicians, statisticians, and epidemiologists to design the study, analyze the data, and interpret the results. Researchers choose a study design based on the research questions, the population available, and the required resources and effort. This chapter will help the clinician understand how to critically review clinical research and apply the results in the clinical practice of ophthalmology.

Researching Answers to Clinical Questions

Formulating the clinical question is the first step in resolving a diagnostic or management issue. Examples of clinical questions in ophthalmology include: What is the prevalence of glaucoma in African Americans? Do racial and ethnic minority populations in the United States have a higher risk of proliferative vitreoretinopathy after pars plana vitrectomy? What is the expected survival of a corneal graft in a patient with Fuchs dystrophy?

Clinicians can use several sources of information to research the answers to their questions. These include general textbooks on ophthalmology (eg, *Duane's Ophthalmology*), journals with detailed reviews on specific subjects (eg, *Survey of Ophthalmology* [www.surveyophthalmol.com]), and educational material from the American Academy of Ophthalmology (www.aao.org/one) (eg, Preferred Practice Pattern guidelines, *Focal Points* modules). In addition, clinicians can use the Cochrane Library (www.thecochranelibrary.com) to access high-quality meta-analyses regarding specific management issues (eg, surgery for nonarteritic ischemic optic neuropathy, intervention for involutional lower-eyelid ectropion).

For more specific questions and data, clinicians can search online for primary sources of information using PubMed (www.ncbi.nlm.nih.gov/pubmed). PubMed provides detailed instructions on using appropriate keywords. PubMed usually identifies the type of study: from laboratory-based studies of basic science (eg, cell culture, molecular biology) to animal studies (eg, testing of new drugs or specific surgical techniques) to clinical studies (eg, case reports, case series, randomized controlled trials). The search can be narrowed based on the type of study desired.

In evaluating a published study, and before committing time to critical reading, the clinician should review the abstract for the study purpose and methods to ascertain whether the study addresses the question of interest. For example, if the clinician is interested in determining whether use of a prostaglandin is beneficial in patients with open-angle glaucoma (OAG), examining data from the Early Manifest Glaucoma Trial (EMGT) would not be useful because prostaglandins were not used in the EMGT. Data from specific drug trials, on the other hand, would be pertinent. However, if the question is whether lowering intraocular pressure (IOP) is beneficial in patients with OAG, then both types of studies might be useful.

Crucial Questions in Study Evaluation

This section describes the steps to take to discern whether the study is valid and applicable to the clinician's specific patients rather than applicable to only specific types of patients. Also, it is necessary to consider the recruitment strategy and characteristics of the study participants, sample size, intervention, outcomes of interest, and statistical methods used.

Are the results generalizable to my patients?

Is there a clear description of the process of selecting study participants (which patients were included or excluded)? This description lays the groundwork for understanding the setting of the study. Was it a clinic-based, multicenter, or community-based trial? For therapeutic trials, patient inclusion and exclusion criteria outline characteristics of those who were or were not treated with an intervention. Specific patient groups may have been excluded because they were considered a vulnerable population. For example, most trials of ocular hypotensive drugs exclude children and pregnant women; as a result, there are minimal data on the safety and efficacy of most ocular hypotensive agents in these 2 groups of patients. Thus, if the clinician must decide whether to use a specific ocular hypotensive agent in a pregnant woman or in a child, most of the evidence can be found only in individual case reports or retrospective case series.

The clinician must next ascertain whether the results can be directly applied to particular patients. The first step in this process is exploring whether the study created selection bias by assigning the intervention to certain participants. Was the intervention randomly assigned? Was the treated group comparable to the control group? The purpose of randomly assigning an intervention to participants is to minimize bias on the part of the investigators and the patient. For example, an investigator may create selection bias by inadvertently enrolling less complex patients for a new surgery, potentially biasing their outcomes toward better results.

Random allocation reduces the likelihood of selection bias. However, it does not always ensure that the participants assigned to each group are similar. To answer this question, the clinician must examine baseline participant characteristics that may affect the outcome. For example, when evaluating a study assessing the effect of lasers for treatment of diabetic retinopathy, the clinician should examine whether patients' hemoglobin A_{1c} levels, blood pressure, and other factors are similar between study groups, as these factors may alter the progression of retinopathy. Use of a control group is also important because it indicates whether the results of the intervention are above and beyond the effects of participants' enrollment in a trial.

The severity of disease is another factor to consider to establish whether the results can be applied to the clinician's patients. Did the study include only a single disease severity group, or did it include different stages of disease, such as mild, moderate, and severe disease? Clinical trials may study a narrow subset of a disease, making the results applicable and generalizable only to similar patients. A common error is extrapolating such data to all patients and their varying degrees of disease severity. For example, if a particular treatment effect size is noted in patients with mild glaucomatous damage who underwent trabeculectomy but not in those with advanced glaucomatous damage, the study results should be applied only to similar patients—in this case, patients with mild glaucomatous damage.

Was the sample large enough to detect a difference?

Was the sample size (the number of participants in the study) established before the trial began and, if so, what criteria were used to determine the sample size? The sample size must have enough power to reject the null hypothesis. The *null hypothesis* is no difference (in the outcome of interest) exists in the group that received the intervention compared with the group that did not receive the intervention. A study must have enough power to reject the null hypothesis if a true difference exists between the groups. *Power* depends on the sample size, the expected difference in the outcome of interest (eg, improvement in visual acuity, resolution of macular edema) in the intervention group compared with the control group, and the variability (eg, standard deviation) of the outcome of interest. In general, an intervention with a larger treatment effect and smaller variability requires a smaller sample size.

Is the intervention reproducible?

The study should describe the intervention in enough detail to allow the experiment to be replicated. For example, a surgical study should explain all the steps of the procedure to allow different surgeons to perform it in the same manner in each case. Did all surgeons involved in the study perform it similarly, and were all of their results similar? Did the study include a training session before the start of the study, monitor specific aspects of the surgical procedure, and standardize postoperative care? In general, a study should avoid differences in study procedures except in regard to the intervention of interest.

Is the outcome clearly defined and reliable?

The outcomes of interest are usually specific to the disease being studied. At the outset of a study, the primary and secondary outcomes should be clearly stated. These outcomes are then used to determine whether the study was able to prove or disprove the null hypothesis. In most studies, the outcome of interest, as well as the expected change in this outcome, must be defined. For example, if the primary outcome is improvement in visual acuity, the study should indicate the logMAR value that represents improvement, the range, the distribution of results (eg, normal, skewed to the right or left), and the variability.

Many outcomes (eg, visual acuity, IOP, macular thickness as measured with optical coherence tomography [OCT]) will have measurement error. This measurement error will increase the variability of the outcome of interest or create a difference in results when no true difference in outcomes exists. Therefore, a study should standardize measurement of the outcome of interest for all investigators. For example, the Ocular Hypertension Treatment Study created a standardized method to check IOP. The "recorder" placed the tonometry dial at 20 mm Hg while an "observer" measured the IOP and adjusted the dial to the intersection of the tonometry mires without viewing the dial. Finally, the recorder recorded the IOP measurement and changed the dial back to 20 mm Hg, then repeated the measurement sequence. The sequence was repeated a third time if the measurements differed by 2 mm Hg. By using a masked recorder and observer and repeating testing, the study created a standardized method intended to decrease measurement error and the variability of IOP measurement.

Also, the study should try to mask the observer to the intervention to decrease the risk of investigator bias. *Investigator bias* may occur when the investigator expects a different result in the intervention group and adjusts his or her measurement of the outcome of interest to satisfy this expectation. Instead, a study should measure the outcome of interest as accurately and reliably as possible. If it does not, the study may underestimate or overestimate the effect of the intervention or encounter higher variability in the outcome of interest, affecting the conclusion of the study.

Was the follow-up long enough?

The validity of a study is anchored on (1) adequate duration of follow-up and (2) follow-up of all participants. Thus, in evaluating a study, the clinician should ask, How many of the participants completed follow-up? Did the study report outcomes for all participants? For example, in a study assessing the use of atropine eyedrops versus patching for treatment of amblyopia, a follow-up of 3–6 months may be adequate; similar follow-up periods may be appropriate for tracking macular edema resolution after laser or drug therapy or visual acuity improvement after cataract extraction. Conversely, glaucoma progresses over long periods; therefore, trials assessing visual field loss in glaucoma would require longer follow-up, such as 5 years. Consequently, the typical rate of disease progression is an important guide in establishing the duration of follow-up required.

The study should report the results for all participants. This may not be practical or feasible in all cases because of dropout from a study (eg, due to death during follow-up). The study should report the reasons for loss to follow-up and report any differences in reasons between the study groups. For example, participants in the intervention group of a drug trial may be more likely to drop out than those in the placebo group if they experience ocular adverse effects from the drug, such as burning or stinging.

Are the treatments and outcomes clinically relevant?

The clinician should ascertain whether the study's results can be applied to his or her patients. Questions to consider include the following:

- Is the intervention available and applicable to the current practice environment?
- Are the outcomes clinically important?

- Are all clinically important outcomes evaluated?
- Is the treatment difference clinically significant?

It is important to consider whether the intervention is useful in practice. It may be too expensive, too difficult to perform, or no longer in general use. If so, the study may pose little benefit to current clinical care.

Is the analysis appropriate for the outcome?

Statistical tests depend on the type of data used to determine the difference between 2 treatment groups. If the data are normally distributed (ie, they conform more or less to a bell-shaped curve) and are continuous (eg, macular thickness in a trial assessing the use of intravitreal corticosteroids for treatment of diabetic macular edema), then a Student *t*-test comparing the intervention and control groups can be performed. For continuous data that are not normally distributed, researchers can utilize nonparametric tests such as the Wilcoxon rank sum test. For categorical data (present or absent; small, medium, or large), the study may use a chi-square test. All of these tests provide a *P* value, which indicates the likelihood that a difference between the 2 groups is due to chance alone. Thus, a *P* value of <.05 suggests that the likelihood that the difference between the 2 groups is due to chance alone is less than 5%. The lower the *P* value, the less likely it is that the difference is due to chance and the more likely it is that the difference represents a true difference.

Is the difference between the groups clinically significant?

It is important to consider whether the difference in results between the 2 groups is clinically significant. For example, if a statistically significant difference in visual acuity is only 2 letters on a Snellen chart, this difference may not be clinically noticeable to patients and may be within the margin of measurement error for visual acuity. Thus, even though a statistical test may suggest a statistically significant difference, the clinician should consider whether the magnitude and nature of the difference are clinically meaningful. In addition to evaluating these primary outcome variables, the study should evaluate secondary clinically important variables related to the safety of the intervention. These variables include dropout rates, pain, and allergic reactions.

Understanding Study Design

Clinical research uses a wide array of study designs. In *observational studies,* also known as *nonexperimental studies,* investigators evaluate characteristics, behaviors, and exposures in participants with a particular disease, condition, or complication. The study only reports the characteristics of the study population; it does not directly manipulate behaviors (eg, cigarette smoking) or exposures (eg, use of a medication, laser treatment). In *experimental studies,* typically clinical trials, the study assigns subjects to a particular treatment, such as a prescribed behavior (eg, eating a diet high in antioxidant foods), or a therapeutic or preventive intervention (eg, use of an oral neuroprotective agent for patients with glaucoma, antioxidant vitamin supplementation for patients with early age-related macular degeneration [AMD]).

Each type of study design may provide valuable information when conducted and interpreted appropriately. Researchers employ observational studies when describing the presentation and progression of disease, generating hypotheses, and efficiently assessing data that may already exist for testing a hypothesis about an intervention. These include case reports, case series, case-control studies, cross-sectional studies, and cohort studies. In contrast, prospective randomized controlled trials provide the best evidence regarding the effects of an intervention. Finally, meta-analyses provide a methodology to summarize the results of multiple clinical trials addressing similar research questions. Figure 1-1 depicts the levels of evidence that can be obtained from different study designs; note that meta-analyses and controlled trials offer the highest levels of evidence.

Case Reports

A case report describes a finding in regard to a single patient to help others recognize a rare condition or unusual treatment result. For example, Friedman reported retinal vasculitis in an apparently healthy patient with none of the common causes of vasculitis, such as toxoplasmosis, syphilis, Behçet disease, sarcoidosis, lupus, or herpes. A magnetic resonance imaging scan of the brain revealed findings typical of multiple sclerosis (MS). Although clinicians recognize that retinal vasculitis develops in MS patients, this study was the first to report retinal vasculitis as the initial presentation of MS. This case report demonstrated that clinicians should consider MS when they have tested for more common causes of vasculitis, but the etiology remains unclear.

Case reports cannot provide information on treatment efficacy or assert whether a disease is caused by an exposure. At most, they can suggest a previously unsuspected finding or mechanism of disease.

Friedman SM. Retinal vasculitis as the initial presentation of multiple sclerosis. *Retina.* 2005;25(2):218–219.

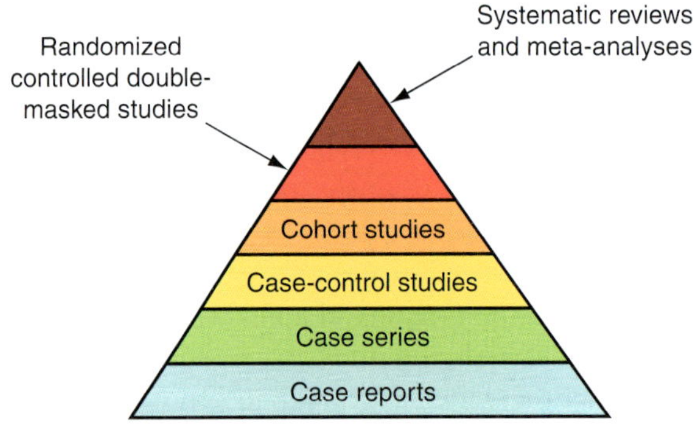

Figure 1-1 The pyramid of evidence, which illustrates the relative strength of different study designs. *(Modified with permission from Medical Research Library of Brooklyn. Guide to Research Methods: the Evidence Pyramid. EBM Tutorial.* http://library.downstate.edu/EBM2/2100.htm.*)*

Case Series

Case series investigate the presentation, history, and/or follow-up of a group of patients and provide valuable information on the natural history or prognosis of a disease. Case series may differ in regard to patient selection, patient characteristics, and length and completeness of follow-up; these characteristics may establish the quality and applicability of a case series.

Case series may include patients with severe disease from tertiary referral centers such as university-based clinics. For example, Margherio and colleagues retrospectively described consecutive patients with choroidal neovascularization secondary to AMD and evaluated the benefit of thermal laser treatment compared with photodynamic therapy using verteporfin. However, eye care providers referred to the authors patients whose macular degeneration lesions were too large to be treated with a thermal laser. Therefore, the case series included a higher proportion of patients who may not have benefited from thermal laser treatment, creating selection bias favoring photodynamic therapy.

Case series might not standardize the collection of patient information, measurements, tests, and other evaluations. This may result in underreporting or overreporting of results. For example, the technicians, examination rooms, lighting, and charts used to measure visual acuity may differ within clinics. Or study personnel may record visual acuity differently; for example, some may record the nearest whole line (20/25) while others record to the letter (20/25 + 2).

Lengths of follow-up may vary within a single case series. For example, follow-up periods for a case series of patients enrolled from 1996 to 2000 that includes a chart review in 2005 will range from 5 to 9 years. This difference in follow-up time requires that the study report specific follow-up times, such as 1, 2, and 3 years after the initiation of treatment. When the outcome being measured is an event, such as corneal graft failure, survival analysis can account for the varying lengths of follow-up. If not all patients are followed for the full length of the possible follow-up period, the reported outlook for the case series may be biased because of losses to follow-up. When a case series is based on review of medical records, losses to follow-up may be strongly related to how the patient fares over time. For example, in a case series of patients with macular edema from branch retinal vein occlusion, some patients may choose not to return because their macular edema has resolved and their vision has improved, some patients may experience further loss of vision and seek care from another ophthalmologist, and some patients may move to another location. When a large percentage of patients have not returned for complete follow-up, the study results may not be valid because the remaining subjects may have had an unusually good or unusually bad course compared with the subjects lost to follow-up. Despite these caveats, case series may provide critical preliminary data for a clinical trial.

Margherio RR, Margherio AR, DeSantis ME. Laser treatments with verteporfin therapy and its potential impact on retinal practices. *Retina.* 2000;20(4):325–330.

Case-Control Studies

Figure 1-2 illustrates the structure of case-control studies. Case-control studies investigate a hypothesis about the association between exposures or potential risk factors (eg,

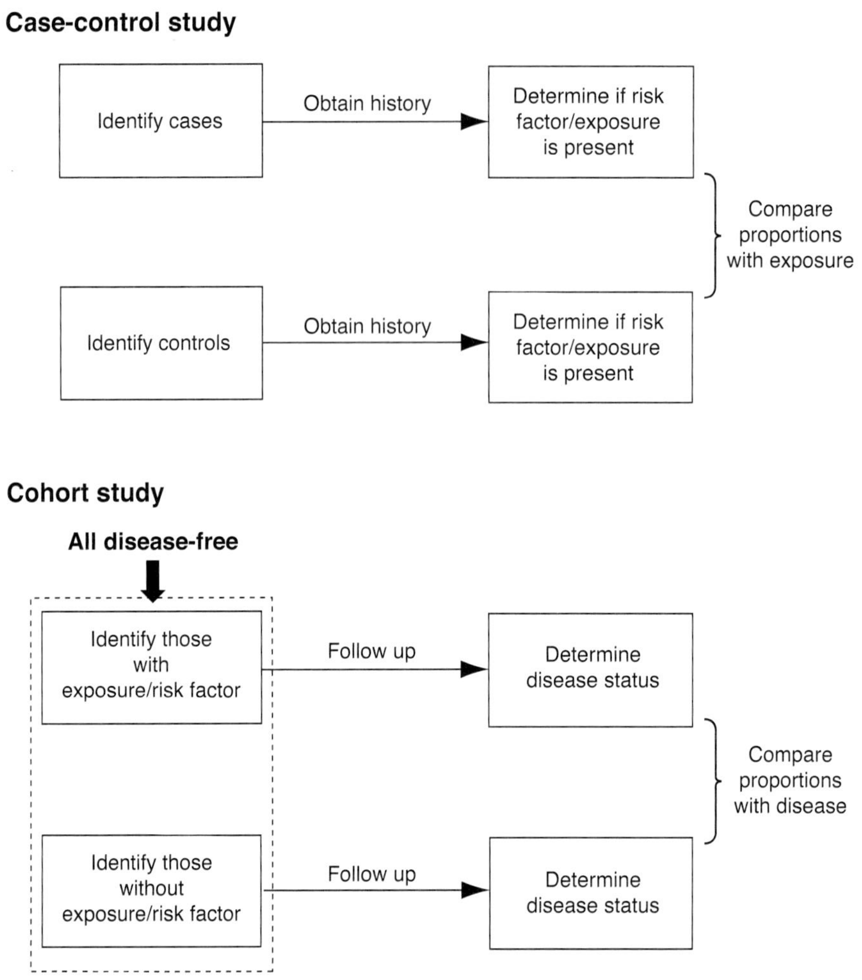

Figure 1-2 Simplified schematics of observational study designs.

smoking, medical conditions, therapies) and outcomes of interest (eg, loss of visual acuity, development of glaucoma, corneal graft failure, complications of cataract surgery). Case-control studies select a group of participants with the disease of interest (cases) and a group of comparable individuals who are free of disease (controls). The study compares the past exposures and characteristics of the 2 groups to determine whether differences exist between the groups. If so, the study will conclude that the exposures or characteristics that differ are associated with the disease.

Researchers select cases and controls from a current database and obtain the history of exposures through patient survey and/or review of medical records. Thus, researchers can perform case-control studies more quickly and inexpensively than cohort studies (discussed later in the chapter) because cohort studies require extra time and money to follow participants. At the time of record review or patient interview, case-control studies can collect data on many potential risk factors simultaneously.

However, exposure data may be less accurate in case-control studies than in cohort studies. For example, patients with retinal vein occlusion (cases) may be more likely than control patients to recall taking medications (eg, aspirin) in the past because control patients do not have a disease to motivate them to scrutinize their past behavior. Therefore, a higher proportion of cases than controls might report use of aspirin in the past 6 months, even if in truth the proportion of aspirin users was the same in both cases and controls. This *recall bias* in cases may strengthen the association between aspirin use and vein occlusion.

Case-control studies may be subject to selection bias if they do not have an appropriate control group. For example, a study may show a protective effect of myopia on retinal vein occlusion if it collects cases from a retinal group but collects controls from a general ophthalmology practice that offers refractive surgery for myopia. The proportion of individuals with myopia would be smaller among the cases (from the retinal group) than among the controls (from the general practice). The study may conclude that myopia is protective against retinal vein occlusion, but the apparent association would be attributable to selection bias. The interested reader may consult general epidemiology textbooks such as the following to learn more about other sources of bias.

Rothman KJ, Greenland S, Lash TL. *Modern Epidemiology.* 3rd, mid-cycle revision ed. Philadelphia: Lippincott Williams & Wilkins; 2012.

Cross-sectional Studies

Cross-sectional studies correlate exposures and risk factors with the presence of disease without the benefit of knowing the timing or sequence of exposure and disease development. An example of a cross-sectional study is one in which a researcher collects a blood sample from patients and records their lens status (phakic, pseudophakic, or aphakic) at the same time. The study could evaluate the association between a history of cataract surgery (case status) and cholesterol level and gender (potential risk factors). However, if the mean cholesterol level is higher in cases than in those without a history of cataract surgery, the researcher would not know whether the elevated cholesterol level occurred before cataract surgery. With this study design, it is also important to consider whether a *confounding factor* may be affecting the association. For this study, age could be a confounding factor, because cholesterol levels increase with age, as does the likelihood of cataract surgery. The researcher could use data analysis tools such as stratification and/or regression analysis to adjust for age and then determine whether the cholesterol–cataract surgery association is still present in each of the age strata.

Cohort Studies

Researchers may use cohort, or follow-up, studies to investigate the association between exposures or potential risk factors and patient outcomes. These studies identify subjects who are free of the disease of interest and classify them by the presence or absence of potential risk factors. Then, the study follows them for subsequent development of the disease of interest (see Fig 1-2).

The Beaver Dam Eye Study is an example of a population-based cohort study with prospective data collection. This study examined and interviewed approximately 5000 residents of Beaver Dam, Wisconsin, and followed them longitudinally for the incidence of ocular disease. Researchers explored potential risk factors for diseases such as AMD, diabetic retinopathy, glaucoma, and cataract using the residents' exposures at the beginning of the study and the incidence of the diseases 10 years later. For example, the investigators classified participants who did not develop advanced AMD according to a number of potential risk factors (age, gender, presence of pigmentary changes, drusen characteristics) and examined the association between these risk factors and progression to advanced AMD over 10 years. The 10-year incidence of advanced AMD was 15.1% among eyes with pigmentary changes in the retina and 0.4% among eyes without pigmentary changes; the incidence was 20.0% among eyes with soft, indistinct drusen and 0.8% among eyes without such drusen. This is an example of prospectively assessing the risk factor (retinal findings) for an outcome of interest (advanced AMD).

Cohort studies may also collect data retrospectively. For example, Strahlman and colleagues examined risk factors for choroidal neovascularization in the second eye of patients who already had neovascularization in the first eye. They captured retinal photographs for the fellow eye when the patient presented with neovascularization in the first eye. After several years, the investigators examined patients for the development of neovascularization in the second eye. The study found that large, confluent drusen were associated with a higher risk of neovascularization in the second eye. Because they used retinal photographs from the patients' medical records, their cohort study is considered retrospective. Also, the study is a cohort study (rather than a retrospective case series) because it classified patients based on their earlier fellow-eye drusen status and compared the incidence of neovascularization between the groups with and without confluent drusen.

Cohort studies can provide associations between risk factors and disease. The primary weakness of this study design is that participants with the risk factor of interest may differ in many ways from those without the risk factor, and those other characteristics may affect the incidence of the disease. One example relates to the higher incidence of graft failure among patients with interrupted sutures. It would be inaccurate to conclude that use of interrupted sutures increases the risk of graft failure because ophthalmologists use interrupted sutures in patients with a preexisting risk of graft failure, such as stromal vascularization. In this example, stromal vascularization is a confounding factor. Statistical analysis techniques, such as stratified analysis and regression analysis, can adjust for the effect of known confounding factors. However, quite often, investigators do not understand all of the factors that affect the incidence of disease. For this reason, cohort studies may identify associations and disease incidence, but these associations are not considered causal.

Klein R, Klein BE, Tomany SC, Meuer SM, Huang GH. Ten-year incidence and progression of age-related maculopathy: the Beaver Dam Eye Study. *Ophthalmology.* 2002;109(10): 1767–1779.

Strahlman ER, Fine SL, Hillis A. The second eye of patients with senile macular degeneration. *Arch Ophthalmol.* 1983;101(8):1191–1193.

Clinical Trials

Figure 1-3 demonstrates the major difference between clinical trials and cohort studies: clinical trials randomly assign patients to different treatment groups (exposure groups). Random assignment yields treatment groups with similar characteristics in regard to variables that may alter outcomes or the risk of complications from the treatment. This control of confounding factors is a major advantage of clinical trials over other study designs.

However, randomization does not necessarily make the study results valid. All of the previously mentioned features of high-quality observational studies, such as the following, should also be applied to randomized controlled trials:

- a well-defined research question and objectives
- explicit inclusion and exclusion criteria
- an adequate sample size
- standardized procedures
- predefined, objective primary and secondary outcomes
- masking of patients, treating clinicians, and evaluators to the assigned treatment
- complete follow-up of all patients

The CONSORT (Consolidated Standards of Reporting Trials) Statement, an evidence-based set of recommendations, includes a checklist of features that should be included in the design and reporting of clinical trials.

When evaluating a clinical trial, the clinician should consider 2 issues in addition to the other features of high-quality studies. The first is whether the study excluded patients from data analysis because they did not meet all of the eligibility criteria, experienced adverse effects and stopped treatment, or did not adhere to the treatment regimen. Exclusion of these types of patients creates biased results because the excluded patients' results may differ from those of the patients included in the analysis. For this reason, clinical

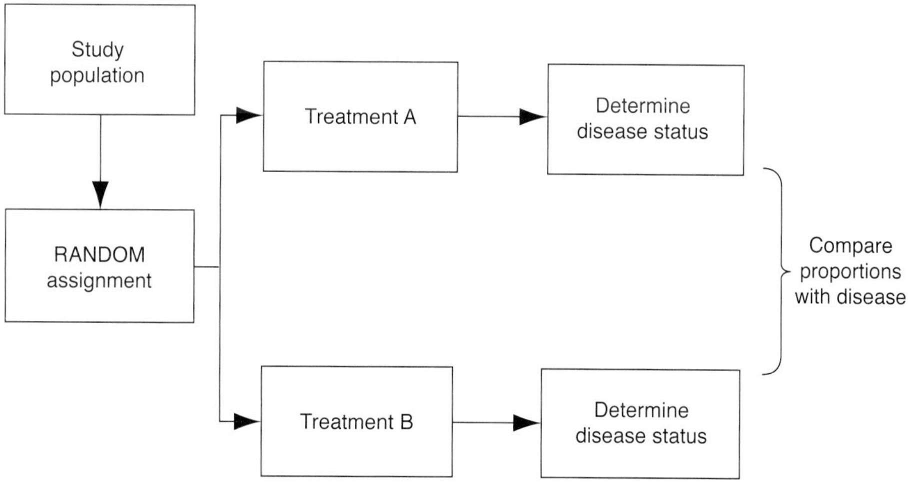

Figure 1-3 Simplified schematic of a randomized controlled trial.

trials should include an intention-to-treat analysis, which includes the data from all enrolled participants, and separate analyses of those who completed the trial and those who did not.

Results from subgroups of patients (eg, young vs old, hypertensive vs nonhypertensive) should be regarded with suspicion. By statistical chance alone, a study can identify a subgroup of patients for whom the benefit of treatment is statistically significant. A subgroup evaluation may be considered valid if the investigators identified the subgroup a priori in the study design, treatment results vary similarly across subgroups (eg, success steadily decreases in each age stratum as the participants become younger), and a biologically plausible explanation exists for the finding.

Systematic Reviews and Meta-analyses of Clinical Trials

Figure 1-1 shows that systematic reviews and meta-analyses provide the strongest evidence for assessing interventions for a particular condition. They do so by combining evidence from 2 or more clinical trials. For example, Calladine and colleagues reviewed the results of multicenter and single-center randomized controlled trials of the use of multifocal versus monofocal intraocular lenses after cataract extraction. Using special statistical methods for combining data from multiple trials, they found no statistically significant difference between use of the 2 lens types in distance visual acuity. However, they found the following statistically significant differences: better near vision and less need for glasses but a higher prevalence of glare, halos, and reduced contrast sensitivity with the use of multifocal lenses.

Calladine D, Evans JR, Shah S, Leyland M. Multifocal versus monofocal intraocular lenses after cataract extraction. *Cochrane Database Syst Rev.* 2012;9:CD003169.

Schulz KF, Altman DG, Moher D; CONSORT Group. CONSORT 2010 statement: updated guidelines for reporting parallel group randomised trials. *Ann Intern Med.* 2010;152(11): 726–732.

Interpreting Diagnostic and Screening Tests

The subsequent paragraphs will help the reader interpret diagnostic and screening tests. The first example is a relatively straightforward case; it involves a screening test with a binary (yes/no) outcome, a disease that the patient definitely either has or does not have, and a patient about whom nothing is known at the time of screening. The subsequent discussions examine complicating features that often occur in ophthalmic practice and in research. The reader should consider these complicating features when evaluating results of diagnostic and screening tests.

The Straightforward Case

A fictitious study evaluates use of a strabismus test in 100 children and finds, using examination for comparison, that 30 children have strabismus and 70 do not. But using the screening test, 60 children have abnormal results and 40 children have normal results. Table 1-1 shows the screening test result data. The screening test performance is described as follows:

- *Sensitivity:* The test correctly identifies 20 of every 30 children who have strabismus (67%). The denominator is all those with the disease (strabismus).
- *Specificity:* The test correctly identifies 30 of every 70 children who do not have strabismus (43%). The denominator is all those without the disease (normal).
- *Positive predictive value (PPV):* If a child has abnormal test results, there is only a 1 in 3 chance (20/60) that the child actually has strabismus (33%). The denominator is all those with abnormal results.
- *Negative predictive value (NPV):* If a child has normal test results, the child has a 3 in 4 chance (30/40) of actually being disease-free (75%). The denominator is all those with normal results.
- *Accuracy:* The screening test is correct in 50 of 100 cases (50%).

Sensitivity is the percentage of those who have the disease of interest and have abnormal results, and *specificity* is the percentage of disease-free people who have normal results. Confidence limits can be stated for both sensitivity and specificity, based in large part on the sample size used. However, an important caveat is that neither sensitivity nor specificity takes into account the prevalence of disease in the study population.

Table 1-2 illustrates the performance of the hypothetical strabismus test if it finds the same results (60 children with abnormal results and 40 children with normal results) when performed in a shopping center where the prevalence of strabismus is only 3% (much lower than in the situation previously discussed). The sensitivity is still 67%, and the specificity is about the same at 41%. However, because of the high number of falsely abnormal results, 58 disease-free children and only 2 truly strabismic children would be referred for complete examinations. In this example, the PPV is only 3% (2/60). The NPV is 98% (39/40). Because of the low prevalence of strabismus in this setting, most children

Table 1-1 Results for Strabismus Screening Test in Clinic

Screening Test Result	Strabismus	No Strabismus	Totals
Abnormal	Truly abnormal (20)	Falsely abnormal (40)	60
Normal	Falsely normal (10)	Truly normal (30)	40
Totals	30	70	100

Table 1-2 Results for Strabismus Screening Test in Shopping Center

Screening Test Result	Strabismus	No Strabismus	Totals
Abnormal	Truly abnormal (2)	Falsely abnormal (58)	60
Normal	Falsely normal (1)	Truly normal (39)	40
Totals	3	97	100

whose results were abnormal were actually disease-free. This increases the cost of unnecessary follow-up testing and increases anxiety for the parent. Clearly, the prevalence of disease in the population of interest and the screening test's PPV and NPV should be considered before the test is used for screening a population.

Complicating Features

Using ROC curves to compare different screening thresholds with a continuous predictive variable

It is more complicated when the screening test measures a continuous value, such as IOP. Figure 1-4 uses data from the Baltimore Eye Survey to graphically display sensitivity and specificity for each value of IOP. The figure shows that the usual cutoff for normal IOP, 21 mm Hg, has a sensitivity of 91% but a specificity of only 47%. The intersection of the sensitivity and specificity is the optimal threshold for maximum sensitivity and specificity in a screening test. This occurs at 18 mm Hg, where the sensitivity is 65% and the specificity is 66%. Figure 1-4 also shows that continuous variables, like IOP, have a trade-off between sensitivity and specificity: a higher sensitivity results in a lower specificity and vice versa.

Figure 1-5 shows a *receiver operating characteristic (ROC) curve*—another graphical representation of sensitivity and specificity. By convention, an ROC curve plots sensitivity on the y-axis and (1 – specificity) on the x-axis. The larger the area under the curve, the more diagnostically precise is the screening test. The line with the diamond-shaped symbols represents a hypothetical optimal screening test, the line with the triangles represents a poor screening test with an ROC area of only 50%, and the line with the circles—the

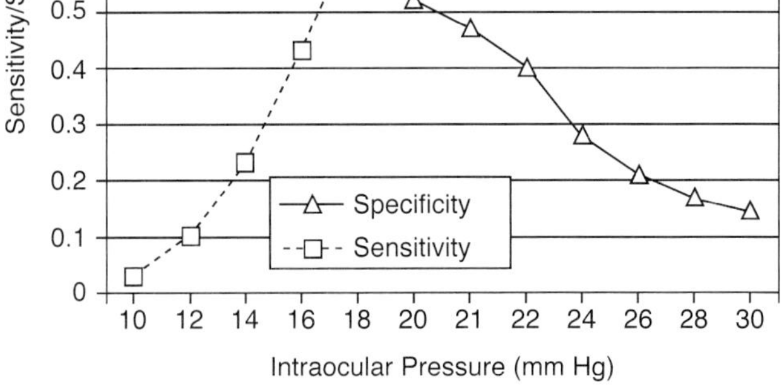

Figure 1-4 Sensitivity and specificity of intraocular pressure (IOP) as a screening tool for glaucoma. For each IOP level (along the x-axis), the values for sensitivity and specificity are plotted. *(Used with permission from Tielsch JM, Katz J, Singh K, et al. A population-based evaluation of glaucoma screening: the Baltimore Eye Survey.* Am J Epidemiol. *1991;134(10):1102–1110.)*

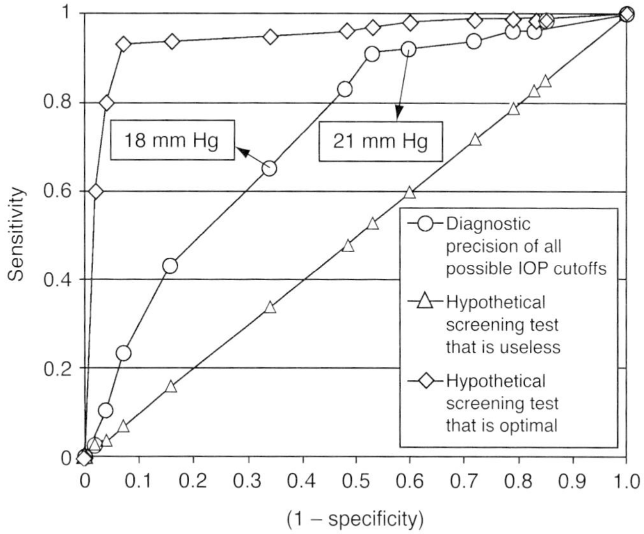

Figure 1-5 Receiver operating characteristic (ROC) curve of IOP as a screening tool for glaucoma with sensitivity on the y-axis and (1 – specificity) on the x-axis. The middle line replots the data from Figure 1-4, showing all combinations of IOP. Two boxes identify the diagnostic precision of IOP ≥18 mm Hg and IOP ≥21 mm Hg. The other lines represent an optimal and a useless screening test, respectively. *(Data from Tielsch JM, Katz J, Singh K, et al. A population-based evaluation of glaucoma screening: the Baltimore Eye Survey.* Am J Epidemiol. *1991;134(10):1102–1110.)*

middle curve—represents the Baltimore Eye Survey data from Figure 1-4. An ROC curve can inform selection of an optimal cutoff point for a screening test by identifying the sensitivity–specificity pair located closest to the upper left of the ROC plot.

Overall, these figures demonstrate that IOP measurement is not a very good screening tool for glaucoma. Other significant factors in choosing a cutoff point for a screening test are the population to be screened and the relative importance of sensitivity and specificity. If the consequence of missing a diagnosis is blindness, an investigator may choose a test with high sensitivity but poor specificity. For example, a low cutoff for erythrocyte sedimentation rate might be chosen for a person who has recent vision loss and who is suspected of having giant cell arteritis.

Tielsch JM, Katz J, Singh K, et al. A population-based evaluation of glaucoma screening: the Baltimore Eye Survey. *Am J Epidemiol.* 1991;134(10):1102–1110.

Using ROC curves to compare different screening devices

In this next example, the disease, glaucoma, is a continuum from no damage to severe damage and cannot be diagnosed with the first loss of a ganglion cell. But even without the benefit of longitudinal follow-up to diagnose glaucoma using a change in the visual field or optic disc, studies can compare new diagnostic tests using ROC curves. ROC curves can be used to compare tests using different units or different scales. Figure 1-6 depicts ROC curves illustrating the ability of 3 devices to discriminate between healthy eyes and eyes with glaucomatous visual field loss using imaging of the optic disc and nerve fiber layer. The area under the ROC curve represents a summary measure of the relative

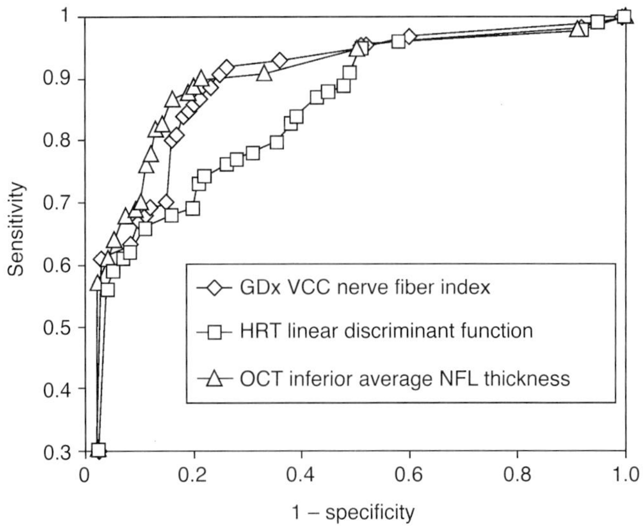

Figure 1-6 ROC curve of 3 glaucoma imaging devices. The single parameter chosen for display for each instrument was the one that performed the best in the authors' study. There was no statistically significant difference in the area under the ROC curves for these 3 parameters. *(The HRT linear discriminant function is from a paper by Bathija et al, referenced by Medeiros et al; the GDx and OCT parameters are standard test outputs provided by the manufacturers. Graph drawn with data from Medeiros FA, Zangwill LM, Bowd C, Weinreb RN. Comparison of the GDx VCC scanning laser polarimeter, HRT II confocal scanning laser ophthalmoscope, and Stratus OCT optical coherence tomograph for the detection of glaucoma.* Arch Ophthalmol. *2004;122(6):827–837.)*

efficacy of screening tests. The ROC curves appear similar for inferior average nerve fiber layer thickness as measured with OCT and scanning laser polarimetry with variable corneal compensation (GDx VCC nerve fiber index), while the ROC curve for confocal scanning laser ophthalmoscopy (HRT linear discriminant function) is lower. Overall, the figure suggests a higher diagnostic precision for scanning laser polarimetry and OCT than confocal scanning laser ophthalmoscopy.

Medeiros FA, Zangwill LM, Bowd C, Weinreb RN. Comparison of the GDx VCC scanning laser polarimeter, HRT II confocal scanning laser ophthalmoscope, and Stratus OCT optical coherence tomograph for the detection of glaucoma. *Arch Ophthalmol.* 2004;122(6):827–837.

The effect of pretest probability of disease

This case uses knowledge of the patient before performance of the screening or diagnostic test. For example, the investigator may know that the patient has a first-degree relative with glaucoma and has a thinner-than-average central corneal thickness (both risk factors for glaucoma). Overall, this information suggests a pretest probability of glaucoma 3 times as high as that of a person picked at random from the general population. How much does a diagnostic test improve the ability to diagnose glaucoma in this patient? How much higher is the relative risk of glaucoma if the test result is positive?

Bayes theorem allows the pretest probability of disease to be combined with the diagnostic precision of a screening test to produce a posttest probability of disease. To use this theorem, the *likelihood ratio* must be calculated. The likelihood ratio of a positive test is the sensitivity divided by (1 – specificity). For a test with 80% sensitivity and 90% specificity (0.8/[1 – 0.9]), the positive likelihood ratio is 8. The likelihood ratio of a negative test is (1 – sensitivity) divided by specificity. For the same test, the negative likelihood ratio is (1 – 0.8)/0.9, or 0.22. Positive likelihood ratios start at 1 and continue to infinity—the bigger, the better. Negative likelihood ratios range from 0 to 1; the smaller, the better. If the goal is to diagnose disease, the test with the larger positive likelihood ratio is the better test; conversely, if the goal is to rule out disease, the test with the smaller negative likelihood ratio is better.

If the positive likelihood ratio is multiplied by the pretest probability of disease, the result is the *posttest probability of disease.* Thus, for the example patient with the positive family history, thin cornea, and pretest probability of 3, a positive test with a positive likelihood ratio of 8 will result in a posttest probability of glaucoma that is 24 times that of a person drawn at random from the population.

Table 1-3 demonstrates another important consideration regarding pretest probability of disease. Consider the case of a 65-year-old woman with no risk factors for glaucoma and a pretest probability of disease of 1.0%. A positive test result for glaucoma would raise her probability of disease to 7.5%. Most patients with a positive test result would not actually have the disease! Similarly, an 85-year-old man with a strong positive family history, thin central corneal thickness, and an IOP of 30 mm Hg might have a pretest probability of disease of 50.0%. If his test result were negative, he would still have a posttest probability of disease of 18.2%, greater than that of the 65-year-old woman! This example illustrates the importance of considering the pretest probability of disease in deciding whether to employ a diagnostic test. In general, screening tests do not perform well when the prevalence of disease is low.

Intermediate diagnostic categories, such as "glaucoma suspect," are often encountered in clinical practice. Likelihood ratios can account for this category in analysis, while sensitivity–specificity and ROC curves cannot because they require that borderline subjects be categorized as either having the disease (eg, glaucoma) or not having it (eg, no glaucoma). However, a likelihood ratio can be calculated for a borderline category, which reflects the risk of patients exhibiting that characteristic (eg, "glaucoma suspect").

Use of tests in combination

Studies can combine tests in series or in parallel. An example of combining 2 tests *in series* is when a clinician performs the second test only if the first is positive. Consider the following case. OCT is used as a diagnostic test, and if the result is positive, scanning laser

Table 1-3 Changes in PPV and NPV Depending on Pretest Probability in a Test With 80% Sensitivity, 90% Specificity

Pretest Probability of Disease, %	Positive Predictive Value (PPV), %	Negative Predictive Value (NPV), %
1	7.5	99.8
10	47.1	97.6
50	88.9	81.8
90	98.6	33.3

polarimetry with variable corneal compensation is employed. Medeiros and colleagues provide likelihood ratios for each test. Although it may be tempting to use the product of the 2 likelihood ratios and the pretest probability to calculate a posttest probability, the predictive ability will appear artificially higher if the screening tests are correlated with one another. Since OCT and scanning laser polarimetry both measure nerve fiber layer thickness, albeit using different technologies, they are highly correlated. Because the 2 tests are not independent, the actual performance of the 2-test strategy is likely to be disappointing in comparison with the posttest probability calculated from the product of the 2 likelihood ratios and the pretest probability. The correlation between 2 tests must be considered when they are used in series.

Other researchers have combined 2 tests *in parallel* and considered the result positive if either test result is positive. This strategy works best when the 2 tests have good specificity (because combining tests this way makes overall specificity deteriorate) and address different aspects of a disease. A clinical example is combining a structural test (eg, optic nerve imaging test) and a functional test (eg, visual field test) to determine whether glaucoma is present.

Medeiros FA, Zangwill LM, Bowd C, Weinreb RN. Comparison of the GDx VCC scanning laser polarimeter, HRT II confocal scanning laser ophthalmoscope, and Stratus OCT optical coherence tomograph for the detection of glaucoma. *Arch Ophthalmol.* 2004;122(6):827–837.

Clinical acceptance and ethics of testing

Clinicians should avoid tests that provide a small increment in the likelihood ratio of detecting disease or that are expensive or painful. In addition, all tests carry some burden, including the potential for adverse effects (eg, corneal abrasion from tonometry), psychological fear of a disease (eg, related to a screening test for glaucoma), and additional testing and follow-up examinations for abnormal or unusual results. A clinician should avoid a test if it will not change the management of the patient. Similarly, screening for eye disease should include a process for follow-up of those who have abnormal results, regardless of their insurance status. Screening provides little value to participants who are told they might have a disease but are given no method of obtaining follow-up evaluation and treatment.

Generalizability

Most studies investigate new screening or diagnostic tests in a clinic setting before evaluating them in a population-based sample (largely because of the high cost of performing population-based research). Clinicians should consider whether the data for a new test will apply to their screening population. Even a clinic-based study may not have patients similar to those of another practice. For example, a study may include only young glaucoma patients without other eye diseases, such as macular degeneration. This leads to excellent sensitivity and specificity, but the results may differ in a sample of patients who have borderline glaucoma and are older.

Summary

Researchers use a variety of measures to evaluate the diagnostic precision of screening and diagnostic tests. Sensitivity and specificity are the simplest and easiest to understand, but their disadvantage is that they do not account for the prevalence of disease in the target population. PPV and NPV are more useful in that regard. ROC curves provide a comprehensive view of the relationship between the sensitivity and specificity of a continuous test result (eg, IOP) and can be used to compare diagnostic tests. Clinicians can use likelihood ratios and pretest probability of disease to critically evaluate screening and diagnostic tests in their clinical setting.

Riegelman RK. *Reading Evidence-based Health Research.* 6th ed. Philadelphia: Lippincott Williams & Wilkins; 2012.

Discussing Benefits, Risks, Probabilities, and Expected Outcomes With Patients

Physicians and their clinical team members need to educate patients regarding their disease, including potential preventive measures, treatments, and outcomes. Although increasingly complex scientific analyses have made the interpretation of findings challenging at times, physicians must be able to interpret them for patients.

Most clinical studies present research findings as a percentage or absolute measure of change in a disease status (eg, presence of AMD) or in a continuous outcome (eg, IOP). Concrete findings such as these can easily be discussed with patients. However, discussing odds ratios and concepts such as absolute and relative risk is more difficult. In everyday language, risk is defined as an expected loss within a distribution of possible outcomes; for example, homeowners buy insurance to guard against the risk of fire damage. However, clinical research defines *risk* as the conditional probability of an event, usually an adverse event. The condition might be as basic as survival to a particular point or exposure to some phenomenon—for example, persons "at risk" for disease or "in the risk set."

In research, 2 measures are commonly used to compare risk between groups of individuals. *Risk difference* is the absolute difference in the risk between the groups. *Relative risk* is the ratio of 2 risk measures. The risk difference depends on the unit of measure, whereas relative risk is dimensionless because it involves division of 2 risk measurements. In the Ocular Hypertension Treatment Study (OHTS), the risk difference of glaucoma development for subjects who were not treated compared with those who were treated was 5% (9.5% – 4.5%) across 5 years. The relative risk of not being treated compared with receiving treatment was 211% (9.5%/4.5%). Both of these measures are consistent with the data, but clinicians may interpret them very differently. Numerically, a 5% increased risk of glaucoma (if ocular hypertension is not treated) might seem small to a patient, while a 211% increased risk might seem large. A key piece of information that may help in the interpretation is the *baseline probability of the outcome.* In everyday life, people may be willing to board an airplane, doubling their relative risk of accidental death, because the baseline probability of an adverse outcome is so low. In this context, if there is a choice between 2 airlines and the risk difference is 5% per million miles flown, the risk difference would not seem small. Thus, baseline probabilities or expected outcomes can help people make decisions. This is especially true when the risk ratio is less than 100% and may be wrongly interpreted as a risk difference. For example, if the adverse outcome rate is 10%

in Group 1 and 13% in Group 2, the relative risk is approximately 1.3 (13%/10%) of having an adverse outcome in Group 2, but to those unfamiliar with the baseline probabilities, this 30% increase in risk may make it sound as though the comparison were between 10% and 40%, when the risk difference was much smaller at 3% (13% – 10% = 3%).

In observational studies, investigators may present their results as *odds ratios*. In an odds ratio, the odds of a subject with the disease (case) having an exposure (eg, smoking) are compared with the odds of a subject without the disease (control) having the exposure. When the disease is rare, the odds ratio approximates the relative risk of the exposure, because the denominators for both the odds being compared are close to 1. For example, in the meta-analyses on potential risk factors for late AMD, which occurs relatively infrequently, the odds ratio for smoking is 2.35. This means that smokers have a 235% risk for development of late AMD compared with nonsmokers.

A *risk factor* is a factor that patients are exposed to, either voluntarily or not, and that is associated with an increased or decreased likelihood of disease. Thus, risk factors may influence the occurrence of a disease. Exposure to specific factors may or may not be clinically significant. For example, use of seat belts may not be a clinically significant exposure for AMD, whereas smoking is. One of the subsets of risk factors is *causal risk factors*, which are root causes of the disease. Because it is difficult to distinguish causal risk factors from noncausal risk factors in observational studies, researchers often use causal criteria to identify which risk factors are causal and which are not.

When interpreting research findings from clinical trials or observational studies, clinicians should consider the generalizability of the findings to individual patients. Questions include the following: Do the study inclusion criteria contain elements that apply to the patient? Can the findings be extrapolated to the patient? The distinction between an *individual effect* and an *average effect* is important. For example, in the OHTS, the investigators reported that a 1 mm Hg increase in IOP was associated with an approximately 10% increase in the risk of glaucoma development. Does this necessarily mean that lowering IOP by 1 mm Hg in all patients with ocular hypertension would decrease the overall risk of glaucoma in each patient by 10%, or does it mean that some patients would experience a risk reduction of more than 10% and others, less? The study results suggest an average effect on the overall population of patients with ocular hypertension and not on an individual patient. However, risk calculators may use population data to estimate risks in individual patients.

Medical providers use *risk calculators* to predict an individual patient's risk of cardiovascular disease, risk of having a child with Down syndrome, likelihood of survival from an intensive care unit, and likelihood of experiencing other medical conditions. Recently, ophthalmologists have used risk calculators to help simplify complex study results and apply them to individual patients. For example, the OHTS regression equation predicted the risk of developing glaucoma from ocular hypertension by using the 5 variables of cup–disc ratio, central corneal thickness, untreated IOP, pattern standard deviation from the visual field, and age. The OHTS risk calculator is available for free online (http://ohts.wustl.edu/risk/calculator.html). Other risk calculators include those for macular degeneration, keratoconus, and glaucoma progression. Also, many risk calculators can be downloaded onto a mobile device. Overall, the advantage of risk calculators is that they simplify complex results to provide an estimate of the mean probability of disease development in individual patients.

Kass MA, Heuer DK, Higginbotham EJ, et al. The Ocular Hypertension Treatment Study: a randomized trial determines that topical ocular hypotensive medication delays or prevents the onset of primary open-angle glaucoma. *Arch Ophthalmol.* 2002;120(6):701–713.

Mansberger SL. A risk calculator to determine the probability of glaucoma. *J Glaucoma.* 2004; 13(4):345–347.

Rubin DB. Bayesian inference for causal effects: the role of randomization. *Ann Stat.* 1978; 6(1):34–58.

Smoking and Health: Report of the Advisory Committee to the Surgeon General of the Public Health Service. Washington, DC: Public Health Service, US Dept of Health, Education, and Welfare; 1964. Public Health Service publication 1103.

Tomany SC, Wang JJ, Van Leeuwen R, et al. Risk factors for incident age-related macular degeneration: pooled findings from 3 continents. *Ophthalmology.* 2004;111(7):1280–1287.

Applying Statistics to Measure and Improve Clinical Practice

Studies have demonstrated large regional differences in practice and in the quality of eye care in the United States and worldwide. These differences suggest opportunities to measure and improve eye care. Donabedian created an organizational framework for quality by separating it into 3 distinct elements—structure, process, and outcomes. *Structure* refers to how the care system is designed, such as whom the patient sees initially; what pathways exist for obtaining various diagnostic tests; and what the financial arrangements are for care reimbursement. *Process* is the content of care: what the provider does or does not do. The principle that drives process quality is "doing the right thing at the right time," to which structure adds "by the right person at the right place." *Outcomes* are the results of care, or the completion of the principle "so that the right results occur." The final component of system improvement is a process for providing feedback to the group to improve performance over time.

Committee on Quality of Health Care in America, Institute of Medicine. *Crossing the Quality Chasm: A New Health System for the 21st Century.* Washington, DC: National Academies Press; 2001.

Donabedian A. Evaluating the quality of medical care. *Milbank Mem Fund Q.* 1966;44(3): Suppl:166–206.

Issues in Designing a Measurement System

A useful measurement system includes indicators that reflect the quality or characteristic to be assessed. This is called *validity.* One question ophthalmologists commonly face is whether they have dilated a diabetic patient's eye at least once every 2 years. What might indicate that a valid dilated eye examination was performed? Several options may be cumbersome to obtain. One method would be to video-record an ophthalmologist performing examinations and review the recording for completion of the dilated eye examination. Other options may include (1) documentation indicating that dilating drops were placed in the eye; (2) notations in the medical record indicating that a peripheral dilated eye examination was performed, such as "P" or "periphery," and noting whether it was normal or abnormal; and (3) a diagram or drawing of the retina, on which the periphery or peripheral findings are indicated. All of these would be valid measures. Their absence in the medical record would suggest that the ophthalmologist did not dilate the eye.

Once a valid measure has been chosen, *reliability* needs to be determined—that is, whether the measure produces the same results when it is repeated under a different set of assessment conditions but without a change in the underlying document or service being assessed. How exactly might conditions change? First, the analysis should yield the same results if performed by the same clinician at a different time. For example, a clinician reviewing a medical record may be distracted or tired. Are the same results obtained when the measure is made with the same instrument the second time and the third? Measures that are designed to minimize errors when repeated are described as having good *test–retest reliability,* or reproducibility. Second, the analysis should yield the same results if performed on the same subject multiple times. If the person doing the measurement gets the same results on the same subject, with multiple attempts, there is good *intrarater reliability.* Third, the analysis should yield the same results if performed by different clinicians. Organizations should design measures (and the training system and support system that will capture and analyze the data) to allow different people to use the same measure and obtain similar results. Measures that have this characteristic are said to have good *interrater reliability.*

In research, 2 statistical techniques are commonly used to determine the degree of agreement between 2 different tests that detect a particular disease in a group of patients. One method is to simply tally the number of times that the results of the 2 tests agree (both tests indicate disease present, both tests indicate no disease) and then divide that number by the total number of items being assessed, thereby yielding the *percent agreement.* Another method, the κ (kappa) statistic, measures the agreement between 2 or more individuals or entities while taking into account the potential for agreement via chance alone. Kappas greater than 0.75 represent excellent agreement; those from 0.40 to 0.75, fair to good agreement; and those below 0.40, poor agreement. However, experts do not agree on these kappa cutoff points and may recommend other cutoffs for agreement.

Once a valid and reliable measure has been established, the organization should first consider the population of interest and the inclusion and exclusion criteria. For example, a study of the quality of cataract surgery might exclude retina specialists (exclusion criterion) and include only comprehensive ophthalmologists who spend at least 50% of their time seeing patients (inclusion criterion).

Second, the organization needs to determine whether the population of interest experiences the studied event at a frequency that will allow meaningful differences to be found. Or are the events so rare ("floor effect") or so common ("ceiling effect") that little value is to be gained in using such a measurement system? Organizations should consider conducting a pilot analysis to investigate these issues before they implement their system.

Third, organizations should use measures that are easily obtained, yet are valid and reliable, whenever possible. Systems that do not require much additional work are more practical for the purpose of monitoring practices. Thus, billing files may provide sufficient information on the completion of specific process quality steps, such as the performance of regular visual field testing in patients with glaucoma, and outcomes, such as suprachoroidal hemorrhage after intraocular surgery.

Implementation of a Monitoring System

An ideal monitoring system would capture data regarding every patient of interest for a given practitioner. Doing so collects the maximum number of cases for statistical analyses and provides maximum statistical power for reliable estimates of uncommon or rare events. In addition, a 100% analysis minimizes bias due to missing patients. For example, electronic billing data could identify every patient who had intraocular surgery (identified by specific Current Procedural Terminology [CPT] codes) in a practice during a specified period and any subsequent surgeries (again identified by CPT codes) within the next 30 or 90 days to identify a specific complication (identified by International Classification of Diseases code), such as retinal detachment or endophthalmitis.

In contrast, questions about process quality—such as whether a target pressure range was set for every patient with glaucoma—are not amenable to a 100% review because that type of data may not be entered in current administrative databases and may need to be extracted from medical records by a trained reviewer. Billing databases may allow assessment of other process quality measures, such as gonioscopy.

An organization's next step is to review the records. What standards should be used for a review? What criteria should be used? Explicit criteria with a yes/no outcome or limited categories (eg, optic nerve documentation could include a statement regarding the nerve's condition, the vertical cup–disc ratio, or a drawing or photograph) have higher reliability than implicit criteria (the reviewer's judgment that overall quality was good or not good), particularly for interrater reliability. For ophthalmology, the American Academy of Ophthalmology (AAO) provides the Preferred Practice Pattern guidelines and summary benchmarks series, both of which can be used to obtain explicit criteria. Similarly, the American Board of Ophthalmology has explicit criteria in its Practice Improvement Modules for maintenance of board certification. These are available at http://one.aao.org/guidelines-browse and at www.abop.org, respectively.

In reviews, medical records may be unavailable or may be missing data or visits. Every effort should be made to obtain unavailable records. If these records remain unavailable, the number of unavailable records is recorded, and replacement records from the randomization should be reviewed. A high proportion of missing medical records may suggest bias. For records with missing visits, it may be possible to capture important data from other available visits. If the review criteria require that every visit be checked, the options are to (1) exclude that patient, (2) exclude that patient only for analyses needing that missing-visit data, (3) impute the missing values through statistical modeling of available data, or (4) treat the missing visit as either meeting or not meeting the criteria (generally the latter). The key steps are to decide what to do and then apply that decision consistently over time (and report the decision with the data and results). Finally, studies usually consider missing data as not meeting the review criteria—which is, in essence, determining whether something is or is not documented in the medical record.

An important element of establishing a system for monitoring quality of care is performing power calculations to determine sample sizes, as these calculations provide confidence that a nonsignificant difference is truly that (and is not due to having an insufficient sample size). See the section "Was the sample large enough to detect a difference?"

One consideration is the validity of the method used to determine whether a quality measure was met. Using chart review, McGlynn and colleagues determined that the rate of annual dilated eye examination among patients with diabetes mellitus was only 19%. But when they used billing codes, they found that the rate was 50%. Was the discrepancy due to poor documentation of the procedure or inaccurate billing practices? These may be systematic errors. The data may have been recorded incorrectly, by either the observer or the person abstracting the data from the data source. Errors related to administrative databases include coding issues, data entry problems, and incorrect diagnoses. Errors related to record review approaches, in addition to those already mentioned, include those made by the abstractor and those made during calculation of quality scores. These errors can be minimized by (1) training all personnel in advance, (2) reviewing cases with values outside the expected range, and (3) duplicating review of a 5%–10% sample of cases.

AAO introduced its IRIS (Intelligent Research in Sight) Registry in 2013. The registry is a centralized system for collecting electronic eye care data from ophthalmology practices; it abstracts data from modern electronic medical record systems automatically. Goals for the registry are to provide benchmark reports for quality of care and identify opportunities for improvement. It also creates large data sets for diseases such as AMD, cataract, and glaucoma, facilitating exploration of trends in treatment, costs, and other factors. It also allows collection of data regarding rare diseases, such as retinitis pigmentosa. This may be an important tool to help ophthalmologists continually monitor and improve their quality performance.

McGlynn EA, Asch SM, Adams J, et al. The quality of health care delivered to adults in the United States. *N Engl J Med.* 2003;348(26):2635–2645.

Analysis of the Results

Once the results have been compiled, organizations must interpret the data correctly. For projects designed to detect important deviations from expected performance, it is important to use statistical tests that determine statistical significance. For many measures, comparisons of mean performance are satisfactory—as in the percentage of AAO benchmark process indicators for cataract that every provider has achieved. However, for others, the best way to compare performance may be to use the number of patients whose care meets a given threshold. For example, investigators may want to know the percentage of patients who have at least a 90% quality score. Once they have obtained that measure, they can compare it among providers.

Even if differences are found to be statistically significant, they still may not be clinically meaningful. The greater the sample size, the more likely it is that a statistically significant difference can be found. For example, one provider may document the optic nerve 78% of the time; another provider, 81% of the time. With a large enough sample size, this difference can be statistically significant. However, is it clinically meaningful? Does this difference show that one doctor is technically of higher quality than the other? Indeed, an appreciation of clinically significant differences is very useful for calculating the sample sizes in the first place.

In addition, investigators should consider factors beyond the provider's control when evaluating quality results. Patients could refuse the cost of additional tests or refuse to be dilated because they need to drive. Outcomes of chronic diseases are even more difficult to evaluate than process measures such as dilation of a diabetic patient. For example, the rate of blindness from glaucoma over 20 years is subject to the physiologic severity on presentation and the risk for progression among the pool of patients. Quality of care for chronic diseases like glaucoma may be affected by patients' ability to return for regular care and use their recommended treatments regularly, as well as their socioeconomic status. Thus, measuring whether the provider performs specific examination steps, such as examining the optic nerve (process), is appropriate, whereas looking at rates of blindness over 20 years (outcomes) may not be appropriate.

Organizations can use statistical analyses to evaluate potential differences in quality between providers. They can control for patients' socioeconomic status and demographic characteristics, as well as other factors that may be related to the outcome of interest. These analyses may show that a factor that cannot be "treated" by the provider (eg, socioeconomic status) is the issue and is outside the provider's control. Even with these caveats, quality improvement is critical to medicine. In addition, the purpose is not to be punitive but to encourage improvement in all providers and improvement in individual providers from year to year.

Methods of Presenting Data to Facilitate Continuous Improvement

The next step in improving care processes and structures is to graphically display and disseminate the results. Studies suggest that just measuring and reporting results improves performance indicators by up to 6%. However, organizations that continually incorporate quality improvement activities demonstrate significantly greater performance gains than organizations that do not. Further information about continuous quality improvement and total quality management can be obtained from other sources.

There are many ways to present data. First, the data can be displayed using a frequency distribution such as a histogram (Fig 1-7) or using a scatter diagram (Fig 1-8). Are the data *normally distributed* (ie, distributed in a bell-shaped curve), or are they skewed? The answer to this question affects the selection of statistical tools and analyses, and it can provide important insights into potential underlying factors. Or, 2 distinct subgroups may be found in the data and need to be defined. For example, care in solo practices may differ from care in large single-specialty groups for a particular disease area.

Second, use of a Pareto chart (Fig 1-9) provides insights into the cumulative distribution of key factors of interest. The chart combines a histogram with a cumulative frequency line, making it possible to assess performance across the range of values for the variable of interest.

Third, use of run charts or control charts (Fig 1-10) can help organizations understand changes over time. Rates of events, especially uncommon ones, can fluctuate over time. Are the fluctuations significant, both statistically and clinically, compared with those of prior periods or other institutions or practices? In run and control charts, event rates are plotted over time with both upper and lower control limits and averages. This enables reviewers to determine (1) whether an aberrant data point is really a meaningful finding

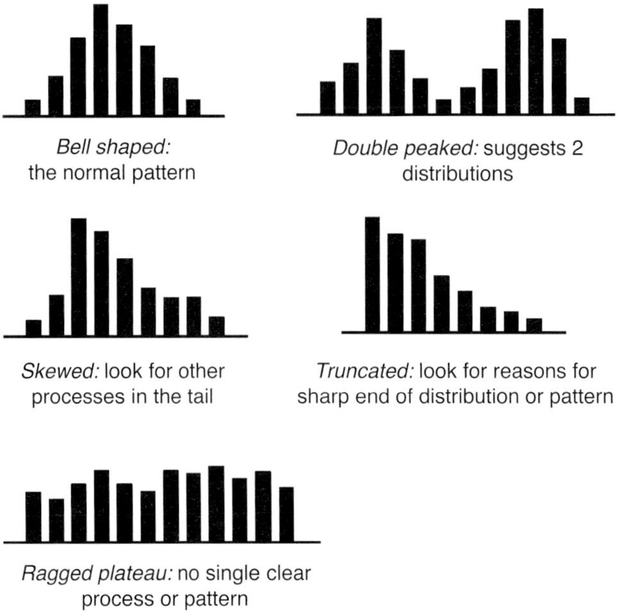

Figure 1-7 Types of histograms. *(Reproduced from the Quality Assurance Project.)*

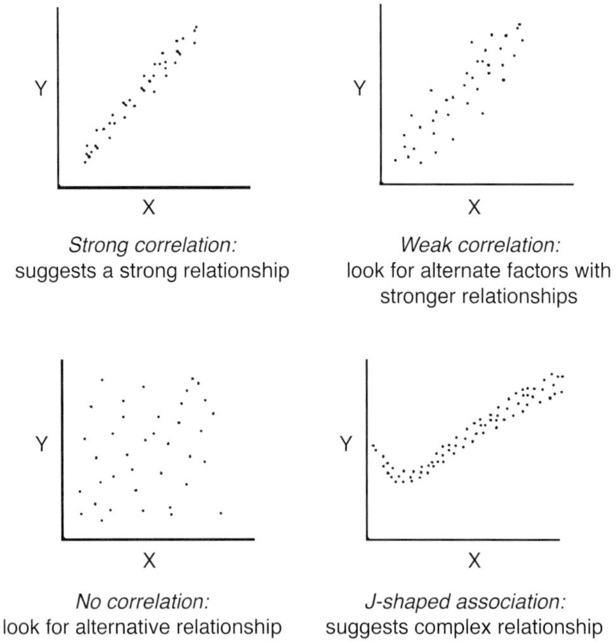

Figure 1-8 Scatter diagram interpretation. *(Reproduced from the Quality Assurance Project.)*

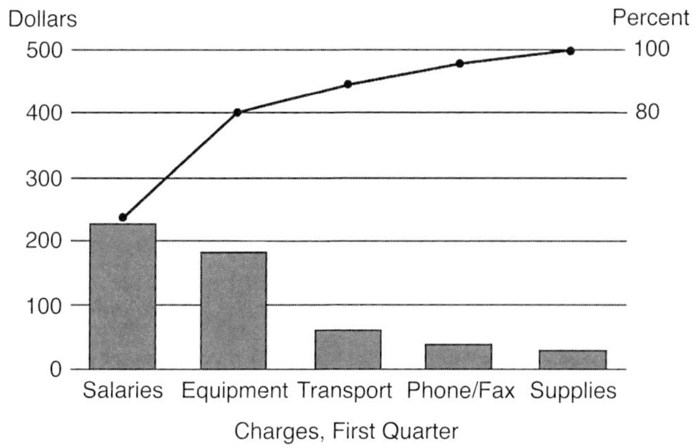

Figure 1-9 Pareto chart. *(Reproduced from the Quality Assurance Project.)*

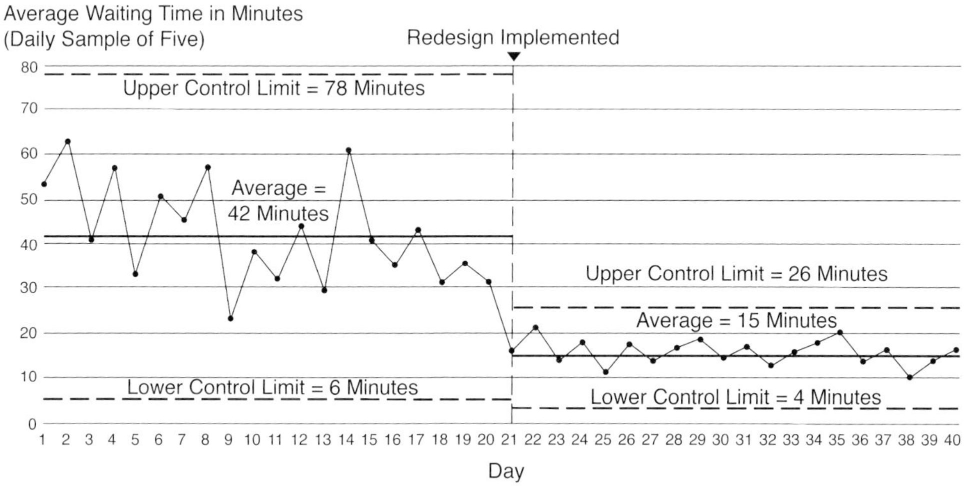

Figure 1-10 Control chart of average wait time before and after a redesign. *(Reproduced from the Quality Assurance Project.)*

or is due to random error and (2) how the organization is faring compared with peer organizations, if data from peers are available.

The purpose of these data analyses is to identify variation in the factor of interest. Factors that are due to the way the system is established and that are inherent in its current state of operations are called *common cause factors.* To improve performance in this area, the organization will have to redesign and reengineer the system. For example, there may be a known rate of "unreliable" visual fields in glaucoma, despite the best training of technicians and screening of patients. In contrast, there are "special causes" of variation that are due to a specific, identifiable factor, often a specific provider or person. Rapid identification of "special cause" variance allows for quick correction of variation that exceeds normal rates. However, it is improving the performance of the overall system and reducing the common cause variation that can improve care and affect the most patients. By "shifting the curve," the organization can improve care for every patient, as opposed to just identifying the outlier providers and assisting in their rehabilitation.

Fremont AM, Lee PP, Mangione CM, et al. Patterns of care for open-angle glaucoma in managed care. *Arch Ophthalmol.* 2003;121(6):777–783.

Other Features of Continuous Quality Improvement

Use of continuous quality improvement tools requires significant thought regarding how to improve care structures and processes. An essential step in improving care processes, before or after initial analysis, is developing a checklist of the steps and parties involved and then creating a flowchart (Fig 1-11) of the care system involved. By looking at the overall process for a specific outcome (eg, making sure a patient with diabetes mellitus gets an annual eye examination), the organization can identify opportunities for improving the process.

Another tool is the fishbone, or cause-and-effect, diagram (Fig 1-12). This diagram provides detailed information on the different factors that are significant inputs in each step of the care process, including personnel. Mapping each of these important factors can help clarify where problems may occur and where work may be improved. Changes in those factors can then be measured and the results monitored. This provides continuous feedback to those interested in improving the quality of care.

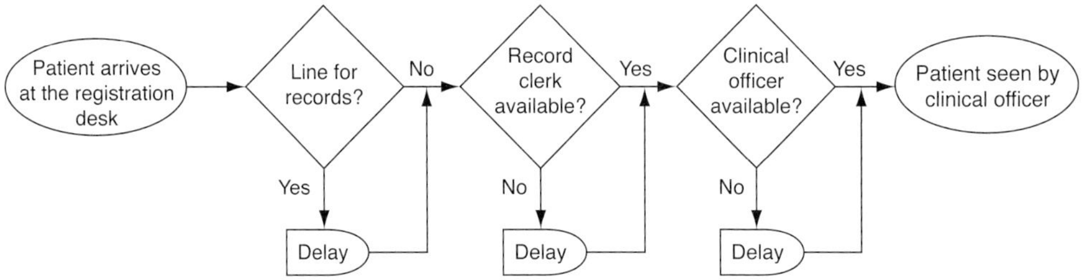

Figure 1-11 Flowchart of patient registration. *(Reproduced from the Quality Assurance Project.)*

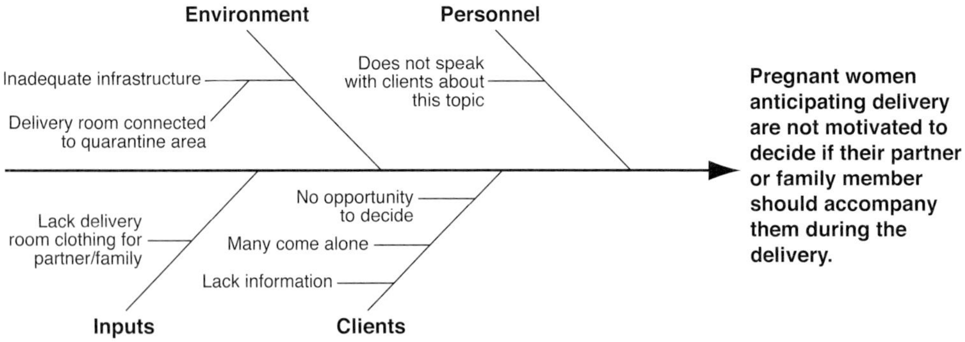

Figure 1-12 Fishbone diagram used at a hospital. *(Reproduced from the Quality Assurance Project.)*

Summary

Efforts to improve the quality of care—and ensure that fair and meaningful quality measures are part of this endeavor—bring key statistical concepts to the forefront. Because quality is likely to become an important component of reimbursement under federal government programs (eg, Physician Quality Reporting System) as well as private managed-care companies, creation and maintenance of appropriate systems are essential. Indeed, to the extent quality measures are also used to select providers for participation in insurance company provider panels, having meaningful systems that entail appropriate statistical approaches in their design and implementation is even more important. Thus, statistics is useful not only for understanding the scientific literature and providing care for patients but also for influencing the practices and livelihoods of providers, including ophthalmologists.

Giaconi JA, Coleman AL. Evidence-based medicine in glaucoma. *Focal Points: Clinical Modules for Ophthalmologists.* San Francisco: American Academy of Ophthalmology; 2008, module 3.

Schuster MA, McGlynn EA, Brook RH. How good is the quality of health care in the United States? *Milbank Q.* 1998;76(4):517–563.

Sloan FA, Brown DS, Carlisle ES, Picone GA, Lee PP. Monitoring visual status: why patients do or do not comply with practice guidelines. *Health Serv Res.* 2004;39(5):1429–1448.

CHAPTER 2

Endocrine Disorders

Recent Developments

- Moderate exercise and weight loss can prevent the onset of type 2 diabetes mellitus in patients at risk for development of the disease.
- Several drugs have recently been approved in the United States for the treatment of diabetes mellitus. They include glucagon-like peptide-1 agonists, dipeptidyl-peptidase IV inhibitors, and sodium-glucose transporter-2 inhibitors.
- Poor glucose control is only one of several risk factors contributing to the complications of diabetes. Equal attention must be paid to other factors, such as hypertension and lipid abnormalities.

Diabetes Mellitus

The prevalence of diabetes mellitus in the United States is estimated to be as high as 8%. Obesity is a major contributing factor and continues to increase in prevalence yearly. In 2012, the total economic impact of diabetes in the United States was $254 billion, due to both direct medical costs and costs related to work loss, disability, and early mortality. Diabetes remains the leading cause of new cases of blindness among adults aged 20–74 years; the ophthalmologist plays a crucial role as a member of a multidisciplinary team engaged in prevention, treatment, and management of this disease.

American Diabetes Association. Economic costs of diabetes in the U.S. in 2012. *Diabetes Care.* 2013;36(4):1033–1046.

Basics of Glucose Metabolism

The plasma glucose level is reduced by a single hormone, insulin. In contrast, 6 hormones increase the plasma glucose level: somatotropin, adrenocorticotropin, cortisol, epinephrine, glucagon, and thyroxine. All of these hormones are secreted as needed to maintain normal serum glucose levels in the face of extremely variable degrees of glucose intake and utilization. In the fed state, *anabolism* is initiated by increased secretion of insulin and growth hormone. This leads to conversion of glucose to glycogen for storage in the liver and muscles, synthesis of protein from amino acids, and combination of fatty acid and glucose in adipose tissue to form triglycerides.

In the fasting state, *catabolism* results from the increased secretion of hormones that are antagonistic to insulin. In this setting, glycogen is reduced to glucose in the liver and muscles, proteins are broken down into amino acids in muscles and other tissues and transported to the liver for conversion to glucose or ketoacids, and triglycerides are degraded into fatty acids and glycerol in adipose tissue for transport to the liver for conversion to ketoacids and glucose (or for transport to muscle for use as an energy source).

A lean adult without diabetes secretes approximately 33 units of insulin per day. If the pancreatic β-cell mass is reduced (as in type 1 diabetes), then insulin production falls. The relative excess of catabolic hormones results in fasting hyperglycemia, and persistent catabolism may lead to fatal diabetic ketoacidosis if insulin therapy is not started. Thus, insulin-dependent diabetic patients require a continuous baseline dose of insulin, even in the fasting state: some level of insulin is needed to offset the effect of all the other hormones.

In an obese adult, insulin secretion can increase almost fourfold, to approximately 120 units per day. In this state, the plasma glucose level may rise only slightly, but pancreatic β-cell mass increases. When serum insulin levels are elevated, the number of insulin receptors on the surface of insulin-responsive cells actually decreases, and formerly insulin-sensitive tissues become resistant to the glucose-lowering effects of both endogenous and exogenous insulin. This condition may progress to fasting hyperglycemia and type 2 diabetes. The risk of hyperglycemia is 2 times as great in individuals who are 20% above ideal body weight, compared with those at ideal body weight; the risk is 4 times, 8 times, 16 times, and 32 times as great in those 40%, 60%, 80%, and 100% above ideal body weight, respectively.

Definition, Diagnosis, and Screening

Diabetes mellitus is now defined as a group of metabolic diseases characterized by hyperglycemia resulting from defects in insulin secretion, insulin action, or both. Several tests are available to screen for diabetes, including the fasting plasma glucose (FPG) test and the oral glucose tolerance test (OGTT). Although the OGTT is more sensitive than the FPG, it is not recommended for routine use because it is more costly, inconvenient, and difficult to reproduce. In 2009, an international expert committee including representatives from the International Diabetes Federation, the American Diabetes Association, and the European Association for the Study of Diabetes issued a consensus recommendation supporting hemoglobin A_{1c} (HbA_{1c}) measurement as a means to diagnose diabetes. The test reflects chronic glycemia levels and does not require patients to alter their dietary intake before testing, making it more convenient.

The American Diabetes Association Expert Panel recommends a diagnosis of diabetes mellitus when 1 of the following 4 criteria are met and confirmed with retesting on a subsequent day:

- HbA_{1c} ≥6.5% (<5.7% = normal)
- FPG level ≥126 mg/dL (7.0 mmol/L)
- 2-hour plasma glucose level ≥200 mg/dL (11.1 mmol/L) with 75-g OGTT
- random plasma glucose level ≥200 mg/dL (11.1 mmol/L) in a patient with classic symptoms of hyperglycemia, including polyphagia, polyuria, and polydipsia

Criteria for diabetes testing in asymptomatic individuals are given in Table 2-1.

American Diabetes Association website; www.diabetes.org.
American Diabetes Association. Diagnosis and classification of diabetes mellitus. *Diabetes Care.* 2010;33(Suppl 1):S62–S69.
International Diabetes Federation website; www.idf.org.
International Expert Committee. International Expert Committee report on the role of the A1C assay in the diagnosis of diabetes. *Diabetes Care.* 2009;32(7):1327–1334.

Classification

Diabetes mellitus can be caused by a number of mechanisms. Although this chapter emphasizes types 1 and 2, which are most frequently seen in clinical practice, many diseases and drugs can be associated with secondary development of diabetes. For instance, diabetes can be seen with pancreatitis, endocrinopathies such as Addison disease, and genetic diseases such as Down syndrome. Drug-induced diabetes may result from use of glucocorticoids, thiazide-type diuretics, and atypical antipsychotic medications.

Type 1 diabetes

Type 1 diabetes was previously called *insulin-dependent diabetes mellitus* or *juvenile-onset diabetes*. Although incidence peaks around the time of puberty, approximately 25% of cases present after 35 years of age. This form of diabetes is due to a deficiency in endogenous insulin secretion secondary to destruction of insulin-producing β-cells in the pancreas.

Most type 1 diabetes is due to immune-mediated destruction characterized by the presence of various autoantibodies. The rate of destruction varies, but it is usually rapid in children and slow in adults. One or more autoantibodies are present in 90% of patients

Table 2-1 Criteria for Testing for Diabetes Mellitus in Asymptomatic Patients in Whom Diabetes Has Not Been Diagnosed

1. Testing for diabetes should be considered in all persons at age 45 years and older; if results are normal, testing should be repeated at 3-yr intervals.
2. Testing should be considered at younger ages or performed more frequently in persons who
   - are obese (≥120% desirable body weight or a BMI ≥25 kg/m^2)*
   - have a first-degree relative with diabetes
   - are members of a high-risk ethnic population (eg, African American, Hispanic American, Native American, Asian American, Pacific Islander)
   - have delivered a baby weighing >9 lb or have a diagnosis of gestational diabetes mellitus
   - are hypertensive (≥140/90 mm Hg)
   - have an HDL cholesterol level ≤35 mg/dL (0.90 mmol/L) and/or a triglyceride level ≥250 mg/dL (2.82 mmol/L)
   - were shown to have impaired glucose tolerance or impaired fasting glucose
   - have polycystic ovarian syndrome
   - have history of cardiovascular disease
   - are habitually physically inactive

BMI = body mass index; HDL = high-density lipoprotein.
*May not be correct for all ethnic groups.

Data from American Diabetes Association. Standards of medical care in diabetes—2014. *Diabetes Care.* 2014;37(Suppl 1):S14–S80.

at initial presentation of fasting hyperglycemia. Studies have shown that patients newly diagnosed with type 1 diabetes can avoid the use of insulin if they are placed on systemic immunosuppressive agents to prevent further β-cell destruction. Unfortunately, this treatment is too toxic to be practical. Some human leukocyte antigens (HLAs), namely HLA-DR3 and HLA-DR4, are strongly associated with type 1 diabetes, and multiple genetic predispositions exist. These patients are also prone to other autoimmune disorders, such as Graves disease, Addison disease, vitiligo, and pernicious anemia. Extragenetic factors may also play a role, as studies of monozygotic twins have shown that diabetes develops in both twins only 30%–50% of the time. Cytotoxic chemicals and viral respiratory infections in the first year of life have been associated with increased risk of type 1 diabetes development.

A subset of adult patients present with islet cell autoantibodies typical of type 1 diabetes without need for insulin in the first 6 months of diagnosis. Referred to as latent autoimmune diabetes in adults (LADA), this disease has an atypical onset, with slow, progressive autoimmune β-cell dysfunction, unlike the rapid onset of type 1 diabetes.

Type 2 diabetes

Type 2 diabetes was formerly known as *non–insulin-dependent* or *adult-onset diabetes mellitus*. It accounts for 90% of US adults with diabetes. Patients with type 2 diabetes are usually, but not always, older than 40 years at presentation. Obesity is a frequent finding and, in the United States, is present in 80%–90% of these patients. Other risk factors for type 2 diabetes include hypertension, a history of gestational diabetes, physical inactivity, and low socioeconomic status. This form of diabetes mellitus is frequently undiagnosed for years because hyperglycemia develops slowly and patients are often asymptomatic. Despite minimal symptoms, these patients are at increased risk for microvascular and macrovascular complications.

Although genetic predisposition is strongly linked to development of type 2 diabetes, no unique genetic locus has been identified. Type 2 diabetes is likely a function of a variable number of abnormal genes that combine to create a tendency for obesity and abnormal glucose metabolism, as well as a predisposition to complications of the disease.

Autoimmune destruction of β cells does not usually occur in type 2 diabetes. The β cells function at first, but their ability to control hyperglycemia gradually diminishes, in part secondary to *glucose toxicity*. Glucose toxicity occurs when chronically elevated glucose levels result in increasing insulin resistance in target tissues and progressive impairment of compensatory insulin production due to β cell damage. The result is a vicious cycle, as elevated glucose levels thus lead to even higher glucose levels. It is therefore crucial to encourage the patient to try to break this cycle by decreasing the glucose level. In a significant number of these patients, the elevated plasma glucose level can revert to normal simply with caloric restriction and weight loss.

Although gestational diabetes is a separate entity, it is metabolically similar to type 2 disease in that a decline in insulin sensitivity occurs as gestation progresses. In 30%–50% of affected women, type 2 diabetes develops within 10 years of initial diagnosis. Defined as any degree of glucose intolerance with onset or first recognition during pregnancy, gestational diabetes complicates approximately 4% of all pregnancies in the United States.

It is also significant for the risk it poses to the fetus, including intrauterine mortality, high birth weight, birth trauma, neonatal mortality, and metabolic problems.

Prediabetic disorders

Impaired glucose tolerance (IGT) is the diagnosis when a standard 75-g OGTT yields a 2-hour plasma glucose level of ≥140 mg/dL to <200 mg/dL. A separate category, *impaired fasting glucose (IFG),* requires a fasting plasma glucose level of ≥110 mg/dL to <126 mg/dL. Both conditions can be considered early stages of type 2 diabetes and are often called *prediabetic states.* For instance, type 2 diabetes develops in 30%–50% of patients with IGT within 10 years of diagnosis. Although there is a great deal of overlap, IGT and IFG are not identical states. An HbA_{1c} value of at least 6.0% but below 6.5% also denotes prediabetes.

Patients with these conditions have an elevated risk of macrovascular disease compared with persons with normal glucose tolerance. Accumulating evidence also suggests an increased risk of microvascular disease, including nephropathy and retinopathy.

Metabolic syndrome

Closely associated with type 2 diabetes, *metabolic syndrome* is not a disease but a collection of disorders. The clinical syndrome includes obesity, lipid abnormalities, hypertension, and some type of glucose intolerance (see Chapter 4), risk factors common to both diabetes and cardiovascular disease. An estimated one-fourth of the adult population in the United States and Europe has metabolic syndrome. Thus, awareness of this syndrome is becoming increasingly important. Men with a majority of metabolic syndrome features have roughly 4 times the risk of coronary heart disease and 25 times the risk of diabetes as those without these abnormalities. Metabolic syndrome represents a profound public health risk, and treatment of the syndrome may have a significant impact on preventing diabetes and cardiovascular diseases.

Clinical Presentation of Diabetes Mellitus

The classic symptoms of diabetes mellitus are polyuria, polydipsia, and polyphagia. Type 1 diabetes tends to present more acutely than type 2, and the diagnosis is usually made based on the presence of these classic symptoms in association with an elevated plasma glucose level. The diagnosis of type 2 diabetes often depends more on laboratory testing, as patients may have abnormal glucose metabolism long before overt symptoms develop. Other important historical findings that suggest the diagnosis of diabetes include complications during pregnancy or birth of large babies, reactive hypoglycemia, family history, advanced vascular disease, impotence, leg claudication, and neuropathy symptoms.

Physical findings, particularly in type 2 diabetes, may include obesity, hypertension, arteriopathy, neuropathy, genitourinary tract abnormalities (especially recurrent *Candida* infections or bacterial bladder or kidney infections), periodontal disease, foot abnormalities, skin abnormalities, and unusual susceptibility to infections.

Prevention of Diabetes Mellitus

Several clinical trials have recently shown that the risk of progression from IGT to type 2 diabetes can be markedly reduced (by approximately 50% over several years) with lifestyle modifications such as a combination of diet and exercise therapy. The amount of weight loss and exercise required to achieve this result is surprisingly modest. For instance, in the Diabetes Prevention Program, patients who were asked to perform only 150 minutes of brisk walking a week (a little over 20 minutes a day) lost only about 12 pounds of weight on average but reduced their risk of diabetes development by 50%. Other studies have suggested that early pharmacologic intervention with oral hypoglycemic agents also decreases the risk of progression to diabetes. There are, as yet, no known ways to prevent type 1 diabetes, but trials of interventions to regulate immune response are under way.

Beyerlein A, Wehweck F, Ziegler AG, Pflueger M. Respiratory infections in early life and the development of islet autoimmunity in children at increased type 1 diabetes risk: evidence from the BABYDIET Study. *JAMA Pediatr.* 2013;167(9):800–807.

Jeon CY, Lokken RP, Hu FB, van Dam RM. Physical activity of moderate intensity and risk of type 2 diabetes: a systematic review. *Diabetes Care.* 2007;30(3):744–752.

Knowler WC, Barrett-Connor E, Fowler SE, et al; Diabetes Prevention Program Research Group. Reduction in the incidence of type 2 diabetes with lifestyle intervention or metformin. *N Engl J Med.* 2002;346(6):393–403.

Noble JA, Valdes AM. Genetics of the HLA region in the prediction of type 1 diabetes. *Curr Diab Rep.* 2011;11(6):533–542.

The importance of glucose control

For patients diagnosed with either type 1 or type 2 diabetes mellitus, glucose control is of the utmost importance. The Diabetes Control and Complications Trial showed that intensive therapy aimed at maintaining near-normal glucose levels had a large and beneficial effect on delaying the development and progression of long-term complications for patients with type 1 diabetes. Intensive therapy decreased the risk of the development and progression of retinopathy, nephropathy, and neuropathy by 40%–76%. The beneficial effects increased over time but came with a threefold increased risk of hypoglycemia. Thus, intensive therapy is recommended for most patients with type 1 disease, but with careful self-monitoring of blood glucose levels to prevent hypoglycemic episodes. A related study, the United Kingdom Prospective Diabetes Study, was designed to assess the effect of intensive control on patients with type 2 diabetes. This study used a combination of diet, sulfonylureas, and insulin to achieve a median HbA_{1c} of 7.0% and a reduction in complications in the intensive therapy group. See also BCSC Section 12, *Retina and Vitreous.*

Tight control has a tremendous effect on the development of complications. As Figure 2-1 shows, the risk of retinopathy progression rises almost exponentially as the HbA_{1c} level increases. However, patients who decrease their HbA_{1c} by 1 percentage point (eg, from 8.0% to 7.0%) decrease the risk of retinopathy by approximately 30%, and this benefit holds for other complications of diabetes, such as nephropathy and neuropathy. When working with patients with diabetes, health care providers need to emphasize the importance of tight control and encourage patients to achieve it.

For patients with type 1 diabetes, intensive control also provides protection against macrovascular complications, such as cardiovascular disease. For patients with type 2 diabetes, however, the role of glycemic control in reducing cardiovascular risk has not been established. In this group, macrovascular disease may be affected more by other risk factors,

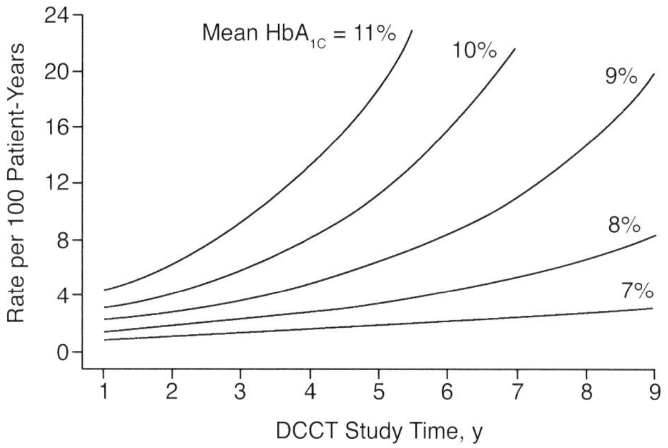

Figure 2-1 Rate of retinopathy progression relative to mean hemoglobin A_{1c}. *(Redrawn with permission from the DCCT Research Group. The relationship of glycemic exposure (HbA_{1C}) to the risk of development and progression of retinopathy in the Diabetes Control and Complications Trial.* Diabetes. *1995;44(8):968–983.)*

such as smoking, obesity, and lipid abnormalities. The Action to Control Cardiovascular Risk in Diabetes (ACCORD) trial even suggested that intensive glycemic control in patients with type 2 diabetes might actually increase the risk of cardiovascular mortality. Although this result received wide coverage in the lay press, the finding may be related more to the study's methodology; the result has not been confirmed in other trials. Nevertheless, based on this, some experts suggest that a target HbA_{1c} of 7.0%–7.9% may be safer for patients with long-standing type 2 diabetes who are at high risk for cardiovascular disease.

Action to Control Cardiovascular Risk in Diabetes Study Group; Gerstein HC, Miller ME, Byington RP, et al. Effects of intensive glucose lowering in type 2 diabetes. *N Engl J Med.* 2008;358(24):2545–2559.

Kravetz JD, Federman DG. Implications of new diabetes treatment trials: should current clinical practice be altered? *Postgrad Med.* 2009;121(3):67–72.

Management

Glucose surveillance

Probably the most important advance in glycemic control is self-monitoring of blood glucose using finger sticks. Newer blood-testing devices require smaller amounts of blood and are less painful. The glucose values are stored in memory and downloaded to give an accurate assessment of glucose control without depending on the patient to recall or reconstruct the data.

Continuous blood glucose–monitoring systems, which measure the glucose content of interstitial fluid through either a subcutaneous needle sensor or a fully implanted device, are also available. The efficacy of these systems compared with that of finger-stick monitoring is uncertain, making it necessary to continue the latter. The greatest potential of continuous blood glucose monitoring is for patients with hypoglycemic unawareness; unfortunately, currently available meters are most inaccurate in the low range of glucose. The technology is also expensive.

The ability to measure *glycosylated hemoglobin levels* has significantly improved long-term surveillance of glucose control. When exposed to glucose, hemoglobin undergoes modification that results in the attachment of glucose (glycosylation). Higher concentrations of glucose and longer periods of exposure result in a higher concentration of glycosylated proteins. The time period reflected by the glycosylated protein concentration depends on the particular protein's turnover rate. Red blood cells and hemoglobin have a half-life of 60 days; thus, the glycosylated hemoglobin level reflects the mean blood glucose concentration during the preceding 2 months. The amount of glycosylated hemoglobin is expressed as a percentage of total hemoglobin.

The test for HbA_{1c}, the most abundant of the glycosylated hemoglobins, is the assay most commonly performed. The HbA_{1c} assay is used to monitor the level of long-term glucose control in both type 1 and type 2 disease and is especially useful in uncooperative or unreliable patients. Patients with diabetes mellitus should aim for levels below 7.0%, while levels above 7.0% indicate that further interventions are warranted. The American Diabetes Association and International Diabetes Federation recommend measuring HbA_{1c} levels at least twice a year for patients with well-controlled diabetes and quarterly for those with suboptimal control.

Diet and exercise

Adherence to nutrition and meal-planning principles is a challenging but essential component of successful diabetes management. In insulin-dependent patients, insulin requirements are matched to the patient's diet and metabolic needs, not vice versa. Meals should be consistent, regularly spaced, and low in cholesterol, with less than 7% of calories coming from saturated fat and with 15%–20% of calories derived from protein. If type 2 diabetes is diagnosed and the patient is overweight, a low-fat and low-cholesterol diet should be started and an exercise routine initiated, with the goal of approaching ideal weight. A modest weight loss of even 10–20 pounds may ameliorate the diabetes or cause its remission. A good exercise program augments the weight-loss program and improves fitness. However, before an exercise program is prescribed for anyone older than 35 years, a clinician must determine that the heart is normal and that no contraindications exist. Anyone who has been sedentary or who is out of shape should start slowly and work up to more demanding physical activities.

Unfortunately, it may be difficult for patients with type 2 diabetes to maintain these lifestyle changes, especially those involving weight loss. This difficulty should not simply be attributed to a lack of willpower; it may well represent a central nervous systems (CNS) manifestation of this disease. Psychiatric counseling can play an important role in treating patients with type 2 diabetes. Studies suggest that efforts directed toward treating the stress and depression often associated with this disease may help improve glucose control.

Bariatric surgery to reduce stomach size and thus promote weight loss has grown in popularity. The US National Institutes of Health recommends considering bariatric surgery for well-informed and motivated patients with severe obesity for whom conventional treatment modalities have failed or for those who have multiple comorbidities or severe lifestyle limitations. Bariatric surgery is not without risk. Morbidity can include venous thrombosis, infection, vitamin deficiencies, and complications related to the surgery itself;

mortality, which is steadily declining with improvements in surgical technique, has decreased to 0.5%. Significant counseling and lifestyle changes are required, as patients can undermine the benefits of surgery by eating small amounts of food frequently, especially high-carbohydrate liquids such as milk shakes.

Thomas D, Elliott EJ. Low glycaemic index, or low glycaemic load, diets for diabetes mellitus. *Cochrane Database Syst Rev.* 2009;1:CD006296.

Insulin therapy

Approximately 1 million North Americans require insulin therapy. Such therapy is indicated for diabetic patients who are pregnant or who are at or below ideal body weight with sustained hyperglycemia, ketoacidosis, or a hyperosmotic state. The use of insulin in type 2 diabetes actually decreases the number of target-cell insulin receptors, increases food intake, and promotes weight gain. Therefore, patients who are above ideal body weight, have not experienced ketoacidosis, and are not pregnant should not be treated with insulin initially.

The goal of therapy is to simulate the physiologic changes in insulin levels that would normally occur in response to food intake and activity level. This therapy usually involves use of a longer-acting insulin to maintain a baseline level and additional use of a rapid-acting insulin to cover meals. Because insulins can be created with different rates of absorption by substituting amino acids or complexing with zinc, patients can fine-tune glucose control with combinations of various types of insulins (Table 2-2). In the past, most insulin was derived from animals, but currently, recombinant human insulin is used almost exclusively.

Motivated patients can adjust injection dosages based on preprandial glucose level, activity level, and amount of food to be ingested, provided they understand the carbohydrate types and overall nutritional value of each meal. Intensive insulin therapy requires that patients become very involved with their own management and underlying disease

Table 2-2 Pharmacokinetics of Commonly Used Insulin Preparations

Insulin Type	Onset of Action	Time to Peak Effect
Rapid acting Insulin aspart Insulin glulisine Insulin lispro	15 min	60 min
Regular/short acting Insulin regular human	30 min	2–3 hr
Intermediate acting Insulin isophane suspension	2–4 hr	4–12 hr
Long acting Insulin detemir Insulin glargine	Several hours	No discernible peak
Ultralong acting Insulin degludec*	30–90 min	No discernible peak

*Not available in the United States.

pathophysiology. Premixed combinations of various insulins are also available for patients less able to work with all these variables.

In addition to exercise and intake, 2 physiologic phenomena may need to be accounted for with insulin therapy. The *Somogyi phenomenon* is the occurrence of rebound hyperglycemia after hypoglycemia. Mild hypoglycemia (plasma glucose level of 50–60 mg/dL), which may be asymptomatic, can activate counterregulation. Recognition of this process is important because patients may incorrectly decide to increase their dose of longer-acting insulin to treat the hyperglycemia and inadvertently increase the hypoglycemia that precipitated the problem. The incidence of the Somogyi phenomenon is not known, but it is probably not frequent.

The second phenomenon is the *dawn phenomenon,* which occurs when a normal physiologic process is exaggerated, resulting in substantial hyperglycemia. Characterized by early-morning hyperglycemia not preceded by hypoglycemia or waning of insulin, this phenomenon is thought to be caused by a surge of growth hormone secretion shortly after the patient falls asleep. It can occur with equal frequency in type 1 and type 2 diabetes, with variable severity. Management consists of increasing a patient's before-dinner intermediate-acting insulin or delaying insulin administration until just before bedtime.

Continuous subcutaneous insulin infusion (CSII) pumps allow more physiologic levels of insulin than do traditional injections. The CSII pump can infuse continuous rapid-acting insulin at a programmed basal rate and additional boluses with meals. CSII is not a simple treatment, however, as patients must be able to understand the more sophisticated demands of using a pump, and improvement in glucose control is not automatic. In the Diabetes Control and Complications Trial, the overall rate of control was not better in patients using the pump than in patients receiving multiple injections; however, more recent studies using very rapid–acting insulins demonstrate better glycemic control with a pump than with multiple-injection therapy.

The pump tends to be used when multiple-injection therapy fails, but some endocrinologists consider using it as initial therapy with motivated patients. Disadvantages include a higher cost, potential for infection at the infusion site, and infusion failure. Infusion failure is significant, because diabetic ketoacidosis can develop if the pump fails for as little as 4–6 hours. Hypoinsulinemia develops, with resulting hyperglycemia and possible ketoacidosis if it is not recognized. Finally, because patients need to wear the pump on an almost constant basis, some patients discontinue use simply because it interferes with activities such as bathing and sexual intercourse. CSII technology is continually improving, however, and for many patients the pump is preferred over multiple injections.

A surgically implanted programmable insulin pump is available in the European Union and is under investigation in the United States. Compared with injection regimens and external pumps, this pump is associated with a lower incidence of severe hypoglycemia and less day-to-day fluctuation in blood glucose concentrations. These advantages may occur, in part, because implantable pumps deliver insulin into the peritoneal cavity or intravascularly, where rapid absorption provides more physiologic insulin levels. However, such pumps are more prone to catheter blockage, and antibodies to insulin develop more commonly with continuous intraperitoneal insulin infusion than with CSII.

Complications of insulin therapy *Hypoglycemia* is the most significant complication of insulin therapy. Stimulation of the adrenal medulla with resulting hyperepinephrinemia may result in anxiety, palpitations, perspiration, pallor, tachycardia, hypertension, and dilated pupils. Neurologic dysfunction is manifested as headache, paresthesia, blurred vision, drowsiness, irritability, bizarre behavior, mental confusion, combativeness, and a variety of other symptoms. Short-term hypoglycemia can lead to accidental injury and even criminal behavior. Prolonged hypoglycemia can result in irreversible brain damage or death. Unfortunately, the epinephrine response to hypoglycemia can diminish over time, often in association with the global autonomic neuropathy that occurs in diabetes mellitus. As a result, patients have fewer warning symptoms of hypoglycemia, as well as a decreased ability to metabolically respond to the hypoglycemia. Thus, the first clinical manifestation of a hypoglycemic episode is CNS dysfunction, and by then it may be too late for the patient to recognize and self-treat the episode. This is the clinical syndrome of *hypoglycemia unawareness.* The result may be a very rapid deterioration from normal functioning to dangerous hypoglycemia in patients with long-standing diabetes mellitus.

Hypoglycemia is usually caused by inadequate carbohydrate intake secondary to a missed or delayed meal, vigorous exercise, decreased hepatic gluconeogenesis, or an excessive dose of insulin. The condition needs to be promptly verified by testing for a venous plasma glucose level lower than 50 mg/dL. Patients who are still able to swallow should be given candy, soft drinks, juice, or glucose. For those unable to swallow, 25 g of intravenous glucose or 1 mg of subcutaneous or intramuscular glucagon is administered. The patient needs to be observed until recovery is complete, and the plasma glucose test is repeated with additional food given.

Other complications of insulin therapy include lipoatrophy (loss of fat) and lipohypertrophy (accumulation of fat) at sites of insulin injection. Local insulin allergy can occur and usually clears as therapy continues. Generalized anaphylaxis, hives, and angioedema may also develop and may need to be treated with desensitization techniques. Immunologic insulin resistance may occur because of production of insulin-neutralizing antibodies. All of these immunologic phenomena have become much less frequent with the use of human insulins.

Oral agents

The general approach to treating type 2 diabetes begins with diet and exercise modifications. If unsuccessful, the patient is given an oral agent, usually metformin. If this is insufficient, a second agent with a different mechanism of action is usually added. If more aggressive control is required, insulin is usually added to the current 1- or 2-drug oral therapy. This regimen is less expensive and more effective than 3-drug oral therapy. If patients are underweight or ketotic at any point, or if they are losing weight, insulin may need to be started earlier. See Figure 2-2 and Table 2-3. Figure 2-2 shows an algorithm for treating hyperglycemia in type 2 diabetes.

Sulfonylureas The sulfonylureas act by stimulating pancreatic insulin secretion. They provide the greatest efficacy of any oral agent for glycemic lowering.

The major problem with sulfonylurea therapy is that approximately one-third of treated patients are primary failures and do not become normoglycemic. Furthermore,

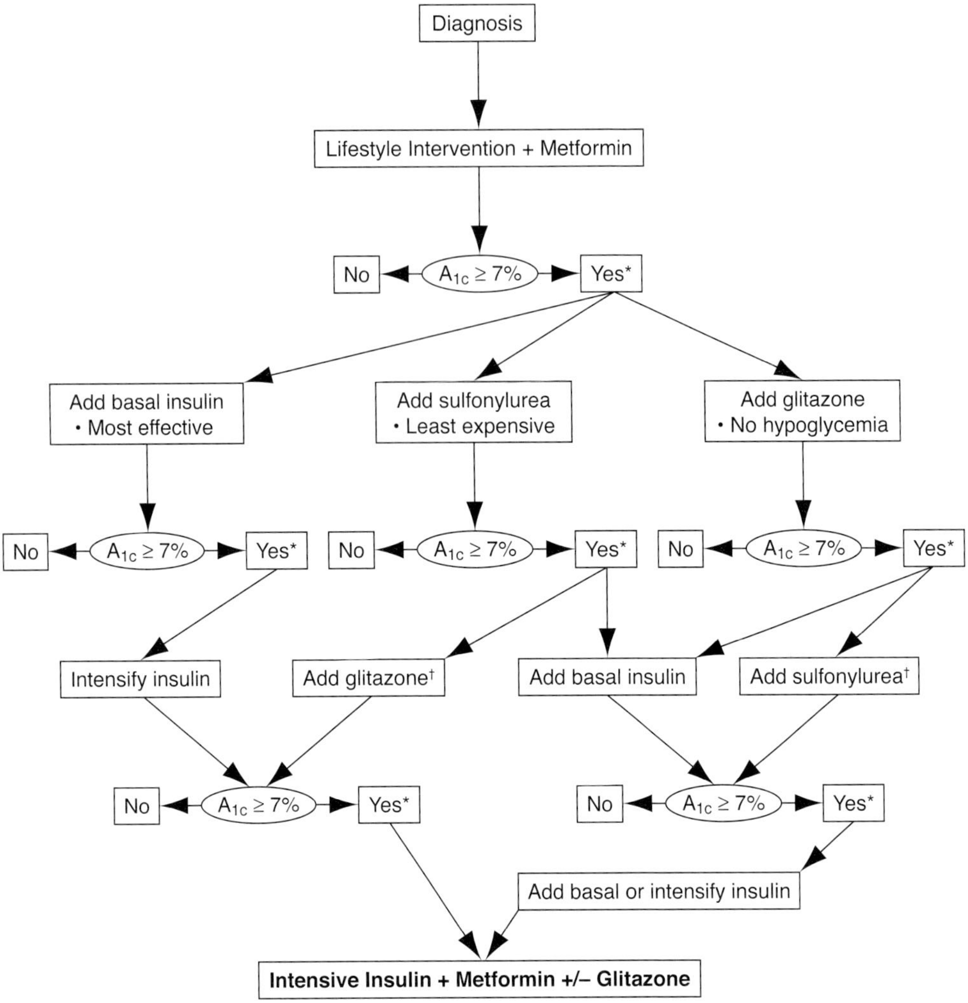

*Check A_{1c} every 3 months until <7% and then at least every 6 months.
†Although 3 oral agents can be used, initiation and intensification of insulin therapy is preferred based on effectiveness and expense.

Figure 2-2 Management of hyperglycemia in type 2 diabetes. *(Used with permission from Nathan DM, Buse JB, Davidson MB, et al. Management of hyperglycemia in type 2 diabetes: a consensus algorithm for the initiation and adjustment of therapy. A consensus statement from the American Diabetes Association and the European Association for the Study of Diabetes.* Diabetes Care. *2006;29:1963. Copyright © 2006 The American Diabetes Association.)*

during a 5-year period, 85% of those who initially respond to the drug experience secondary failure to control blood glucose. The sulfonylureas are contraindicated in diabetic patients who are pregnant and in those who have had ketoacidosis.

The most significant adverse effect of the sulfonylureas is hypoglycemia, which, though infrequent, may be severe and life-threatening (see "Complications of insulin therapy"). First-generation sulfonylureas compete for carrier protein–binding sites with many

Table 2-3 **Efficacy of Commonly Used Oral Hypoglycemic Agents**

Drug Class/Agents	HbA_{1C} Reduction, %
First-generation sulfonylureas	
Acetohexamide, chlorpropamide, tolbutamide	0.5–1.5
Second-generation sulfonylureas	
Glimepiride, glipizide, glyburide	1.0–2.0
Biguanide	
Metformin	1.5
α-Glucosidase inhibitors	
Acarbose, miglitol	0.5–0.8
Thiazolidinediones	
Pioglitazone, rosiglitazone	0.5–1.4
Meglitinides	
Nateglinide, repaglinide	0.5–1.5
Glucagon-like peptide-1 (GLP-1) agonists	
Exenatide, liraglutide, lixisenatide	0.5–1.0
Dipeptidyl-peptidase IV (DPP-IV) inhibitors	
Linagliptin, saxagliptin, sitagliptin, vildagliptin	0.7–1.2
Sodium-glucose transporter-2 (SGLT2) inhibitors	
Canagliflozin, dapagliflozin	0.6–1.0

other drugs, including sulfonamides, salicylates, and thiazide-type diuretics. Because the pharmacologic effect of the sulfonylureas may be increased when they are displaced from their albumin-combining sites, combination drug therapy may have unforeseen toxic consequences. Another adverse effect is weight gain.

Second-generation sulfonylurea agents (*glipizide*, *glyburide*, and *glimepiride*) differ from the first-generation agents in structure and potency. The newer sulfonylureas are more potent than first-generation agents and are generally dosed daily. Complications are less frequent with the second-generation agents because of their nonionic binding to albumin, and patients may be less susceptible to drug interactions. Although these newer agents are more potent than the first-generation sulfonylureas in facilitating insulin release, they are not associated with better control of hyperglycemia. As a result, in most cases the choice of initial sulfonylurea depends on cost and availability; the efficacy of the various agents tends to be similar.

Biguanides A major advance occurred with the development of *metformin,* currently the only available biguanide. Metformin improves insulin sensitivity. Metformin may also lead to modest weight loss or at least weight stabilization (in contrast to the weight gain that may occur with use of insulin or sulfonylureas). In addition, it is less likely to cause hypoglycemia and can be used in nonobese patients. Metformin is generally the first agent used in patients whose hyperglycemia cannot be controlled with lifestyle changes alone (see Fig 2-2).

Although metformin is generally safe, patients may report gastrointestinal tract symptoms, including a metallic taste, nausea, and diarrhea. A more severe potential problem is lactic acidosis. Though rare, this problem is more likely to occur in patients with renal insufficiency. Metformin should therefore not be prescribed to patients with elevated serum creatinine levels, and the drug should be discontinued before patients take part in any studies involving iodinated contrast materials, given the risk of renal failure. The same precaution should be taken before major surgery when there is a possibility of circulatory compromise and secondary renal insufficiency. Metformin is also available as a combination pill with glyburide, glipizide, or rosiglitazone maleate.

α-Glucosidase inhibitors *Acarbose* and *miglitol* delay the absorption of carbohydrates by inhibiting the enzymes that convert complex carbohydrates into monosaccharides. Though relatively safe, these agents often cause flatulence, which limits patient adherence, and they are to be avoided in patients with intestinal disorders.

Thiazolidinediones This newer class of drugs, represented by *rosiglitazone* and *pioglitazone,* is thought to increase insulin sensitivity in muscle and adipose tissue and to inhibit hepatic gluconeogenesis. The first available agent of this class, *troglitazone,* was withdrawn from the market in 2000, when the US Food and Drug Administration (FDA) noted a higher rate of liver toxicity associated with this drug than with other class members. In 2010, the FDA restricted the use of rosiglitazone because of an increased risk of fluid retention and resulting cardiovascular complications. Patients who continue on thiazolidinediones may gain weight, and they have increased rates of diabetic macular edema.

Meglitinides *Repaglinide* and *nateglinide* are meglitinides, whose mechanism of action and side effect profile are similar to those of the sulfonylureas. They are more expensive and generally no more efficacious. Because of their rapid onset of action and short duration, these agents are taken daily with meals. They can be used as single agents or in combination therapy with other oral hypoglycemic agents.

Other pharmacologic therapies

Besides injectable and infusable insulin therapy, an inhaled form of rapid-acting insulin is currently in development. Previously, lack of interest led to discontinuation of the production of inhaled insulin in 2007.

Incretins are gut-derived factors that are released when nutrients enter the stomach; they help to stimulate postprandial insulin release. *Incretin mimetics* improve glycemic control by enhancing pancreatic insulin secretion, inhibiting glucagon secretion, and promoting satiety. Two recently approved injectable incretin mimetics, or glucagon-like peptide-1 (GLP-1) agonists, are available worldwide; they are exenatide and liraglutide. They are used as adjunctive therapy for patients with type 2 diabetes whose condition is inadequately controlled by oral agents. The most common adverse effects are gastrointestinal; however, liraglutide has been associated with pancreatitis as well as thyroid C-cell tumor development. Lixisenatide is a once-daily injectable GLP-1 agonist available in Europe that is currently under US FDA review.

Dipeptidyl-peptidase IV (DPP-IV) is an enzyme that deactivates bioactive peptides, including incretins; therefore, inhibiting this enzyme can enhance glucose regulation. Sitagliptin, saxagliptin, and linagliptin are 3 oral DPP-IV inhibitors approved by the

US FDA that require daily dosing. Unfortunately, they are expensive, only modestly effective, and thus not commonly used. Vildagliptin, another DPP-IV inhibitor, is available in the European Union.

The US FDA recently approved a novel group of agents, sodium-glucose transporter-2 inhibitors. Glucose is filtered in the renal glomerulus and reabsorbed in the proximal tubule. Beyond a certain threshold (usually 160–180 mg/dL), it is excreted in the urine. Glucose transport inhibitors lower the renal glucose threshold, increasing urinary glucose excretion. The lost calories then cause weight loss and improve blood glucose values. Canagliflozin and dapagliflozin have been approved for use in the United States. Potential adverse effects of such agents include hypotension and dehydration.

Pancreatic transplantation

For patients with type 1 diabetes, pancreas transplantation can be performed in conjunction with renal transplantation. With modern techniques and immunosuppression, the transplant survival rate is high, and the majority of patients become euglycemic without the need for insulin. Although quality of life is usually improved, the patient faces the risks of both surgery and long-term immunosuppression. Pancreas transplantation alone is therefore used only in certain situations, such as in patients with frequent metabolic complications or patients for whom standard insulin therapy consistently fails to control disease. When combined with renal transplantation in a patient with end-stage renal disease, however, the benefits of pancreas transplantation far outweigh the risks.

Transplantation of pancreatic islet cells is currently under investigation; the cells can be injected directly into the liver without the need for formal transplantation. This procedure has been attempted in humans, but the failure rate is high due to rejection. A newly discovered hormone holds promise as an alternative therapy. Betatrophin, a peptide hormone, increases the rate of pancreatic β-cell division. Injection of mice with betatrophin lowered blood glucose levels, raising the possibility that betatrophin or its homologue may become a treatment for diabetes mellitus.

Yi P, Park JS, Melton DA. Betatrophin: a hormone that controls pancreatic β cell proliferation. *Cell.* 2013;153(4):747–758. Epub 2013 Apr 25.

Complications of Diabetes Mellitus

Acute complications of diabetes mellitus

The acute complications of diabetes mellitus are *nonketotic hyperglycemic hyperosmolar coma* and diabetic *ketoacidosis.* Either of these, if not recognized promptly and treated aggressively, can lead to death. These complications should be considered part of a continuum of hyperglycemia rather than separate entities; the main difference between the 2 is whether ketoacids accumulate. Both are often precipitated by some sort of stress, such as an infection, that leads to increased production of glucagon, catecholamines, and cortisol, which in turn enhances gluconeogenesis. If insufficient amounts of insulin or oral hypoglycemic agents are used, the resulting elevated glucose level will lead to osmotic diuresis and volume depletion. If insulin levels are extremely low or absent (eg, in a patient with type 1 diabetes), then catabolic processes (eg, conversion of lipids to ketones) prevail and ketoacids are produced, superimposing severe metabolic acidosis on the hyperosmotic volume-depleted state.

The treatment of both entities involves correcting precipitating factors and addressing metabolic abnormalities. The treatment is complex and usually involves admission to an intensive care unit and careful monitoring of all metabolic parameters.

Long-term complications of diabetes mellitus

The long-term complications of diabetes mellitus are usually secondary to vascular disease. Nephropathy, neuropathy, peripheral arterial disease, coronary atherosclerosis, secondary cerebral thrombosis, cardiac infarction, and retinopathy are all important causes of morbidity and mortality. The precise mechanism for the development of diabetic complications is elusive, but hyperglycemia plays some central role by triggering a number of mechanisms that ultimately cause vascular damage. (Diabetic retinopathy is discussed in BCSC Section 12, *Retina and Vitreous.*)

Glucose control is not the only risk factor that can be modified to minimize the development of complications. In particular, hypertension and lipid abnormalities seem to be inextricably intertwined with glucose control. Thus, any attempt to minimize complications must include aggressive control of these other factors. Studies have found that candesartan, an angiotensin II receptor antagonist, and fenofibrate, a cholesterol-lowering agent, may mildly slow the progression of retinopathy. Additional risk factors for diabetic complications include duration of disease, smoking, pregnancy, and genetic predisposition. Risk factors that seem to exacerbate diabetic retinopathy in particular include early renal disease and anemia.

Nephropathy Approximately 40% of patients who have had diabetes mellitus for 20 or more years have nephropathy. Albuminuria greater than 300 mg/24 hours, which is about the level at which a standard urine dipstick test becomes positive, is the hallmark of diabetic nephropathy. Renal failure eventually occurs in approximately 50% of patients in whom diabetes develops before age 20 and in 6% of those with onset after 40 years of age. Diabetic nephropathy is the leading cause of end-stage renal disease, and the 5-year survival rate of diabetic patients on maintenance dialysis is less than 20%. Almost invariably, nephropathy and retinopathy develop within a short time of each other.

The progression of diabetic nephropathy is as follows: microalbuminuria (urine albumin levels of 30–300 mg/24 hours), macroalbuminuria (urine albumin levels over 300 mg/24 hours), nephrotic syndrome, and finally end-stage renal disease. Tight control of blood glucose can delay and perhaps prevent the development of microalbuminuria. Controlling hypertension (particularly with angiotensin-converting enzyme inhibitors) and adhering to low-protein diets may help decrease the rate of decline in glomerular filtration rate.

Neuropathy Diabetic neuropathy is a common problem. After 30 years of diabetes mellitus, half of patients have signs of neuropathy, and 15%–20% have symptoms of distal symmetric polyneuropathy. Changes in nerve metabolism and function are thought to be mediated in part through increased aldose reductase activity; Schwann cell synthesis of myelin is impaired, and axonal degeneration ensues. In addition, microangiopathy of the endoneural capillaries leads to vascular abnormalities and microinfarcts of the nerves, with multifocal fiber loss. Symptoms in the feet and lower legs are most common. Foot pain, paresthesias, and loss of sensation occur frequently and probably result from both ischemic and metabolic nerve abnormalities. Weakness may occur as part of mononeuritis or a mononeuritis multiplex and is usually associated with pain. Cranial neuropathies may also occur (see BCSC Section 5, *Neuro-Ophthalmology*). Additional morbidity stemming from autonomic dysfunction can occur, including male and female sexual dysfunction, impaired urination, delayed gastric emptying, orthostatic hypotension, and tachycardia due to loss of vagal tone.

There is no specific treatment for diabetic neuropathy. Aldose reductase inhibitors (not yet commercially available) may improve nerve conduction slightly but do not result in major clinical improvement. The pain may respond to tricyclic antidepressants or capsaicin cream. Anticonvulsant drugs such as carbamazepine and gabapentin may also be useful.

Large-vessel disease The risk of coronary artery disease is 2–10 times higher in patients with diabetes mellitus than that in the general population, and the mortality rate in diabetic patients with an anterior myocardial infarction is twice that in nondiabetic patients. Because myocardial infarction in patients with diabetes may present without the classic symptom of chest pain, an increased index of suspicion is required to make the diagnosis. Hypertension increases the risk of cardiovascular disease for persons with diabetes. Cerebral thrombosis is approximately twice as prevalent in the diabetic population as it is in the nondiabetic population, and peripheral arterial disease is 40 times as prevalent.

Ophthalmic considerations Management of patients with diabetes mellitus can be challenging. The ophthalmologist may be the first to identify a complication related to a patient's diabetes, whether a transient refractive change due to glucose elevation or actual diabetic retinopathy. Sometimes the ophthalmologist is a patient's only regular health care provider. Thus, it is important that both the patient and the ophthalmologist be aware of the patient's HbA_{1c} level, a specific and objective measure of glucose control.

Patients may need to be educated about the glucose test, the great importance of maintaining good control, and the possible consequences of poor control. In addition, patients should be reminded that other modifiable risk factors for retinopathy progression, including hypertension, lipid abnormalities, early renal failure, and anemia, are also important.

From an ophthalmic perspective, awareness of a patient's control is important as it may affect the rate of retinopathy progression and in turn affect decisions regarding treatment and follow-up frequency. Studies have shown that poor control can increase the rate of retinopathy progression after cataract surgery and blunt response to laser treatment for diabetic macular edema. Educating patients with poorly controlled diabetes about their prognosis before surgical intervention may facilitate more realistic expectations. However, attempting to rapidly improve glucose control in a patient with poor control at the same time that cataract surgery is performed may actually contribute to retinopathy progression and a poorer visual outcome.

The importance of all the risk factors for retinopathy progression should be conveyed to the patient's primary care physician so that all potential exacerbating factors are controlled as much as possible. The ophthalmologist should strive to monitor how well these issues are being controlled, because a patient with significant problems in any of these areas is likely to have less-than-optimal results with any ophthalmic surgical intervention. (Perioperative management in ocular surgery is reviewed in Chapter 15.)

Suto C, Hori S, Kato S, Muraoka K, Kitano S. Effect of perioperative glycemic control in progression of diabetic retinopathy and maculopathy. *Arch Ophthalmol.* 2006; 124(1):38–45.

Thyroid Disease

Physiology

Functionally, the thyroid gland can be thought of as having 2 parts. The *parafollicular* (or C) cells secrete calcitonin and play a role in calcium homeostasis; they do not affect thyroid physiology. Thyroid *follicles* are made up of a single layer of epithelial cells surrounding colloid, which consists mostly of thyroglobulin, the storage form of the thyroid hormones T_4 and T_3.

T_4 (thyroxine), the main secretory product of the thyroid gland, contains 4 iodine atoms. Deiodination of T_4, which occurs mainly in the liver and kidneys, gives rise to T_3 (triiodothyronine), the metabolically active form of thyroid hormone. Eighty percent of serum T_3 is derived through deiodination; the remainder is secreted by the thyroid. Only a small fraction of the hormones circulate freely in the plasma (0.02% of total T_4 and 0.30% of total T_3); the remainder is bound to the proteins thyroxine-binding globulin (TBG), transthyretin, and albumin.

Thyroid function is regulated by the interrelationships of hypothalamic, pituitary, and thyroid activity. Thyrotropin-releasing hormone (TRH), which is secreted by the hypothalamus, causes the synthesis of thyrotropin (or thyroid-stimulating hormone, TSH) and its release from the anterior pituitary. TSH, in turn, stimulates the thyroid, leading to the release of T_4 and T_3. In this negative-feedback loop, increased levels of T_4 and T_3 inhibit the release of TSH and the TSH response to TRH at the level of the pituitary.

The main role of the thyroid hormones is regulation of tissue metabolism through their effects on protein synthesis. Normal development of the CNS requires adequate amounts of thyroid hormone during the first 2 years of life. Congenital hypothyroidism results in irreversible cognitive disabilities (cretinism). Normal growth and bone maturation also depend on sufficient hormone levels.

Testing for Thyroid Disease

Detection of thyroid disease and evaluation of the efficacy of therapy require the use of various combinations of laboratory tests. The American Thyroid Association recommends initial screening with TSH and free T_4.

Measurement of serum TSH

Thyroid-stimulating hormone secretion by the pituitary is tightly controlled by negative-feedback mechanisms regulated by serum T_4 and T_3 levels. TSH levels begin to rise early in the course of hypothyroidism and fall in hyperthyroidism, even before free T_4 levels are outside the reference range. Therefore, the serum TSH level is a sensitive indicator of thyroid dysfunction.

The concentration of TSH is very low, and previous tests were not sensitive enough to differentiate between normal TSH levels and the reduced TSH levels seen in hyperthyroidism. In recent years, extremely sensitive assays of TSH have been developed that can detect levels down to 0.005 mIU/L, making it possible to differentiate low normal values from abnormally low values. The TSH test is useful for (1) screening for thyroid disease, (2) monitoring replacement therapy in hypothyroid patients (TSH levels respond 6–8 weeks after changes in hormone replacement dosage), and (3) monitoring suppressive therapy for thyroid nodules or cancer. In screening for thyroid disease, the combination of free T_4 and sensitive TSH assays has a sensitivity of 99.5% and a specificity of 98.0%. As a result, the combination of both TSH and free T_4 is used for screening in most situations. There is presently some controversy about the upper limit of normal for TSH, so endocrinologic consultation is indicated in borderline cases.

Measurement of serum T_4

Total serum T_4 comprises 2 parts: the protein-bound fraction and the free hormone. Total T_4 levels can be affected by changes in serum TBG levels, while euthyroidism is maintained and free T_4 levels remain normal. Levels of TBG and total T_4 are elevated in pregnancy and with use of oral contraceptives, while free T_4 levels remain normal. Low TBG and total T_4 levels are associated with chronic illness, protein malnutrition, hepatic failure, and use of glucocorticoids.

Measurement of serum T_3

Serum T_3 levels may not accurately reflect thyroid gland function for 2 reasons: first, T_3 is not the major secretory product of the thyroid; and second, many factors influence T_3 levels, including nutrition, medications, and mechanisms regulating the enzymes that convert T_4 to T_3. Determination of T_3 levels is indicated in patients who may have T_3 thyrotoxicosis, an uncommon condition in which clinically hyperthyroid patients have normal T_4 and free T_4 but elevated T_3 levels.

Thyroid hormone–binding protein tests

Thyroxine-binding globulin concentrations can be measured directly by immunoassay. However, it is rarely necessary to determine the levels of circulating TBG and transthyretin in the clinical setting. The T_3 resin uptake test can be used to estimate thyroid hormone binding.

Radioactive iodine uptake test

A 24-hour test of the thyroid's ability to concentrate a dose of radioactive iodine, the radioactive iodine uptake (RAIU) test is not always accurate enough to assess thyroid metabolic status. The RAIU test is used mainly to determine whether a patient's hyperthyroidism is due to Graves disease (elevated RAIU, >30%–40%), toxic nodular goiter (normal to elevated), or subacute thyroiditis (low to undetectable, <2%–4%).

Thyroid antibody tests

Several antibodies related to thyroid disease can be detected in the blood. The most common is *thyroid microsomal antibody,* found in approximately 95% of patients with Hashimoto thyroiditis, 55% of those with Graves disease, and 10% of adults with no apparent thyroid disease. Antibodies to thyroglobulin are also found in thyroid disease of various causes, including Hashimoto thyroiditis, Graves disease, and thyroid carcinoma. Patients with Graves disease usually have antibodies directed at TSH receptors. These antibodies generally stimulate the release of thyroid hormone, but in rare cases patients have antibodies that block thyroid hormone release. High serum levels of thyroid-stimulating immunoglobulin and the absence of thyroperoxidase antibody are both risk factors for ophthalmopathy in Graves disease. Assays are available to detect antibodies against antigens present on extraocular muscles in thyroid eye disease, but the significance of these antibodies is unclear.

Thyroid scanning

Scanning with iodine 123 reveals concentration and binding; using technetium-99m demonstrates iodide-concentrating capacity. Thyroid scanning is useful in distinguishing functioning ("hot") from nonfunctioning ("cold") thyroid nodules and in evaluating chest and neck masses for metastatic thyroid cancer.

Thyroid ultrasonography

Ultrasonography is used to establish the presence of cystic or solid thyroid nodules when palpation is inconclusive in suspicious cases. This modality detects nodules as small as 1 mm, although nodules of this size are not of clinical significance.

Biopsy or fine-needle aspiration biopsy

Biopsy or fine-needle aspiration techniques are used to obtain tissue samples for the evaluation of thyroid nodules. Fine-needle aspiration specimens require interpretation by an experienced cytopathologist. Fine-needle aspiration is recommended for obtaining samples from nodules larger than 1 cm and draining fluid from cystic thyroid nodules. Although nodules deemed benign are followed with annual thyroid ultrasonography, an increase in size demands a second fine-needle aspiration for evaluation.

Hyperthyroidism

Hypermetabolism caused by excessive quantities of circulating thyroid hormones results in the clinical syndrome of *hyperthyroidism (thyrotoxicosis).* Clinical findings include exophthalmos, chest palpitations, excessive sweating, diarrhea, weight loss, and sensitivity to heat. Graves hyperthyroidism accounts for approximately 85% of cases of thyrotoxicosis.

Toxic nodular goiter and thyroiditis account for most of the remaining cases. *Thyroid storm* is a rare, acute hypermetabolic state that is fatal if untreated. It is often precipitated by surgery, infection, or trauma in a patient with otherwise mild hyperthyroidism. Patients typically present with fever, tachycardia, nausea, vomiting, agitation, and psychosis; patients can become comatose secondary to hypotension. Modern treatments aimed at controlling the process have dramatically reduced mortality.

Graves hyperthyroidism

Thyroid eye disease (TED) is discussed in BCSC Section 5, *Neuro-Ophthalmology,* and Section 7, *Orbit, Eyelids, and Lacrimal System.* This discussion focuses on the thyroid disease.

Patients with Graves hyperthyroidism (also known as *diffuse toxic goiter*) exhibit various combinations of hypermetabolism, diffuse enlargement of the thyroid gland, TED, and infiltrative dermopathy. Graves hyperthyroidism is believed to be an autoimmune disorder. Up to 90% of patients have circulating TSH receptor antibodies; furthermore, the level of thyroid-stimulating immunoglobulin has been shown to correlate with the severity of clinical disease.

Graves hyperthyroidism is common, with a 10:1 female preponderance. The incidence peaks in the third and fourth decades of life, and there is a strong familial component. Risk factors including stress and smoking are associated with increased incidence of thyroid eye disease.

The clinical syndrome consists of nervousness, tremor, weight loss, palpitations, heat intolerance, emotional lability, muscle weakness, and gastrointestinal hypermotility. Clinical signs include tachycardia or atrial fibrillation, increased systolic and decreased diastolic blood pressure (widened pulse pressure), and thyroid enlargement. *Infiltrative dermopathy*—brawny, nonpitting swelling of the pretibial area, ankles, or feet—may be present and is almost always associated with TED. Approximately one-third of patients with Graves hyperthyroidism have clinically obvious TED at the time of diagnosis of the hyperthyroidism.

Treatment of Graves hyperthyroidism is aimed at returning thyroid function to normal. A significant proportion of patients (30%–50%) experience remission in association with drug treatment directed at the thyroid. Later in the course of the disease, patients may experience relapse, hypothyroidism, or both.

The first step in treatment is to control symptoms, if necessary, with a β-blocker. In addition, thyroid secretion is suppressed using one of the thiourea derivatives, propylthiouracil or methimazole. The drugs inhibit the use of iodine by the gland. Treatment is continued until clinical and laboratory indexes show improvement. Adverse effects include rash (common), liver damage (rare), vasculitis (rare), and agranulocytosis (0.02%–0.05% of patients).

There are several options for long-term treatment of Graves hyperthyroidism: the aforementioned antithyroid drugs can be continued for 12–24 months in hopes of remission; part of the gland can be surgically removed, an option that is frequently successful, although approximately half of such patients eventually become hypothyroid; or radioactive iodine can be used, which is the most common choice. Iodine 131 is highly effective, resulting in hypothyroidism in 80% of patients within 6–12 months; some require a second treatment. Adverse effects are minimal, but use of ^{131}I may be associated with worsening of TED. Corticosteroids may be useful in preventing progression of TED related to this treatment.

Toxic nodular goiter

In toxic nodular goiter, thyroid hormone–producing adenomas (either single or multiple) make enough hormone to cause hyperthyroidism. Hot nodules are almost never carcinomatous and often result in hyperthyroidism. Toxic nodules may be treated with radioactive iodine or surgery.

Hypothyroidism

Hypothyroidism is a clinical syndrome resulting from a deficiency of thyroid hormone. *Myxedema* is the nonpitting edema caused by subcutaneous accumulation of mucopolysaccharides in severe cases of hypothyroidism; the term is sometimes used to describe the entire syndrome of severe hypothyroidism.

Primary hypothyroidism accounts for more than 95% of cases and may be congenital or acquired. Most primary cases are due to Hashimoto thyroiditis (discussed in the following section), "idiopathic" myxedema (thought by many to be end-stage Hashimoto thyroiditis), and iatrogenic causes (^{131}I or surgical treatment of hyperthyroidism). *Secondary hypothyroidism,* caused by hypothalamic or pituitary dysfunction (usually after pituitary surgery), is much less common. As in hyperthyroidism, the female preponderance among adults is significant. *Subclinical hypothyroidism* is defined as a normal T_4 concentration and a slightly elevated TSH level. These patients may or may not have symptoms suggestive of hypothyroidism, and some controversy surrounds whether such patients should be treated.

Clinically, the patient with hypothyroidism presents with signs and symptoms of hypometabolism and accumulation of mucopolysaccharides in the tissues of the body. Many of the symptoms are nonspecific—they include weakness, fatigue, memory loss, dry skin, hair loss, deepening of the voice, weight gain (despite loss of appetite), cold intolerance, arthralgias, constipation, and muscle cramps—and their relationship to thyroid dysfunction may not be recognized for some time. Clinical signs include bradycardia, reduced pulse pressure, myxedema, weight gain, loss of body and scalp hair, and menstrual disorders. In severe cases, personality changes ("myxedema psychosis") and death (following "myxedema coma") may occur.

Treatment of hypothyroidism is straightforward, consisting of oral thyroid replacement medication to normalize circulating hormone levels. Levothyroxine is the most commonly used preparation. Serum T_4 and TSH levels are monitored at regular intervals to ensure that euthyroidism is maintained.

Thyroiditis

Thyroiditis may be classified as acute, subacute, or chronic. *Acute thyroiditis,* caused by bacterial infection, is extremely rare. *Subacute thyroiditis* occurs in 2 forms: granulomatous and lymphocytic. Hashimoto thyroiditis is the most common type of *chronic thyroiditis.*

Patients with *subacute granulomatous thyroiditis* present with a painful, enlarged gland associated with fever, chills, and malaise. Thyroid function tests may be helpful because they may reveal the unusual combination of an elevated T_4 level and a low RAIU. Patients may be hyperthyroid because of the release of hormone from areas of thyroid destruction; pathologic examination reveals granulomatous inflammation. The disease is self-limited, and treatment is symptomatic, with use of either analgesics or, in severe cases, oral corticosteroids. After resolution, transient hypothyroidism, which becomes permanent in 5%–10% of patients, may occur.

Patients with *subacute lymphocytic thyroiditis* ("painless" thyroiditis), which commonly occurs 2–4 months postpartum in mothers but may occur in isolation, present with symptoms of hyperthyroidism and a normal or slightly enlarged but nontender thyroid gland. Pathologic investigation shows lymphocytic infiltration resembling Hashimoto thyroiditis, suggesting an autoimmune cause. This disease is also self-limited, generally lasting less than 3 months. Hypothyroidism may ensue. Treatment is symptomatic.

Hashimoto thyroiditis is an autoimmune disease that causes goitrous hypothyroidism. Patients have antibodies to thyroid antigens and an increased incidence of other autoimmune diseases. Patients with Hashimoto thyroiditis may present with hypothyroidism, an enlarged thyroid, or both. Pathologic examination reveals lymphocytic infiltration. Treatment is aimed at normalizing hormone levels with thyroid replacement therapy. Patients with enlarged glands and airway obstruction who do not respond to TSH suppression may require surgery. The risk of primary thyroid lymphoma and papillary thyroid cancer is slightly increased in patients with Hashimoto thyroiditis.

Postpartum thyroiditis occurs in approximately 5% of women after delivery (often in subsequent pregnancies) and can cause hyperthyroidism or hypothyroidism (or first one problem and then the other). Postpartum thyroiditis is usually painless and self-limited and is often associated with antimicrosomal antibodies.

Thyroid Tumors

Virtually all tumors of the thyroid gland arise from glandular cells and are, therefore, adenomas or carcinomas. Functioning adenomas were discussed previously (see "Toxic nodular goiter").

On thyroid scan, 90%–95% of thyroid adenomas are cold nodules and come to attention only if large enough to be physically apparent. Diagnostic testing involves a combination of approaches, including ultrasonography (cysts are benign and simply aspirated), fine-needle aspiration, and surgery, depending on the clinical situation. Treatment options for benign cold nodules are suppressive therapy, in which thyroid hormone replacement is used to suppress TSH secretion and its stimulatory effect on functioning nodules, and surgery.

Carcinomas of the thyroid are of 4 types: papillary, follicular, medullary, and anaplastic (undifferentiated). *Papillary carcinoma* is the most common form of thyroid tumor. Tumors removed before extension outside the capsule of the gland appear to have no adverse effect on survival. *Follicular carcinoma* may also be associated with a normal life span if it is identified before it becomes invasive, but late metastases can occur. *Medullary carcinoma* arises from the C cells and produces calcitonin. The lesion can occur as a solitary malignant tumor or as part of multiple endocrine neoplasia type 2 (discussed at the end of the chapter). *Anaplastic carcinoma,* though rare, is the most malignant tumor of the thyroid gland and is found mainly in patients older than 60 years. For the giant cell form, the survival time is less than 6 months from time of diagnosis; for the small cell form, the 5-year survival rate is 20%–25%.

Ponto KA, Kanitz M, Olivo PD, Pitz S, Pfeiffer N, Kahaly GJ. Clinical relevance of thyroid-stimulating immunoglobulins in Graves' ophthalmopathy. *Ophthalmology.* 2011;118(11): 2279–2285.

Disorders of the Hypothalamic-Pituitary Axis

The hypothalamus is the coordinating center of the endocrine system. It consolidates signals from higher cortical centers, the autonomic nervous system, the environment, and systemic endocrine feedback. The hypothalamus then delivers precise instructions to the pituitary gland, which releases hormones that influence most endocrine systems in the body. The hypothalamic-pituitary axis directly affects the thyroid gland, the adrenal gland, and the gonads, and it influences growth, milk production, and water balance.

Table 2-4 outlines the major hypothalamic hormones and their actions on the anterior pituitary hormones. The hypothalamic hormones are released directly into a primary capillary plexus that empties into the portal venous circulation, travel down the pituitary stalk, and bathe the anterior pituitary gland in a secondary capillary plexus. The hormones released by the hypothalamic neurons, therefore, reach their target cells rapidly and in high concentrations. This proximity allows a rapid, pulsatile response to signals between the hypothalamus and the anterior pituitary. The posterior pituitary is controlled by direct neuronal innervation from the hypothalamus rather than by blood-borne hormones. The main products of the posterior pituitary are vasopressin and oxytocin. Vasopressin (antidiuretic hormone) is primarily involved in controlling water excretion by the kidneys. Oxytocin produces uterine contractions required for delivery.

Table 2-4 Hypothalamic Neurohormones and Neurotransmitters Involved in Anterior Pituitary Function

Thyrotropin-releasing hormone (TRH) → ↑TSH, PRL
Gonadotropin-releasing hormone (GnRH) → ↑FSH, LH
Growth hormone–releasing hormone (GHRH) → ↑GH
Corticotropin-releasing hormone (CRH) → ↑ACTH
Somatostatin → ↓GH, TSH
Dopamine → ↓PRL

ACTH = adrenocorticotrophic hormone; FSH = follicle-stimulating hormone; GH = growth hormone; LH = luteinizing hormone; PRL = prolactin; TSH = thyroid-stimulating hormone; ↑ = stimulates release of; ↓ = inhibits release of.

Pituitary Adenomas

Pituitary tumors account for 10%–15% of intracranial tumors. They are classified as *microadenomas* (<10 mm in widest diameter) or *macroadenomas* (≥10 mm in widest diameter). Typically benign, these tumors arise from hormone-producing cells and may be functionally active (ie, secrete large amounts of hormones) or inactive. The clinical presentation depends on what type of cell the tumor is derived from and whether the tumor produces hormones. Any type of tumor may be clinically inactive; such tumors will become apparent only when they have enlarged enough to cause symptoms, at which time patients may present with headaches, visual symptoms such as visual field loss due to chiasmal compression, cranial neuropathies, and/or hypopituitarism from compression of normal pituitary tissue. (The ophthalmic effects of pituitary adenomas and other parasellar lesions are discussed in BCSC Section 5, *Neuro-Ophthalmology.*)

Accounting for approximately 15% of pituitary tumors, *somatotroph adenomas* produce growth hormone and cause acromegaly in adults and gigantism in prepubertal patients. Acromegaly often develops insidiously over several years. Patients may present with headaches and visual symptoms due to enlargement of the adenoma before the diagnosis is recognized. The characteristic findings include an enlarged jaw, coarse facial features, and enlarged and swollen hands and feet. Patients may also have cardiac disease and diabetes mellitus in addition to the typical bone and soft-tissue changes.

Lactotroph adenomas (prolactinomas) account for approximately 25% of symptomatic pituitary tumors. Hyperprolactinemia produces amenorrhea and galactorrhea in women and decreased libido and impotence in men. The symptoms tend to be gradual in males, and patients may present with compression symptoms due to tumor enlargement before the hormonal effects are recognized.

Thyrotroph adenomas are rare, accounting for less than 1% of pituitary tumors. They may cause hyperthyroidism, hypothyroidism, or no change in thyroid function, depending on how the TSH subunits are processed in the tumor cells. These tumors tend to be large macroadenomas, and patients may present with compressive symptoms in addition to any thyroid changes.

Corticotroph adenomas account for approximately 15% of pituitary tumors. They are associated with Cushing syndrome, which includes the classic features of centripetal obesity, hirsutism, and facial plethora. Fat deposits develop over the thoracocervical spine (buffalo hump) and temporal regions (moon facies). Psychiatric abnormalities occur in 50% of patients, and long-standing Cushing disease can cause osteoporosis. Patients bruise easily and have violet striae on the abdomen, upper thighs, and arms. Hypertension and glucose intolerance leading to diabetes mellitus can also occur. Cushing syndrome can also develop secondary to adrenal gland neoplasms and, most commonly, from iatrogenic administration of glucocorticoids.

Gonadotroph adenomas (approximately 10% of pituitary tumors) may produce serum follicle-stimulating hormone and, in rare cases, luteinizing hormone. Affected patients present with hypogonadism related to gonadal downregulation. Gonadotropin-producing pituitary tumors may also be clinically inactive, and patients may present with compression symptoms.

Accounting for approximately 15% of pituitary tumors, *plurihormonal adenomas,* as the name implies, produce more than one type of hormone. Common combinations include elevated growth hormone with prolactin and growth hormone with TSH.

Null-cell adenomas (approximately 20% of pituitary tumors) do not have any pathologic markers to suggest a certain cell type and do not produce hormone excess. Most tumors that present with signs of enlargement and compression are gonadotroph or null-cell adenomas.

Tumors of the pituitary gland are best diagnosed with contrast magnetic resonance imaging focused on the pituitary region. Endocrinologic testing is warranted when hypersecretion syndromes are suspected or when the patient has evidence of hypopituitarism. The treatment approach is complex and depends on a number of factors, including the size of the tumor and the nature of the hormonal activity. Treatment is discussed further in BCSC Section 5, *Neuro-Ophthalmology.*

Pituitary Apoplexy

Pituitary apoplexy results from hemorrhage or infarction in a pituitary adenoma; it can occur spontaneously or after head trauma. In its most dramatic presentation, apoplexy causes the sudden onset of excruciating headache, visual field loss, diplopia due to pressure on the oculomotor nerves, and hypopituitarism. All pituitary hormonal deficiencies can occur, but cortisol deficiency is the most serious because it can cause life-threatening hypotension. Imaging of the pituitary may show intra-adenomal hemorrhage and deviation of the pituitary stalk. Most patients recover but experience long-term pituitary insufficiency. Signs of reduced vision and altered mental status are indications for transsphenoidal surgical decompression. Ophthalmologists need to be aware of this entity because of the high incidence of visual symptoms on presentation.

Multiple Endocrine Neoplasia Syndromes

Multiple endocrine neoplasia (MEN) syndromes are rare hereditary syndromes of benign and malignant endocrine neoplasms. There are 2 syndromes, MEN 1 and MEN 2. Both are autosomal dominant, but sporadic cases exist. MEN 2 is further divided into types 2A, 2B, and medullary thyroid cancer (MTC) alone.

The most common features of MEN 1 are parathyroid, enteropancreatic, and pituitary tumors. Hyperparathyroidism is the most common endocrine abnormality. Enteropancreatic tumors include gastrinomas, which cause increased gastric acid output (Zollinger-Ellison syndrome), and insulinomas, which cause fasting hypoglycemia. Pituitary adenomas can be present and are usually prolactinomas, but other types can occur. Carcinoid and adrenal tumors can develop as well.

MEN 2A and 2B are characterized by MTC, which occurs in 90%–100% of patients and is the main cause of morbidity. The lifetime incidence of pheochromocytoma is approximately 50%. Hyperparathyroidism is seen in approximately 20%–30% of patients with MEN 2A but is rarely seen in MEN 2B.

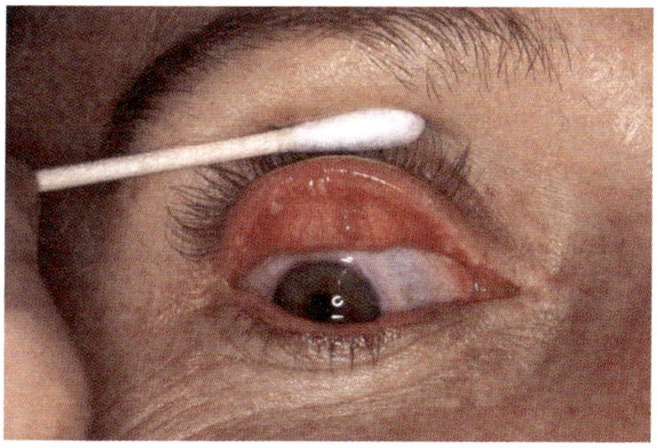

Figure 2-3 Eyelid nodules in multiple endocrine neoplasia (MEN) 2B. *(Courtesy of Jason M. Jacobs, MD, and Michael J. Hawes, MD.)*

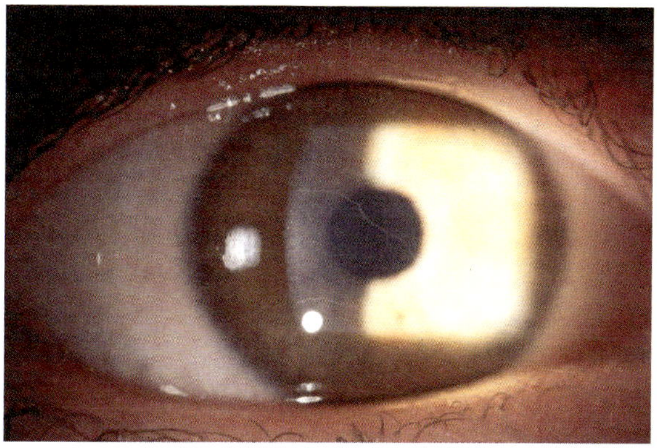

Figure 2-4 Enlarged corneal nerves in MEN 2B. *(Courtesy of Jason M. Jacobs, MD, and Michael J. Hawes, MD.)*

MEN 2B is characterized by ganglioneuromas, which occur in 95% of patients. They can be present on the lips, eyelids, and tongue, giving these patients a characteristic phenotype that can be apparent at birth. Patients with MEN 2B may also have marfanoid features including pectus excavatum and scoliosis but lack lens subluxation and aortic disease. The eyelid margins may be nodular because of the presence of multiple small tumors (Fig 2-3); neuromas have also been reported subconjunctivally. Perhaps the most striking ophthalmic finding is the presence of prominent corneal nerves in a clear stroma (Fig 2-4); this is reported to occur in 100% of cases. Because MTC may not appear until the patient's second or third decade, the ophthalmic manifestations may be the initial indication that a patient has MEN 2B, making ophthalmologists potentially instrumental in diagnosing this disease.

The management of MEN depends on the nature of the tumor and usually involves medical treatment to control hormonal effects and/or surgical excision when possible. The genes that cause all types of MEN have been located, and genetic testing can identify patients at risk. Identification of involved family members is particularly useful in MEN 2 because prophylactic thyroidectomy can decrease the risk of death from MTC. Screening for pheochromocytoma is also warranted in order to identify problems before complications such as hypertension develop.

Melmed S, Polonsky KS, Larsen PR, Kronenberg HM, eds. *Williams Textbook of Endocrinology.* 12th ed. Philadelphia: Elsevier/Saunders; 2012.

CHAPTER 3

Hypertension

Recent Developments

- Normal blood pressure (BP) in adults is less than 120/80 mm Hg, according to guidelines published in 2003 by the Joint National Committee on Prevention, Detection, Evaluation, and Treatment of High Blood Pressure (JNC 7).
- The Eighth Report of the Joint National Committee on Prevention, Detection, Evaluation, and Treatment of High Blood Pressure (JNC 8), published in 2014, significantly alters the treatment algorithms for hypertension.
- JNC 8 and the European Society of Hypertension recommend that the general population aged 60 years or older with systolic BP of 150 mm Hg or higher or diastolic BP of 90 mm Hg or higher be treated to maintain systolic BP below 150 mm Hg and/or diastolic BP below 90 mm Hg. For the general population 18 through 59 years of age, the goals are less than 140 mm Hg for systolic BP and less than 90 mm Hg for diastolic BP.
- The BP goals set by many subspecialty associations continue to be generally in line with those of JNC 7, especially for patients with diabetes mellitus, proteinuria, congestive heart failure, or renal insufficiency.
- The risk of cardiovascular disease, beginning at 115/75 mm Hg, doubles with each 20/10 mm Hg increase in BP.
- Masked hypertension (BP that is normal in the office but elevated when measured at home) carries a worse prognosis than white coat hypertension with regard to development of arteriosclerosis.
- Based on the history and comorbidities of the hypertensive patient, treatment with renin-angiotensin system (RAS) blockade, β-blockers, or calcium channel blockers may be initiated. Thiazide-type diuretics are no longer the primary choice.
- Combination therapy, or 2 or more medications, at onset of hypertension is indicated for patients whose BP is 20/10 mm Hg or more above goal.
- Hypertension in children and adolescents is increasingly common and has substantial long-term health implications.

Introduction

Hypertension affects an estimated 73 million persons aged 20 years or older in the United States and approximately 1 billion people worldwide. Those with hypertension are at greater risk for stroke, myocardial infarction (MI), heart failure, peripheral arterial disease, kidney disease, and retinal vascular complications. The prevalence of hypertension increases with age and tends to be familial. Hypertension is more common in black persons than in white persons, and the incidence of devastating complications is higher in lower socioeconomic groups because of greater prevalence, delayed detection, and poor control rates. Antihypertensive therapy is effective in reducing cardiovascular morbidity and mortality. However, only 59% of patients with hypertension are treated, and only 34% achieve a BP of 140/90 mm Hg or less, according to the National Health and Nutrition Examination Surveys (NHANES) in the United States and similar studies in Canada and Europe.

Classification of Blood Pressure and Diagnosis of Hypertension

A classification of BP for adults aged 18 years or older was published in 2003 by the Joint National Committee on Prevention, Detection, Evaluation, and Treatment of High BP (JNC 7) and reconfirmed by JNC 8 in 2014. Under the guidelines outlined in Table 3-1, normal BP is less than 120/80 mm Hg. *Hypertension* is defined as systolic BP of 140 mm Hg or higher or diastolic BP of 90 mm Hg or higher. *Prehypertension* is systolic BP of 120–139 mm Hg or diastolic BP of 80–89 mm Hg. Stage 1 hypertension is systolic BP of 140–159 mm Hg or diastolic BP of 90–99 mm Hg. Stage 2 hypertension is systolic BP of 160 mm Hg or higher or diastolic BP of 100 mm Hg or higher. The classification is based on the average of 2 or more properly measured seated BP readings on each of 2 or more office visits.

In 10%–15% of patients, BP increases only in a physician's office; these patients are said to have "white coat" hypertension. Home BP monitoring or 24-hour ambulatory BP measurement (ABPM) is warranted in these individuals and in patients with labile hypertension, resistant hypertension, hypotensive episodes, or postural hypotension, as well as in patients with masked hypertension. ABPM, which is more widely used in Europe, provides data on circadian variations of BP. ABPM readings are usually lower than measurements taken in the office, and they correlate better with target-organ injury than do office measurements. BP in most individuals decreases by 10%–20% during sleep (dipping pattern); those without such a decrease (nondipping pattern) are at greater risk for cardiovascular events. Masked hypertension may occur in 10%–30% of patients and was shown to carry a worse prognosis than white coat hypertension with regard to the development of atherosclerosis. Thus, it is important to recognize that a normal office BP does not exclude

Table 3-1 Classification of Blood Pressure for Adults Aged 18 Years or Older

BP Classification	Systolic, mm Hg		Diastolic, mm Hg
Normal	<120	and	<80
Prehypertension	120–139	or	80–89
Stage 1 hypertension	140–159	or	90–99
Stage 2 hypertension	≥160	or	≥100

Adapted with permission from Chobanian AV, Bakris GL, Black HR, et al; National High Blood Pressure Education Program Coordinating Committee. The Seventh Report of the Joint National Committee on Prevention, Detection, Evaluation, and Treatment of High Blood Pressure: the JNC 7 report. *JAMA*. 2003; 289(19):2561. ©2003 American Medical Association.

hypertension. Individuals with a mean self-measured BP above 135/85 mm Hg at home are generally considered to be hypertensive.

Chobanian AV, Bakris GL, Black HR, et al; National Heart, Lung, and Blood Institute Joint National Committee on Prevention, Detection, Evaluation, and Treatment of High Blood Pressure; National High Blood Pressure Education Program Coordinating Committee. The Seventh Report of the Joint National Committee on Prevention, Detection, Evaluation, and Treatment of High BP: the JNC 7 report. *JAMA*. 2003;289(19):2560–2572.

James PA, Oparil S, Carter BL, et al. 2014 Evidence-based guideline for the management of high blood pressure in adults: report from the panel members appointed to the Eighth Joint National Committee (JNC 8). *JAMA*. 2014;311(5):507–520.

Etiology and Pathogenesis of Hypertension

Approximately 90% of cases of hypertension are *primary (essential),* in which the etiology is unknown, and 10% are secondary to identifiable causes. Primary hypertension most likely results from a disregulation of various renal, hormonal, and cellular processes in conjunction with environmental factors such as diet and exercise. These processes include abnormal sodium transport, increased sympathetic nervous system activity, abnormal vasodilation, excess transforming growth factors β (TGF-βs), and abnormalities in the renin-angiotensin-aldosterone system (Fig 3-1).

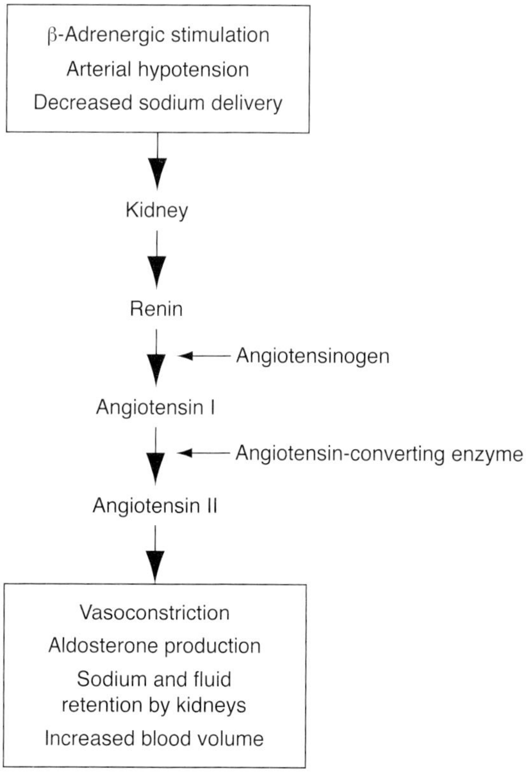

Figure 3-1 Renin-angiotensin-aldosterone system.

Causes of *secondary hypertension* are outlined in Table 3-2. Following are some of these causes, along with signs associated with secondary hypertension:

- *polycystic kidney disease:* flank mass
- *renovascular disease:* unilateral abdominal bruit in a young patient with marked hypertension; new-onset hypertension with severe end-organ disease
- *pheochromocytoma:* markedly labile BP with tachycardia and headache
- *hyperaldosteronism:* persistent hypokalemia in the absence of diuretic therapy or marked drop with low-dose diuretics
- *coarctation of the aorta:* delayed or absent femoral pulses in a young patient
- *Cushing syndrome:* truncal obesity and abdominal striae

Secondary causes of hypertension should be suspected in persons who have accelerating hypertension or hypertension unresponsive to medication or in those who have a sudden change in previously well-controlled BP. Patients with secondary hypertension are more likely to have resistant hypertension.

Resistant hypertension is defined as a failure to achieve goal BP when a patient adheres to the maximum tolerated doses of 3 antihypertensive drugs, including a diuretic. The prevalence of resistant hypertension is currently not known, but indirect population study evidence suggests it is more common than once was thought. This is probably because of the aging population and the increased prevalence of obesity, obstructive sleep apnea syndrome, and chronic kidney disease.

Most cases of diagnosed resistant hypertension are due to inadequate dosing of medication and nonadherence to treatment. Other causes are listed in Table 3-2. These include nonsteroidal anti-inflammatory drugs (NSAIDs), which have volume-retaining effects,

Table 3-2 Causes of Secondary Hypertension and Resistant Hypertension

Chronic kidney disease
Obstructive uropathy
Renovascular disease
Genetic mutations
Primary hyperaldosteronism and other mineralocorticoid excess states
Pheochromocytoma
Cushing syndrome and corticosteroid excess
Coarctation of the aorta
Thyroid or parathyroid disease
Sleep apnea
Drugs (oral contraceptives, sympathomimetics, antidepressants, NSAIDs, erythropoietin-stimulating agents, calcineurin inhibitors [cyclosporine, tacrolimus], over-the-counter medicines, ephedra, ma huang, bitter orange)
Alcohol

NSAIDS = nonsteroidal anti-inflammatory drugs.

Data from Chobanian AV, Bakris GL, Black HR, et al; National High Blood Pressure Education Program Coordinating Committee. The Seventh Report of the Joint National Committee on Prevention, Detection, Evaluation, and Treatment of High Blood Pressure: the JNC 7 report. *JAMA*. 2003;289(19):2563. ©2003 American Medical Association.

and substances such as alcohol, oral contraceptives, licorice, calcineurin inhibitors, and antidepressants. The most common factor contributing to resistant hypertension is excess sodium intake and volume overload and failure to treat this with dietary modification or the proper diuretic and dosage. Resistant hypertension is also discussed later in this chapter, under Special Considerations.

Evaluation of Patients With Hypertension

The evaluation of patients with hypertension should include an assessment of lifestyle and identification of other cardiovascular risk factors (Table 3-3), a search for causes of secondary hypertension, and determination of the presence or absence of target-organ damage and cardiovascular disease.

The physical examination should include measurement of BP in both arms; ophthalmoscopic examination; calculation of body mass index; measurement of waist circumference, which is considered the most important anthropometric factor associated with

Table 3-3 Cardiovascular Risk Factors

Major risk factors

- Hypertension*
- Cigarette smoking
- Obesity (BMI ≥30)*
- Physical inactivity
- Dyslipidemia*
- Diabetes mellitus*
- Microalbuminuria or estimated GFR <60 mL/min in early-morning specimen
- Age (>55 years for men, >65 years for women)
- Family history of premature cardiovascular disease (men <55 years of age or women <65 years of age)

Target-organ damage

- Heart
  - Left ventricular hypertrophy
  - Angina or prior myocardial infarction
  - Prior coronary revascularization
  - Heart failure
- Brain
  - Stroke or transient ischemic attack
- Chronic kidney disease
- Peripheral arterial disease
- Retinopathy

BMI = body mass index, calculated as weight in kilograms divided by the square of height in meters; GFR = glomerular filtration rate.

*Components of the metabolic syndrome.

Adapted with permission from Chobanian AV, Bakris GL, Black HR, et al; National High Blood Pressure Education Program Coordinating Committee. The Seventh Report of the Joint National Committee on Prevention, Detection, Evaluation, and Treatment of High Blood Pressure: the JNC 7 report. *JAMA.* 2003; 289(19):2563. ©2003 American Medical Association.

hypertensive risk; auscultation for carotid, abdominal, and femoral bruits; examination of the thyroid gland; examination of the heart and lungs; examination of the abdomen for masses and aortic pulsation; examination of the lower extremities for edema and pulses; and neurologic assessment.

Laboratory tests to screen for secondary causes and exclude comorbidity (recommended before starting treatment) include an electrocardiogram, urinalysis, complete blood count, and serum chemistry studies, including a fasting lipid profile. More extensive testing for identifiable causes of hypertension is usually not indicated unless BP control is not achieved or there are other clinical findings.

Seidell JC, Han TS, Feskens EJ, Lean ME. Narrow hips and broad waist circumferences independently contribute to increased risk of non-insulin-dependent diabetes mellitus. *J Intern Med.* 1997;242(5):401–406.

Treatment of Hypertension

The primary objective of antihypertensive therapy is to reduce cardiovascular and renal morbidity and mortality. Controlling systolic BP is the major concern because, in patients older than 50 years, systolic BP greater than 140 mm Hg is a more important cardiovascular risk factor than diastolic BP. Diastolic BP is usually controlled when the systolic goal is reached. Maintaining BP at less than 140/90 mm Hg decreases cardiovascular complications. In hypertensive patients with diabetes mellitus or renal disease, the BP goal is less than 130/80 mm Hg. Effective BP control can be attained in most patients with hypertension, but the majority require 2 or more medications. It is important for patients to understand that lifelong treatment is usually necessary and that symptoms are not a reliable indicator of the severity of hypertension.

In considering the appropriate therapy for a patient, the physician should weigh multiple factors: stage of hypertension, target-organ disease, cardiovascular risk factors, cost, adherence, side effects, and comorbid conditions. In general, the higher the BP, the greater the damage to target organs; and the greater the risk factors for cardiovascular disease, the sooner treatment should be initiated. For example, patients with severe hypertension and encephalopathy require emergent treatment, whereas those with mild hypertension may attempt lifestyle modifications before drug therapy is initiated.

Lifestyle Modifications

Obesity, sedentary lifestyle, excessive sodium intake, high daily alcohol consumption, and inadequate intake of vitamins and minerals such as potassium, calcium, magnesium, and folate can contribute to the development of hypertension. Smoking is also important as a major contributor to cardiovascular disease in patients with hypertension. Lifestyle modifications, including reducing weight, adopting the DASH (Dietary Approaches to Stop Hypertension) eating plan, reducing dietary sodium intake, increasing physical activity, and moderating alcohol consumption can decrease BP, enhance the effectiveness of antihypertensive drugs, and lower the risk of cardiovascular disease; see Table 3-4 for

Table 3-4 Lifestyle Modifications to Manage Hypertension*

Modification	Recommendation	Approximate Systolic BP Reduction, Range
Weight reduction	Maintain normal body weight (BMI, 18.5–24.9)	5–20 mm Hg/10 kg weight loss
Adoption of DASH eating plan	Consume a diet rich in fruits, vegetables, and low-fat dairy products with a reduced content of saturated and total fat	8–14 mm Hg
Dietary sodium reduction	Reduce dietary sodium intake to no more than 100 mEq/L (2.4 g sodium or 6 g sodium chloride)	2–8 mm Hg
Physical activity	Engage in regular aerobic physical activity such as brisk walking (at least 30 minutes per day, most days of the week)	4–9 mm Hg
Moderation of alcohol consumption	Limit consumption to no more than 2 drinks per day (1 oz or 30 mL ethanol [eg, 24 oz beer, 10 oz wine, or 3 oz 80-proof whiskey]) in most men and no more than 1 drink per day in women and lighter-weight persons	2–4 mm Hg

BMI = body mass index, calculated as weight in kilograms divided by the square of the height in meters; BP = blood pressure; DASH = Dietary Approaches to Stop Hypertension.

*For overall cardiovascular risk reduction, stop smoking. The effects of implementing these modifications are dose- and time-dependent and could be higher for some individuals.

Adapted with permission from Chobanian AV, Bakris GL, Black HR, et al; National High Blood Pressure Education Program Coordinating Committee. The Seventh Report of the Joint National Committee on Prevention, Detection, Evaluation, and Treatment of High Blood Pressure: the JNC 7 report. *JAMA.* 2003;289(19):2564. ©2003 American Medical Association.

Other Modifications to Manage Hypertension*	
Adequate sleep	Sleep deprivation increases risk twofold in middle-aged adults who sleep ≤5 hours a night.
Treatment of obstructive sleep apnea syndrome (OSAS)	Reduce weight, apply CPAP (continuous positive airway pressure); surgery may be needed in more severe cases.

*For overall cardiovascular risk reduction, stop smoking.

further details. Such healthful lifestyle habits are essential for the prevention and control of hypertension.

Pharmacologic Treatment

Several classes of drugs effectively lower BP and reduce the complications of hypertension. The most commonly prescribed antihypertensive drugs include diuretics, β-blockers, angiotensin-converting enzyme (ACE) inhibitors, angiotensin II receptor blockers (ARBs), and calcium channel blockers (CCBs). Tables 3-5 and 3-6 list these and other types

Table 3-5 Oral Antihypertensive Drugs

Class	Drugs
Thiazide-type diuretics	Chlorothiazide, chlorthalidone, hydrochlorothiazide, indapamide, metolazone, polythiazide
Loop diuretics	Bumetanide, furosemide, torsemide
Potassium-sparing diuretics	Amiloride, triamterene
Aldosterone-receptor blockers	Eplerenone, spironolactone
β-Blockers	Atenolol, betaxolol, bisoprolol, metoprolol, metoprolol extended release, nadolol, nebivolol, propranolol, propranolol long-acting, timolol
β-Blockers with intrinsic sympathomimetic activity	Acebutolol, penbutolol, pindolol
ACE inhibitors	Benazepril, captopril, enalapril, fosinopril, lisinopril, moexipril, perindopril, quinapril, ramipril, trandolapril
Angiotensin II antagonists	Candesartan, eprosartan, irbesartan, losartan, olmesartan, telmisartan, valsartan
Calcium channel blockers: nondihydropyridines	Diltiazem, verapamil
Calcium channel blockers: dihydropyridines	Amlodipine, felodipine, isradipine, nicardipine, nifedipine, nisoldipine
α_1-Blockers	Doxazosin, prazosin, terazosin
Combined α- and β-blockers	Carvedilol, labetalol
Central α_2-agonists and other centrally acting drugs	Clonidine, clonidine patch, guanfacine, methyldopa, reserpine
Direct vasodilators	Hydralazine, minoxidil
Direct renin inhibitor	Aliskiren*

ACE = angiotensin-converting enzyme.
*Aliskiren is an oral renin inhibitor that effectively lowers BP when used either alone or with other antihypertensive agents. It is the first new class of antihypertensive drug approved by the FDA in more than a decade, and its role in the management of patients with hypertension is yet to be established.

Data from Chobanian AV, Bakris GL, Black HR, et al; National High Blood Pressure Education Program Coordinating Committee. The Seventh Report of the Joint National Committee on Prevention, Detection, Evaluation, and Treatment of High Blood Pressure: the JNC 7 report. *JAMA.* 2003;289(19):2565–2566.

of oral antihypertensive drugs. Figure 3-2 provides an algorithm for the treatment of hypertension.

The JNC 8 report focuses more narrowly on the pharmacologic treatment of hypertension, in comparison with JNC 7, which was a more comprehensive discussion of hypertension. In the JNC 7 guidelines, thiazide-type diuretics were recommended as initial drug therapy unless compelling reasons dictated otherwise (Table 3-7); CCBs, ACE inhibitors, ARBs, and β-blockers were alternatives. According to JNC 8 guidelines, the initial drug choice may be selected from 4 drug classes—thiazide-type diuretics, CCBs, ACE inhibitors, and ARBs—for nonblack patients, and from 2 drug classes—thiazide-type diuretics and CCBs—for black patients. β-Blockers are no longer recommended for initial therapy because they may afford less protection against stroke.

Table 3-6 Combination Drugs for Hypertension

Combination Type	Fixed-Dose Combination, mg*
ACE inhibitor and CCB	Amlodipine/benazepril HCl (2.5/10, 5/10, 5/20,10/20)
	Enalapril maleate/felodipine (5/5)
	Trandolapril/verapamil (2/180, 1/240, 2/240, 4/240)
ACE inhibitor and diuretic	Benazepril/hydrochlorothiazide (5/6.25, 10/12.5, 20/12.5, 20/25)
	Captopril/hydrochlorothiazide (25/15, 25/25, 50/15, 50/25)
	Enalapril maleate/hydrochlorothiazide (5/12.5, 10/25)
	Lisinopril/hydrochlorothiazide (10/12.5, 20/12.5, 20/25)
	Moexipril HCl/hydrochlorothiazide (7.5/12.5, 15/25)
	Quinapril HCl/hydrochlorothiazide (10/12.5, 20/12.5, 20/25)
ARB and diuretic	Candesartan cilexetil/hydrochlorothiazide (16/12.5, 32/12.5)
	Eprosartan mesylate/hydrochlorothiazide (600/12.5, 600/25)
	Irbesartan/hydrochlorothiazide (75/12.5, 150/12.5, 300/12.5)
	Losartan potassium/hydrochlorothiazide (50/12.5, 100/25)
	Telmisartan/hydrochlorothiazide (40/12.5, 80/12.5)
	Valsartan/hydrochlorothiazide (80/12.5, 160/12.5)
β-Blocker and diuretic	Atenolol/chlorthalidone (50/25, 100/25)
	Bisoprolol fumarate/hydrochlorothiazide (2.5/6.25, 5/6.25, 10/6.25)
	Metoprolol tartrate/hydrochlorothiazide (50/25, 100/25)
	Nadolol/bendroflumethiazide (40/5, 80/5)
	Propranolol LA/hydrochlorothiazide (40/25, 80/25)
	Timolol maleate/hydrochlorothiazide (10/25)
Centrally acting drug and diuretic	Methyldopa/hydrochlorothiazide (250/15, 250/25, 500/30, 500/50)
	Reserpine/chlorothiazide (0.125/250, 0.25/500)
	Reserpine/hydrochlorothiazide (0.125/25, 0.125/50)
Diuretic and diuretic	Amiloride HCl/hydrochlorothiazide (5/50)
	Spironolactone/ hydrochlorothiazide (25/25, 50/50)
	Triamterene/hydrochlorothiazide (37.5/25, 50/25, 75/50)

ARB = angiotensin II receptor blocker; CCB = calcium channel blocker; HCl = hydrochloride; LA = long-acting.
*Some drug combinations are available in multiple fixed doses. Each drug dose is reported in milligrams.

Adapted with permission from Chobanian AV, Bakris GL, Black HR, et al; National High Blood Pressure Education Program Coordinating Committee. The Seventh Report of the Joint National Committee on Prevention, Detection, Evaluation, and Treatment of High Blood Pressure: the JNC 7 report. *JAMA.* 2003; 289(19):2567. ©2003 American Medical Association.

Table 3-7 Compelling Indications for Individual Drug Classes

High-Risk Condition	Diuretic	β-Blocker	ACE Inhibitor	ARB	CCB	Aldosterone Antagonist
Heart failure	•	•	•	•		•
Post–myocardial infarction		•	•			•
High coronary disease risk	•	•	•		•	
Diabetes	•	•	•	•	•	
Chronic kidney disease			•	•		
Recurrent stroke prevention	•		•			

Adapted with permission from Chobanian AV, Bakris GL, Black HR, et al; National High Blood Pressure Education Program Coordinating Committee. The Seventh Report of the Joint National Committee on Prevention, Detection, Evaluation, and Treatment of High Blood Pressure: the JNC 7 report. *JAMA.* 2003; 289(19):2568. ©2003 American Medical Association.

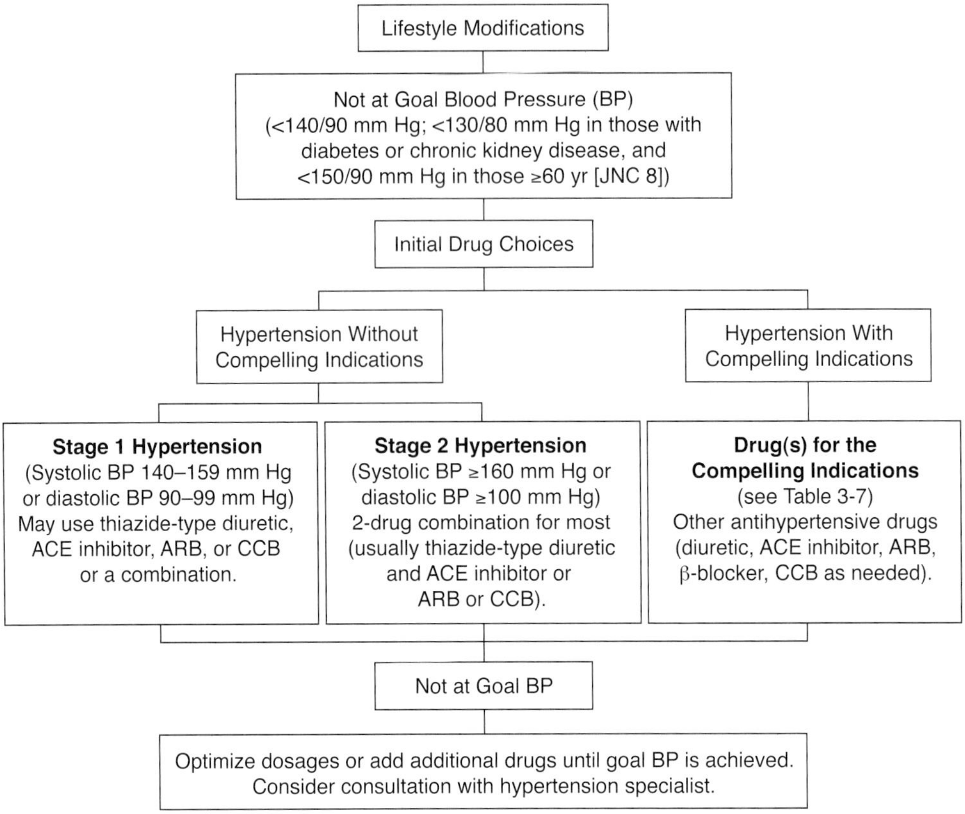

Figure 3-2 Algorithm for treatment of hypertension. ACE = angiotensin-converting enzyme; ARB = angiotensin II receptor blocker; CCB = calcium channel blocker. *(Modified and updated with permission from Chobanian AV, Bakris GL, Black HR, et al; National High Blood Pressure Education Program Coordinating Committee. The Seventh Report of the Joint National Committee on Prevention, Detection, Evaluation, and Treatment of High Blood Pressure: the JNC 7 report.* JAMA. *2003;289(19):2564. ©2003 American Medical Association. Updated with data from James PA, Oparil S, Carter BL, et al. 2014 Evidence-based guideline for the management of high blood pressure in adults: report from the panel members appointed to the Eighth Joint National Committee (JNC 8).* JAMA. *2014;311(5):507–520.)*

Antihypertensive Drugs

Diuretics

Diuretics are categorized by their site of action in the kidney and are divided into thiazide, loop, and potassium-sparing types.

Thiazide-type diuretics increase the sodium load on the kidney's distal tubules and initially decrease plasma volume and cardiac output through natriuresis. As the renin-angiotensin-aldosterone system compensates for a diminished plasma volume, cardiac output returns to normal and peripheral vascular resistance is lowered.

Loop diuretics act on the ascending loop of Henle and block sodium resorption, causing an initial decrease in plasma volume. As with thiazide-type diuretics, BP is eventually lowered because of decreased peripheral vascular resistance. Loop diuretics are used primarily in treating patients with moderate renal insufficiency.

Potassium-sparing diuretics may competitively block the actions of aldosterone to prevent potassium loss from the distal tubule, or they may act directly on the distal tubule to inhibit aldosterone-induced sodium resorption in exchange for potassium. They are often used as adjuncts to the thiazide-type or loop diuretics to counteract potassium depletion, but in some cases they are used alone.

Adverse effects of diuretics vary according to class. Thiazide-type diuretics can cause weakness, muscle cramps, impotence, hypokalemia, hyperglycemia, hyperlipidemia, hyperuricemia, hypercalcemia, hypomagnesemia, hyponatremia, azotemia, and pancreatitis. Thiazide-type diuretics may unmask type 2 diabetes and aggravate lipid disorders. On a positive note, they may also slow the demineralization that occurs with osteoporosis. Loop diuretics can cause ototoxicity, as well as electrolyte abnormalities such as hypokalemia, hypocalcemia, and hypomagnesemia. Potassium-sparing diuretics can cause hyperkalemia, renal calculi, renal tubular damage, and gynecomastia. Diuretics are particularly effective in individuals with salt-sensitive hypertension such as older persons and black patients.

Angiotensin-Converting Enzyme Inhibitors

Angiotensin-converting enzyme (ACE) catalyzes the conversion of angiotensin I to angiotensin II. Angiotensin II, a potent vasoconstrictor, is the primary vasoactive hormone of the renin-angiotensin-aldosterone system, and it plays a major role in the pathophysiology of hypertension. ACE inhibitors block the conversion of angiotensin I to angiotensin II, resulting in vasodilation with decreased peripheral vascular resistance and natriuresis. They also decrease aldosterone production and increase levels of vasodilating bradykinins. Some ACE inhibitors stimulate production of vasodilatory prostaglandins. The efficacy of ACE inhibitors is enhanced when they are used together with diuretics; they can reduce hypokalemia, hypercholesterolemia, hyperglycemia, and hyperuricemia caused by diuretic therapy. ACE inhibitors are beneficial in patients with left ventricular dysfunction and with kidney disease. They may also help improve insulin sensitivity.

Adverse effects of ACE inhibitors include a dry cough (5%–20% of patients), angioneurotic edema, hypotension, hyperkalemia, abnormal taste, leukopenia, proteinuria, and renal failure in patients with preexisting renal insufficiency. ACE inhibitors should be avoided in patients with a history of angioedema. They are contraindicated during pregnancy and in patients trying to become pregnant because of the adverse effects on fetal renal function and fetal death.

Angiotensin II Receptor Blockers

Angiotensin II receptor blockers (ARBs) inhibit the vasoconstrictive and aldosterone-secreting effects of angiotensin II by selectively blocking angiotensin II receptors that are found in such tissues as vascular smooth muscle and the adrenal gland, resulting in decreased peripheral vascular resistance. ARBs are effective in managing hypertension in a variety of situations, including in patients with heart failure who are unable to tolerate

ACE inhibitors. ARBs also have been associated with a reduced incidence of new-onset diabetes mellitus and, like ACE inhibitors, improve insulin sensitivity.

The adverse effects of ARBs are similar to those occurring with ACE inhibitors, though less common. The cough caused by ACE inhibitors generally does not occur with ARBs, and angioedema is rare. Like ACE inhibitors, ARBs are contraindicated in pregnancy.

Calcium Channel Blockers

Calcium channel blockers (CCBs) block the entry of calcium into vascular smooth muscle cells, resulting in reduced myocardial contractility and decreased systemic vascular resistance. CCBs are divided into dihydropyridine and nondihydropyridine types.

Adverse effects of CCBs vary according to the agent but include constipation, headache, fatigue, dizziness, nausea, palpitations, flushing, edema, gingival hyperplasia, arrhythmias, and cardiac ischemia. Because of their negative inotropic effects, CCBs generally should be avoided in patients with cardiac conduction abnormalities or heart failure associated with left ventricular dysfunction and in the setting of acute MI. CCBs may be helpful in Raynaud syndrome and in some arrhythmias.

β-Blockers

There are 2 types of β-adrenergic receptor sites: β_1 is present in vascular and cardiac tissue, and β_2 is found in the bronchial system. Circulating or locally released catecholamines stimulate β sites, resulting in vasoconstriction, bronchodilation, tachycardia, and increased myocardial contractility. β-Blockers inhibit these effects. They also decrease plasma renin, reset baroreceptors to facilitate lower BP, induce release of vasodilatory prostaglandins, decrease plasma volume, and may have a CNS-mediated antihypertensive effect.

β-Blockers are divided into those that are nonselective (β_1 and β_2), those that are cardioselective (primarily β_1), and those that have intrinsic sympathomimetic activity (ISA). The cardioselective agents may be prescribed with caution in patients with pulmonary disease, diabetes mellitus, or peripheral arterial disease, but at higher doses they lose their β_1 selectivity and can cause adverse effects in these patients. Those with ISA minimize the bradycardia caused by other β-blockers. β-Blockers with α-blocking properties such as carvedilol or labetalol have additional vasodilatory effects caused by selective α_1-receptor blockade. In patients with heart failure due to systolic dysfunction, the use of certain β-blockers—particularly carvedilol, metoprolol succinate, and bisoprolol—reduces hospitalizations for heart failure and improves survival. Nebivolol has nitric oxide–potentiating vasodilatory effects.

Adverse effects of β-blockers include bronchospasm, bradycardia, masking of insulin-induced hypoglycemia, insomnia, fatigue, depression, impotence, impaired peripheral circulation, impaired exercise tolerance, nasal congestion, and hypertriglyceridemia (except β-blockers with ISA). Angina pectoris and increased BP can be precipitated by abrupt cessation of β-blocker therapy. β-Blockers should generally be avoided in patients with asthma, reactive airways disease, or second-degree or third-degree heart block. β-Blockers are beneficial in the treatment of atrial fibrillation and tachyarrhythmias, migraine, thyrotoxicosis, and essential tremor.

α_1-Blockers

α_1-Adrenergic antagonists block postsynaptic α-receptors, resulting in arterial and venous vasodilation. Selective α_1-blockers have replaced older nonselective agents in the treatment of hypertension. Although these agents are not as effective as diuretics, CCBs, and ACE inhibitors, they may be prescribed as adjunct therapy in selected cases, not as a primary agent.

Adverse effects include "first-dose effect," in which BP is decreased more with the initial dose than with subsequent doses; orthostatic hypotension; headache; dizziness; and drowsiness.

Combined α-Adrenergic and β-Adrenergic Antagonists

Combined α-adrenergic and β-adrenergic antagonists block the action of catecholamines at both α-adrenergic and β-adrenergic receptor sites. Adverse effects are similar to those of other α-adrenergic and β-adrenergic antagonists.

Centrally Acting Adrenergic Drugs

Centrally acting adrenergic drugs are potent antihypertensive agents that stimulate presynaptic α_2-adrenergic receptors in the central nervous system, causing reductions in sympathetic tone, cardiac output, and peripheral vascular resistance.

Adverse effects include fluid retention, dry mouth, drowsiness, dizziness, orthostatic hypotension, rash, impotence, and hepatitis; positive results on the direct antiglobulin (Coombs) test and the antinuclear antibody (ANA) test; and heart failure in patients with decreased left ventricular dysfunction. There may also be severe rebound hypertension when the drug is abruptly discontinued.

Methyldopa continues to be widely used in pregnancy because of its proven safety. Older centrally acting sympatholytic agents (eg, reserpine) have significant adverse effects and are seldom used.

Direct Vasodilators

Direct-acting vasodilators such as minoxidil and hydralazine decrease peripheral vascular resistance by direct arterial vasodilation. They are generally reserved for special situations, such as pregnancy or intractable hypertension. They should be avoided or used with caution in patients with ischemic heart disease.

Adverse effects include headache, tachycardia, edema, nausea, vomiting, a lupuslike syndrome, and hypertrichosis. Because of the sympathetic hyperactivity and the sodium and fluid retention caused by direct vasodilators, they are often used in conjunction with diuretics or β-blockers.

Combination Therapy

Combination therapy usually includes small doses of a diuretic, which potentiates the effects of other drugs such as ACE inhibitors, ARBs, and β-blockers (see Table 3-6). This therapy may improve patient adherence and reduce BP to target level more quickly than other classes of drugs. Another advantage is that low-dose therapy with 2 antihypertensive drugs is associated with fewer side effects than is higher-dose therapy with a single agent.

Direct Renin Inhibitors

Aliskiren is the first orally active renin inhibitor launched to treat hypertension. It has a high specificity for renin and has a long half-life (approximately 24 hours), which makes it ideal for once-daily treatment of hypertension. Direct renin inhibitors (DRIs) are more likely to be effective in younger white patients, who, in general, have a more active renin system, and in any patients receiving diuretics or CCBs, in whom the renin system has been activated. The main adverse effect is possible diarrhea at higher doses.

Parenteral Antihypertensive Drugs

Parenteral antihypertensive therapy is indicated for immediate reduction of BP in hypertensive emergencies.

Sodium nitroprusside, a direct arterial and venous vasodilator, is the drug of choice for most hypertensive emergencies. Nitroglycerin may be preferable in patients with severe coronary insufficiency or advanced kidney or liver disease. Labetalol is also effective and is the drug of choice in hypertensive emergencies that occur in pregnancy. Esmolol is a cardioselective β-adrenergic antagonist that can be used in hypertensive emergencies when β-blocker intolerance is a concern; it is also useful in treating aortic dissection. Phentolamine is effective in managing hypertension with acute drug intoxication or withdrawal. Nicardipine is a CCB that can be administered intravenously for postoperative hypertension. Intravenous enalapril is an ACE inhibitor that can be effective, although unpredictable results have been reported with its use. Diazoxide and hydralazine are used infrequently now, but hydralazine does have a long-established safety profile and may be useful in pregnancy-related hypertensive emergencies.

Future Treatments and Targets for Hypertension

Data from the Conduit Artery Function Endpoint (CAFE) study showed that different classes of antihypertensive drugs have different effects on brachial versus central aortic systolic and pulse pressures and that central pressures may be a better predictor of cardiovascular outcomes in response to treatment. The Strong Heart Study also showed that central aortic pressures may be a better predictor of target end-organ damage and outcomes than are conventional brachial pressures.

Thus, it is worth mentioning several other drugs, such as soluble guanylate cyclase activators, that would lower central aortic pressures. These increase cyclic guanosine monophosphate levels in target tissues, resulting in vasodilation and an antiproliferative effect. One report found that such an activator lowered BP and inhibited cardiac hypertrophy in rats with angiotensin II–induced hypertension. This new drug may also potentially reduce large-artery stiffness, lowering central aortic systolic pressures beyond the benefits observed on brachial BP.

Other experimental agents, known as *advanced glycation cross-link breakers,* target vascular wall thickness and its effects on BP. We know that increased large-artery stiffness occurs with aging and disease and is associated with increased brachial systolic pressure. This increased pressure is due to the accumulation of advanced glycation end products (AGEs) within the vascular wall. AGEs also impair endothelial function, which also leads to arterial stiffness. Thus, targeting these molecules to reduce their levels or indeed their presence in vascular walls may have an effect on decreasing vessel stiffness and lowering BP.

Other, more intriguing studies have involved attempts to develop a vaccine for hypertension and the use of acupuncture in its treatment.

Masuyama H, Tsuruda T, Kato J, et al. Soluble guanylate cyclase stimulation on cardiovascular remodeling in angiotensin II–induced hypertensive rats. *Hypertension.* 2006;48(5):972–978.

Williams B, Lacy PS, Thom SM, et al; CAFE Investigators; Anglo-Scandinavian Cardiac Outcomes Trial Investigators. Differential impact of blood pressure-lowering drugs on central aortic pressure and clinical outcomes: principal results of the Conduit Artery Function Evaluation (CAFE) study. *Circulation.* 2006;113(9):1213–1225.

Special Considerations

Resistant Hypertension

Catheter-based radiofrequency ablation of the renal sympathetic nerves lowers BP in patients with resistant hypertension (defined earlier in the chapter). The initial results look promising, but it is not yet known whether the antihypertensive effect of radiofrequency ablation is due in part to improved patient adherence to the medication regimen. Poor adherence to the medication regimen is a major factor in resistant hypertension.

Sarafidis PA, Bakris GL. Resistant hypertension: an overview of evaluation and treatment. *J Am Coll Cardiology.* 2008;52(22):1749–1757.

Ischemic Heart Disease

For patients with hypertension and stable angina pectoris, a β-blocker is generally the initial drug of choice; alternatively, CCBs can be used. ACE inhibitors and β-blockers are recommended as first-line drugs in hypertensive patients with acute coronary syndromes (unstable angina or MI). In post-MI patients, β-blockers, ACE inhibitors, and potassium-sparing diuretics (aldosterone antagonists) are beneficial.

Heart Failure

In asymptomatic patients with hypertension and ventricular dysfunction, ACE inhibitors and β-blockers are recommended. In patients with symptomatic ventricular dysfunction or end-stage heart failure, ACE inhibitors, β-blockers—especially carvedilol or nebivolol—ARBs, aldosterone antagonists, and loop diuretics are useful.

Diabetes Mellitus and Hypertension

As mentioned earlier, hypertensive patients with diabetes mellitus usually require 2 or more antihypertensive drugs to achieve a BP goal of less than 130/80 mm Hg. Thiazide-type diuretics, β-blockers, ACE inhibitors, ARBs, and CCBs reduce cardiovascular complications in these patients. ACE inhibitors and ARBs are beneficial for those with diabetic nephropathy.

Chronic Renal Disease

Aggressive treatment, often with 3 or more drugs, may be necessary to achieve a BP goal of less than 130/80 mm Hg and to prevent deterioration of renal function and cardiovascular complications in hypertensive patients with chronic renal disease. ACE inhibitors and ARBs favorably alter the progression of diabetic and nondiabetic nephropathy. However, as the glomerular filtration rate nears 20 mL/min, less aggressive treatment may be appropriate.

Cerebrovascular Disease

The combination of an ACE inhibitor and a thiazide-type diuretic lowers the risk of recurrent stroke. The optimal BP level during an acute stroke remains undetermined, but consensus favors intermediate control in the range of 160/100 mm Hg until patient stabilization is achieved.

Obesity and the Metabolic Syndrome

Obesity (body mass index ≥30) is a risk factor for the development of hypertension and has become a major concern in the United States, where an estimated 122 million adults are overweight or obese. Closely related to obesity is the *metabolic syndrome.* The International Diabetes Federation has developed a consensus definition for this syndrome, which includes presence of central obesity and 2 of the following or treatment for these conditions: elevated triglyceride level (≥150 mg/dL), reduced high-density lipoprotein cholesterol level, systolic BP >130 mm Hg and/or diastolic >85 mm Hg, and elevated fasting blood glucose level (≥100 mg/dL). Patients with these conditions should adopt healthful lifestyle habits and, if necessary, use drug therapy, excepting thiazide-type diuretics, which may aggravate this syndrome. See Chapter 4 for additional discussion of the metabolic syndrome.

Obstructive Sleep Apnea Syndrome

Obstructive sleep apnea syndrome (OSAS) is a sleep-related breathing disorder with cardinal signs, including obstructive apneas; hypopneas; and sleep arousals with snoring, restlessness, or resuscitative snorts. This disrupted sleep leads to daytime fatigue, poor concentration, and sleeplessness and has been associated with the development of hypertension, heart disease, and metabolic syndrome.

Left Ventricular Hypertrophy

Left ventricular hypertrophy is a risk factor for cardiovascular disease, but regression is possible with treatment of hypertension. All antihypertensive drug classes, except the direct vasodilators, are effective in treating left ventricular hypertrophy.

Peripheral Arterial Disease

The risk factors for peripheral arterial disease parallel those for ischemic heart disease in patients with hypertension. All classes of antihypertensive agents are useful in treating hypertensive patients with peripheral arterial disease.

Ophthalmic considerations In most people, a physiological drop in systemic BP (dipping pattern) occurs during sleep; BP normalizes when these individuals awaken. This decrease in BP may be exacerbated when antihypertensive medications are taken at night. Systemic nocturnal hypotension may be a risk factor for low-tension glaucoma. There is also some evidence that nocturnal arterial hypotension may play a role in the development of nonarteritic anterior ischemic optic neuropathy (NAION), which has been associated with obstructive sleep apnea syndrome (OSAS). OSAS may increase the risk of NAION and low-tension glaucoma by several potential mechanisms, including impaired autoregulation of optic nerve head blood flow, optic nerve vascular dysregulation, and direct optic nerve damage due to prolonged hypoxia. OSAS also plays a role in the development of various retinal findings, including microaneurysms, hypertensive retinopathy, and intraocular production of postischemic molecules that are associated with neovascularization, apoptosis, and macular edema.

Orthostatic Hypotension

Orthostatic hypotension is a postural drop in systolic BP of more than 10 mm Hg associated with dizziness or fainting. It occurs more frequently in older patients with systolic hypertension; in patients with diabetes mellitus; and in those taking diuretics, vasodilators, or certain psychotropic drugs. In these individuals, BP should be monitored while they are in the upright position, and hypovolemia should be avoided. Also, medication dosages should be carefully titrated and various shorter-acting drugs considered for these patients.

Hypertension in Older Patients

Hypertension is present in most individuals older than 65 years. Treatment recommendations for this group are generally the same as for others with hypertension. In older patients with isolated systolic hypertension, a diuretic with or without a β-blocker, or a dihydropyridine CCB alone, is the preferred treatment. Diastolic BP less than 75 mm Hg increases these patients' risk of stroke and should be avoided.

Antihypertensive drug therapy in older patients can cause adverse effects such as dizziness and hypotension that increase the risk of falls. Appropriate precautions should be taken to reduce this risk and enhance patient safety.

Dementia occurs more commonly with hypertension. In some patients, antihypertensive therapy may slow the progression of cognitive impairment.

Women and Pregnancy

Women taking oral contraceptives should have regular BP checks, as the use of oral contraceptives increases the risk of hypertension. Hypertension in women who are pregnant may be classified as follows:

- *preeclampsia or eclampsia:* preeclampsia—pregnancy, hypertension, proteinuria, generalized edema, and possibly coagulation and liver function abnormalities after 20 weeks' gestation; eclampsia—those same abnormalities plus generalized seizures

- *chronic hypertension:* BP of more than 140/90 mm Hg before 20 weeks' gestation
- *chronic hypertension with superimposed preeclampsia or eclampsia*
- *transient hypertension:* hypertension without proteinuria or central nervous system manifestations during pregnancy; the return of normal BP within 10 days of delivery

Hypertension in women who are pregnant potentially increases maternal and fetal morbidity and mortality. The possible adverse effects of antihypertensive drug therapy on fetal development must be considered, however, when pharmacologic treatment is planned. Methyldopa, β-blockers, and vasodilators are the recommended drugs for treatment of hypertension in pregnancy. ACE inhibitors and ARBs are contraindicated in pregnancy because of teratogenic effects; they should also be avoided in women who are likely to become pregnant.

Children and Adolescents

Considerable advances have been made in the detection, evaluation, and management of hypertension in children and adolescents. Current evidence indicates that primary hypertension in the young occurs more commonly than previously recognized and has substantial long-term health implications. There is little doubt that obesity in young people predicts the risk of developing hypertension and associated metabolic risk factors. Hypertension in this group is defined as average systolic BP and/or diastolic BP that is in the 95th percentile or higher for sex, age, and height on 3 or more occasions. BP between the 90th percentile and the 95th percentile in childhood is designated as *prehypertension* and is an indication for lifestyle modifications. It is recommended that children older than 3 years have their BP measured when they are examined in a medical setting.

Hypertensive children and adolescents are frequently overweight, and some have sleep disorders. Secondary hypertension occurs more commonly in children than in adults.

Indications for antihypertensive drug therapy in children include uncontrolled hypertension despite nonpharmacologic measures, symptomatic hypertension, secondary hypertension, hypertensive target-organ damage, and hypertension with diabetes mellitus. Acceptable drug choices for treating hypertension in children include diuretics, β-blockers, ACE inhibitors, ARBs, and CCBs.

National High Blood Pressure Education Program Working Group on High Blood Pressure in Children and Adolescents. The fourth report on the diagnosis, evaluation, and treatment of high blood pressure in children and adolescents. *Pediatrics.* 2004;114(2 Suppl 4th report): 555–576.

Racial and Ethnic Variations in Hypertension in the United States

In the United States, there are significant racial and ethnic differences in the awareness, treatment, and control of hypertension. For example, BP control rates are lowest in Mexican Americans and Native Americans. The prevalence and severity of hypertension are increased in black persons, in whom β-blockers, ACE inhibitors, and ARBs are less effective than diuretics and CCBs in lowering BP. In general, the treatment guidelines for hypertension are similar for all demographic groups; unfortunately, for many minority patients, socioeconomic and lifestyle factors continue to be barriers to treatment.

Centers for Disease Control and Prevention (CDC). Racial/ethnic disparities in prevalence, treatment, and control of hypertension—United States, 1999–2002. *MMWR Morb Mortal Wkly Rep.* 2005;54(1):7–9.

Withdrawal Syndromes

Hypertension can be associated with withdrawal from alcohol or drugs such as cocaine, amphetamines, and opioid analgesics. Withdrawal syndromes can occur with acute drug intoxication or as the result of abrupt discontinuation of a drug after long-term use. Phentolamine, sodium nitroprusside, and nitroglycerin are all effective in the immediate management of hypertension in these situations. β-Blockers should not be used, as unopposed α-adrenergic stimulation can exacerbate the hypertension.

Monoamine oxidase inhibitors taken with certain drugs or with tyramine-containing foods can cause accelerated hypertension by increasing catecholamine levels. Phentolamine, sodium nitroprusside, and labetalol are effective for treating this type of hypertension.

Abrupt discontinuation of antihypertensive therapy can cause severe rebound hypertension. This occurs most commonly with centrally acting adrenergic agents (particularly clonidine) and with β-blockers, but it can occur with other drug classes as well, including diuretics. When an acute withdrawal syndrome occurs and parenteral antihypertensive treatment is necessary, sodium nitroprusside is the drug of choice.

Hypertensive Crisis

Patients with severe BP elevation and acute target-organ damage (eg, encephalopathy, MI, unstable angina, pulmonary edema, stroke, head trauma, eclampsia, or aortic dissection) should be admitted to the hospital for emergency parenteral antihypertensive therapy. Patients with marked BP elevation but without target-organ damage may not require admission, but they should be treated urgently with combination oral antihypertensive drugs (see Table 3-6). Identifiable causes of hypertension should be sought, and these patients should be carefully monitored for target-organ damage.

Ophthalmic considerations Retinal vascular complications (hypertensive retinopathy, retinal vein occlusions, retinal arterial occlusions), glaucoma, ischemic optic neuropathy, microvascular cranial nerve palsies, and stroke-related disorders of the afferent and efferent pathways of the visual system are commonly associated with hypertension. Moreover, ophthalmic surgery patients with poorly controlled hypertension may be more susceptible to intraoperative and postoperative complications.

There is strong evidence that certain signs of hypertensive retinopathy, independent of other risk factors, are associated with increased cardiovascular risk. Based on these reported associations, a simplified classification of hypertensive retinopathy was proposed in 2004 (Table 3-8).

Table 3-8 Classification of Hypertensive Retinopathy With Systemic Associations

Grade of Retinopathy	Retinal Signs	Systemic Associations
None	No detectable signs	None
Mild	Generalized and/or focal arteriolar narrowing, arteriovenous nicking, opacity ("copper wiring") due to thickening of arteriolar wall, or a combination of these signs	Modest association with risk of stroke, coronary artery disease, and death
Moderate	Hemorrhage (blot, dot, or flame-shaped), microaneurysm, cotton-wool spot, hard exudates, or a combination of these signs	Strong association with stroke, cognitive decline, and death from cardiovascular causes
Malignant	Signs of moderate retinopathy plus swelling of the optic disc	Strong association with death

Adapted with permission from Wong TY, Mitchell P. Hypertensive retinopathy. *N Engl J Med.* 2004; 351(22):2314. ©2004 Massachusetts Medical Society.

JNC 7 and several societies (European Society of Hypertension, European Society of Cardiology, American Society of Hypertension, International Society of Hypertension) emphasize that control of hypertension is possible only if patients are motivated to take their prescribed medications and to maintain healthful lifestyle habits. Motivation improves when individuals develop empathy with and trust in their physicians. As members of the health care team, ophthalmologists have an important role in the identification, monitoring, and shared management of patients with hypertension.

Wong TY, Mitchell P. Hypertensive retinopathy. *N Engl J Med.* 2004;351(22):2310–2317.

The authors would like to thank Jerry A. Dancik, MD, for his contributions to this chapter.

CHAPTER 4

Hypercholesterolemia and Cardiovascular Risk

Recent Developments

- Therapeutic lifestyle changes remain an essential modality in the management of hypercholesterolemia.
- More aggressive management of cholesterol and risk factors has been emphasized by the US National Cholesterol Education Program (NCEP) and the European Society of Cardiology (ESC).
- Numerous clinical trials have shown that effective reduction of low-density-lipoprotein cholesterol (LDL-C) levels substantially reduces the risk of coronary heart disease.
- A number of tools (eg, Framingham, HeartSCORE, Pooled Cohort Equations) are available to assess the cardiovascular risk for an individual patient.
- Statin therapy is recommended for the vast majority of dyslipoproteinemic adult patients with cardiometabolic risk.
- Use of statins in acute coronary syndromes reduces the risk of recurrent coronary events.

Introduction

Coronary heart disease (CHD) is the leading cause of death in the United States and most of the developed world, accounting for more deaths than all forms of cancer combined. Several major studies have confirmed earlier reports that lowering elevated LDL-C levels reduces the risk of CHD. The NCEP provided 3 updates for treating elevated blood cholesterol levels in adults: Adult Treatment Panel (ATP) I, II, and III. ATP I proposed a strategy for primary prevention of CHD in persons with high levels of LDL-C (≥160 mg/dL) or borderline high levels of LDL-C (130–159 mg/dL) and multiple (at least 2) risk factors (discussed later in the chapter). ATP II added intensive management of LDL-C in persons with established CHD (target cholesterol level <100 mg/dL). ATP III guidelines, which are very similar to those currently used in Europe and the rest of the developed world, recommend the following target levels for adults:

- total cholesterol <200 mg/dL
- LDL cholesterol <100 mg/dL

- HDL cholesterol ≥60 mg/dL (more is better)
- triglycerides <150 mg/dL

In 2013, a series of reports in the United States questioned the value of specific targets for LDL-C levels. These reports instead recommend the assessment of cardiovascular risk, followed by aggressive treatment with statin drugs in those most likely to benefit. These recommendations are discussed later in this chapter.

Lipoproteins, Cholesterol, and Cardiovascular Disease

Cholesterol and triglycerides are transported in the body by *lipoproteins*. The various classes of lipoprotein differ in the relative concentrations of their components: cholesterol, triglycerides, phospholipids, and proteins *(apolipoproteins)*. Chylomicrons carry triglycerides following dietary lipid absorption, whereas *very-low-density lipoproteins (VLDLs)* produced by the liver carry most circulating triglycerides. LDL, or "bad cholesterol," is a product of VLDL and intermediate-density-lipoprotein metabolism and is the primary carrier of cholesterol. High-density lipoprotein (HDL), or "good cholesterol," is the smallest and densest lipoprotein particle. The result of the inflammatory interaction among these lipoproteins, macrophages, and the cellular components of the arterial wall is *atherosclerosis*. Although cholesterol levels are what is typically measured, it is the lipoproteins that interact with the arterial wall, producing plaques. The narrowing of the arterial lumen that occurs as a result of plaque growth or the rupture of a plaque with subsequent thrombosis leads to stroke and cardiovascular disease (CVD), including myocardial infarction (MI) and peripheral arterial disease.

Risk Assessment

The cholesterol level of approximately half the US population puts these persons at significant risk. A fasting lipoprotein profile (total cholesterol, LDL-C, HDL-C, and triglyceride levels) helps determine an individual's risk status. The US Preventive Services Task Force recommends screening for lipid disorders in men 20–35 years of age and women aged 45 years and older when other risk factors exist, and all men aged 35 years and older regardless of other risk factors. Experimental studies directly support the central role of LDL in atherogenesis, and lowering LDL-C levels is associated with a reduction in CVD risk. Conversely, HDL-C appears protective against atherosclerosis because of its anti-inflammatory properties and ability to transport cholesterol from vessel walls to the liver for disposal. In general, current guidelines recommend a high-HDL and low-LDL concentration to decrease CVD risk. Other CHD risk factors, such as hypertension, smoking, diabetes mellitus, obesity, and limited physical activity should be assessed and managed appropriately in all adults (Table 4-1). The INTERHEART study, which involved 15,000 patients with acute MI versus 15,000 controls in 52 countries, found that current smoking, hypertension, diabetes mellitus, abdominal obesity, psychosocial factors, and a raised apo B/apo AI ratio increased the risk of acute MI, while moderate or strenuous exercise, daily consumption of fruits and vegetables, and moderate alcohol consumption were protective.

Table 4-1 Risk Factor Modification Treatment Goals

Risk Factor	Goal	Intervention
Blood pressure	<140/90 mm Hg <130/80 mm Hg with chronic kidney disease or diabetes mellitus	Weight control, increased physical activity, alcohol moderation, sodium reduction, medications
Smoking	Smoking cessation Avoid environmental tobacco smoke	Smoking cessation programs, nicotine replacement, bupropion, varenicline
Lipid management	LDL-C <100 mg/dL (optional goal <70 mg/dL if high CAD risk) Non–HDL-C ≤130 mg/dL	Diet low in saturated fat, weight control, increased physical activity, statins, niacin, fibrates
Diabetes mellitus	HbA_{1c} <7%	Diet, weight control, oral hypoglycemic agents, insulin
Physical activity	30 minutes, 7 days/week Minimum 5 days/week	Walking, biking, swimming, gardening, household work
Weight management	BMI 18.5–24.9 kg/m^2 Waist circumference: ≤40 inches men; ≤35 inches women	Physical activity, caloric intake, behavioral programs

BMI = body mass index; CAD = coronary artery disease; HDL-C = high-density-lipoprotein cholesterol; LDL-C = low-density-lipoprotein cholesterol.

Modified with permission from Bates ER, Babb JD, Casey DE JR, et al; American College of Cardiology Foundation. ACCF/SCAI/SVMB/SIR/ASITN 2007 clinical expert consensus document on carotid stenting. *J Am Coll Cardiol.* 2007;49(1):126–170.

A number of risk assessment tools are available to estimate the 10-year risk of a cardiovascular event, including the Framingham Global Risk and Pooled Cohort Equations (United States); QRISK (United Kingdom); and HeartSCORE (Europe). Physicians are encouraged to use the risk tool best suited to the individual patient, since relative cardiac risk varies among national, ethnic, and racial groups. Use of these tools guides the clinician in identifying patients requiring aggressive treatment and those most likely to benefit.

2013 prevention guidelines tools: CV risk calculator (pooled cohort equations). American Heart Association website. http://my.americanheart.org/professional/StatementsGuidelines/Prevention-Guidelines_UCM_457698_SubHomePage.jsp. Accessed June 23, 2014.

Conroy RM, Pyörälä K, Fitzgerald AP, et al. Estimation of ten-year risk of fatal cardiovascular disease in Europe: the SCORE project. *Eur Heart J.* 2003;24(11):987–1003.

Goff DC Jr, Lloyd-Jones DM, Bennet G, et al. 2013 ACC/AHA guideline on the assessment of cardiovascular risk: a report of the American College of Cardiology/American Heart Association Task Force on Practice Guidelines. *J Am Coll Cardiol.* 2014;63(25 Pt B): 2935–2959. Epub 2013 Nov 12.

HeartScore. European Society of Cardiology website. www.heartscore.org. Accessed June 23, 2014.

QRISK2-2014 risk calculator. ClinRisk website. http://qrisk.org. Accessed June 23, 2014.

Risk assessment tool for estimating your 10-year risk of having a heart attack (Framingham Heart Study). National Heart, Lung and Blood Institute website. http://cvdrisk.nhlbi.nih.gov/calculator.asp. Accessed June 23, 2014.

Management

In its simplest terms, the management of hypercholesterolemia consists of matching the intensity of LDL-lowering therapy with absolute risk: the higher the risk, the lower the target level. This approach is based primarily on data from clinical trials and epidemiological studies, which have suggested that a direct relationship exists between the level of LDL-C and the risk of CHD. The ATP III guidelines suggest measuring fasting lipoprotein levels in patients with hypercholesterolemia, hyperlipidemia, and/or hyperlipoproteinemia. The clinician should also assess the presence of other risk factors (see Table 4-1) and the presence of clinical atherosclerotic disease, including clinical cardiovascular disease, carotid or peripheral arterial disease, or abdominal aortic aneurysm. The patient's 10-year risk for CVD is determined based on these factors on a scale from lower risk to high risk. LDL treatment goals from the ATP III and similar guidelines are determined based on this risk level (Table 4-2). In contrast, the 2013 guidelines from the American College of Cardiology and the American Heart Association (ACC/AHA) recommend that patients be given the maximum tolerated intensity of a statin drug when a statin is indicated.

Table 4-2 ATP III LDL-C Goals and Cutpoints for TLC and Drug Therapy in Different Risk Categories

Risk Category	LDL-C Goal	Initiate TLC	Consider Drug Therapy
High risk: CHD* or CHD risk equivalents† (10-year risk >20%)	<100 mg/dL (optional goal: <70 mg/dL)	≥100 mg/dL	≥100 mg/dL (<100 mg/dL: consider drug options)
Moderately high risk: 2+ risk factors‡ (10-year risk 10%–20%)	<130 mg/dL	≥130 mg/dL	≥130 mg/dL (100–129 mg/dL: consider drug options)
Moderate risk: 2+ risk factors‡ (10-year risk <10%)	<130 mg/dL	≥130 mg/dL	≥160 mg/dL
Lower risk: 0–1 risk factor	<160 mg/dL	≥160 mg/dL	≥190 mg/dL (160–189 mg/dL: LDL-lowering drug optional)

BP = blood pressure; CHD = coronary heart disease; HDL-C = high-density-lipoprotein cholesterol; LDL-C = low-density-lipoprotein cholesterol; TLC = therapeutic lifestyle changes.

*CHD includes history of myocardial infarction, unstable angina, stable angina, coronary artery procedures (angioplasty or bypass surgery), or evidence of clinically significant myocardial ischemia.

†CHD risk equivalents include clinical manifestations of noncoronary forms of atherosclerotic disease (peripheral arterial disease, abdominal aortic aneurysm, and carotid artery disease [transient ischemic attacks or stroke of carotid origin or >50% obstruction of a carotid artery]), diabetes, and 2+ risk factors with 10-year risk for hard CHD >20%.

‡Risk factors include cigarette smoking, hypertension (BP ≥140/90 mm Hg or on antihypertensive medication), low HDL-C (<40 mg/dL), family history of premature CHD (CHD in male first-degree relative <55 years of age; CHD in female first-degree relative <65 years of age), and age (men ≥45 years; women ≥55 years).

Modified with permission from Grundy SM, Cleeman JI, Merz CN, et al. Implications of recent clinical trials for the National Cholesterol Education Program Adult Treatment Panel III guidelines. *J Am Coll Cardiol.* 2004;44(3):720–732.

These groups no longer advocate treatment to a preset generalized goal but instead recognize that any reduction in LDL-C is beneficial, and that some patients should be treated more aggressively because of their higher cardiovascular risk.

Therapeutic lifestyle changes, including dietary modifications, weight management, and increased physical activity, should be initiated. A diet high in fruits, vegetables, fiber, omega-3 fatty acids, and foods with a low glycemic index, and substituting monounsaturated fats for polyunsaturated or trans fats, have repeatedly been shown to lower cardiovascular risk. If LDL goals are not achieved by lifestyle changes alone, drug therapy should be introduced and, if necessary, advanced. Specific drugs, their lipid-lowering effects, and adverse effects are presented in Tables 4-3 and 4-4.

Once the LDL treatment goals have been reached, other lipid and nonlipid risk factors can be modified. Elevated triglyceride levels may respond to increased physical activity or weight management, but if the triglyceride levels are ≥200 mg/dL after the LDL goal is reached, a secondary goal of treatment would be a non–HDL-C (total – HDL) level of 30 mg/dL higher than the LDL goal.

Brunzell JD, Davidson M, Furberg CD, et al. Lipoprotein management in patients with cardiometabolic risk: consensus conference report from the American Diabetes Association and the American College of Cardiology Foundation. *J Am Coll Cardiol.* 2008;51(15):1512–1524.

Table 4-3 Drugs Affecting Lipoprotein Metabolism

Drug Class	Agents	Lipid/Lipoprotein Effects	Adverse Effects
HMG-CoA reductase inhibitors	Statins (see Table 4-4)	LDL ↓ 18%–55% HDL ↑ 5%–15% TG ↓ 7%–30%	Myopathy, increased levels of liver enzymes
Bile acid sequestrants	Cholestyramine Colestipol Colesevelam	LDL ↓ 15%–30% HDL ↑ 3%–5% TG no change or increase	Gastrointestinal distress, constipation, decreased absorption of other drugs
Nicotinic acid	Immediate-release nicotinic acid Extended-release nicotinic acid Sustained-release nicotinic acid	LDL ↓ 5%–25% HDL ↑ 15%–35% TG ↓ 20%–50%	Flushing, hyperglycemia, hyperuricemia (gout), upper gastrointestinal tract distress, hepatotoxicity
Fibric acids	Gemfibrozil Fenofibrate Clofibrate Bezafibrate Ciprofibrate	LDL ↓ 5%–20% (may be increased in patients with high TG) HDL ↑ 10%–20% TG ↓ 20%–50%	Dyspepsia, gallstones, myopathy; unexplained non-CHD deaths in WHO study
Cholesterol absorption inhibitor	Ezetimibe	LDL ↓ 14%–17%	Myopathy, increased liver enzymes, possible increased cancer risk

CHD = coronary heart disease; HDL = high-density lipoprotein; HMG-CoA = 3-hydroxy-3-methylglutaryl coenzyme A; LDL = low-density lipoprotein; TG = triglycerides; WHO = World Health Organization; ↓ = decrease; ↑ = increase.

Table 4-4 Intensity of Statin Therapy With Daily Dosing

High-intensity statin therapy (reduces LDL-C by ≥50%)
Atorvastatin 40–80 mg
Rosuvastatin 20–40 mg
Moderate-intensity statin therapy (reduces LDL-C by 30%–50%)
Atorvastatin 10–20 mg
Fluvastatin 40 mg twice daily
Fluvastatin XL 80 mg
Lovastatin 40 mg
Pitavastatin 2–4 mg
Pravastatin 40–80 mg
Rosuvastatin 5–10 mg
Simvastatin 20–40 mg
Low-intensity statin therapy (reduces LDL-C by <30%)
Fluvastatin 20–40 mg
Lovastatin 20 mg
Pitavastatin 1 mg
Pravastatin 10–20 mg
Simvastatin 10 mg

Modified with permission from Stone NJ, Robinson JG, Lichtenstein AH, et al. 2013 ACC/AHA guideline on the treatment of blood cholesterol to reduce atherosclerotic cardiovascular disease risk in adults: a report of the American College of Cardiology/American Heart Association Task Force on Practice Guidelines. *J Am Coll Cardiol.* 2014;63(25 Pt B):2889–2934. Epub 2013 Nov 12.

Eckel RH, Jakicic JM, Ard JD, et al. 2013 AHA/ACC guideline on lifestyle management to reduce cardiovascular risk. *J Am Coll Cardiol.* 2014;63(25 Pt B):2960–2984. Epub 2013 Nov 12.

Perk J, De Backer G, Gohlke H, et al; European Association for Cardiovascular Prevention & Rehabilitation; ESC Committee for Practice Guidelines. European guidelines on cardiovascular disease prevention in clinical practice (version 2012). *Eur Heart J.* 2012;33(13):1635–1701.

Rosenson RS. Screening guidelines for dyslipidemia. In: *UpToDate,* Freeman MW (ed), Waltham, MA. Available at www.uptodate.com. Accessed June 23, 2014.

The Role of Statins

For virtually all patients whose LDL-C goals cannot be achieved by therapeutic lifestyle changes alone, 3-hydroxy-3-methylglutaryl coenzyme A (HMG-CoA) reductase inhibitors, more popularly known as *statins,* are the first choice for medical therapy. Multiple trials involving the use of statins have reinforced the value of LDL-lowering therapy in reducing cardiometabolic disease. Moreover, the statins are the only class of drugs whose use has been shown to improve overall mortality in primary and secondary prevention. The Heart Protection Study, Myocardial Ischemia Reduction with Acute Cholesterol Lowering (MIRACL) study, and the PROVE IT study, among others, each demonstrated a decreased risk of major cardiovascular events in patients lowering their LDL-C levels with statins. Findings from the JUPITER trial suggest that statins—which are known to lower C-reactive protein levels in addition to having positive effects on hyperlipidemia—may decrease the risk of stroke, coronary artery disease, and death in apparently healthy persons without hyperlipidemia but with a C-reactive protein level of >2.0 mg/L. The beneficial effects of statins arise from the reduction of LDL-C levels, stabilization of atherosclerotic plaques, and decreased atherogenic inflammation.

The 2013 ACC/AHA guidelines identify 4 patient groups likely to benefit from statin use:

- individuals with clinical atherosclerotic cardiovascular disease (ASCVD)
- individuals with LDL-C ≥190 mg/dL
- individuals aged 40–75 years with diabetes (but without ASCVD) and LDL-C 70–189 mg/dL
- individuals aged 40–75 years without diabetes or ASCVD with LDL-C 70–189 mg/dL and estimated 10-year ASCVD risk >7.5%.

In these patients, the ACC/AHA recommendation is the maximum tolerated statin therapy (see Table 4-4), while those intolerant of high-intensity therapy or at lower estimated cardiovascular risk may be treated with a moderate intensity. Current ESC and other international guidelines continue to recommend specific goals similar to those outlined in the NCEP/ATP III studies.

Other drugs used to lower LDL-C levels (see Table 4-3) include nicotinic acid, bile acid sequestrants, fibric acids, and cholesterol absorption inhibitors. While many of these drugs have been shown to lower LDL-C levels, they generally lack large randomized controlled trials demonstrating an effect on ASCVD or mortality. These drugs are often used worldwide; however, the most recent ACC/AHA guidelines do not support the use of these drugs in place of statins when statin therapy is effective and well tolerated. The role of these drugs when added to high-intensity statin use is still to be elucidated.

Adverse effects of statin use are rare but can include elevated hepatic transaminases, diarrhea, liver failure, polyneuropathy, and myopathy. Simvastatin should not be started at or increased to a dose of 80 mg per day because of the high risk of muscle injury. The risk of myopathy is also increased when simvastatin is used in conjunction with other medications, including amiodarone, some fibrates (gemfibrozil), and some calcium channel blockers. Cerivastatin was voluntarily withdrawn from the market after more than 52 reports of rhabdomyolysis and death related to this statin. Although these drugs are largely safe and effective, serious adverse effects must be carefully monitored for, especially in the first few months of treatment. Pregnant women should not take statin drugs due to possible teratogenic effects.

ESC Clinical Practice Guidelines. European Cardiovascular Society website. www.escardio.org/guidelines. Accessed June 23, 2014.

Ridker PM, Danielson E, Fonseca FA, et al; JUPITER Study Group. Rosuvastatin to prevent vascular events in men and women with elevated C-reactive protein. *N Engl J Med.* 2008;359(21):2195–2207.

Rouleau J. Improved outcome after acute coronary syndromes with an intensive versus standard lipid-lowering regimen: results from the Pravastatin or Atorvastatin Evaluation and Infection Therapy-Thrombolysis in Myocardial Infarction 22 (PROVE IT-TIMI 22) trial. *Am J Med.* 2005;118(Suppl 12A):28–35.

Stone NJ, Robinson J, Lichtenstein AH, et al. 2013 ACC/AHA guideline on the treatment of blood cholesterol to reduce atherosclerotic cardiovascular disease risk in adults: a report of the American College of Cardiology/American Heart Association Task Force on Practice Guidelines. *J Am Coll Cardiol.* 2014;63(25 Pt B):2889–2934. Epub 2013 Nov 12.

Waters D, Schwartz GG, Olsson AG. The Myocardial Ischemia Reduction With Acute Cholesterol Lowering (MIRACL) trial: a new frontier for statins? *Curr Control Trials Cardiovasc Med.* 2001;2(3):111–114.

Metabolic Syndrome

Metabolic syndrome comprises a constellation of lipid and nonlipid risk factors of metabolic origin. The International Diabetes Federation has developed a consensus definition for metabolic syndrome, which includes

- central obesity (waist circumference):
  - United States: ≥102 cm (male); ≥88 cm (female)
  - Europe: ≥94 cm (male); ≥80 cm (female)
  - Asia; Central and South America: ≥90 cm (male); ≥80 cm (female)
- plus any 2 of the following, or treatment for the condition listed:
  - raised triglyceride level ≥150 mg/dL
  - reduced HDL cholesterol <40 mg/dL (male), <50 mg/dL (female)
  - elevated blood pressure: systolic >130 mm Hg and/or diastolic >85 mm Hg
  - elevated fasting blood glucose level ≥100 mg/dL

Metabolic syndrome is closely linked to insulin resistance. Excess body fat (particularly abdominal fat) and physical inactivity promote impaired responses to insulin, which may also occur as a genetic predisposition. The risk factors for metabolic syndrome are highly concordant; in aggregate, they increase the risk of CHD at any given LDL level. Management of the metabolic syndrome includes measures previously discussed for elevated LDL and triglyceride levels, as well as treatment of hypertension and the use of aspirin for CHD patients to reduce the prothrombotic state.

Grundy SM, Cleeman JI, Daniels SR, et al; American Heart Association; National Heart, Lung, and Blood Institute. Diagnosis and management of the metabolic syndrome: an American Heart Association/National Heart, Lung, and Blood Institute scientific statement. *Circulation.* 2005;112(17):2735–2752.

IDF worldwide definition of the metabolic syndrome. International Diabetes Federation website. www.idf.org/metabolic-syndrome. Accessed January 8, 2014.

Ophthalmic considerations Hypercholesterolemia is a significant risk factor for ischemic heart disease, cerebrovascular disease, and peripheral arterial disease. The ophthalmologist may be the first physician to detect or recognize manifestations of atherosclerosis, particularly amaurosis fugax, retinal vascular emboli or occlusions, ischemic optic neuropathy, or cortical visual field deficits from a previous cerebral infarction. Detection of atherosclerosis may initiate a diagnostic evaluation that reveals significant carotid artery stenosis or coronary artery disease.

The Action to Control Cardiovascular Risk in Diabetes (ACCORD) trial was designed to assess the effect of tight glycemic, dyslipidemic, and blood pressure control on cardiovascular events in patients with type 2 diabetes. A subset of these patients (ACCORD EYE) was examined to assess the effects of this control on the progression of diabetic retinopathy (DR). Previous studies had shown mixed results of the effect of tight glycemic control on DR. In the ACCORD EYE study, the tight control of glycemia resulted in a 33% reduction in the relative risk of progression of DR. Using simvastatin plus fenofibrate for dyslipidemia control yielded a 40% reduction in the risk of DR progression. Tight blood pressure control did not appear to affect DR progression in ACCORD. Previous studies (eg, FIELD) have also suggested a possible protective effect of fenofibrate in DR.

Statin use may be associated with a reduction in intraocular pressure and potentially a protective effect against glaucoma. Additional clinical research is needed. Patients with ocular hypertension or glaucoma being treated with topical timolol have a small but significant elevation of serum LDL and reduction in HDL, but do not appear to have increased mortality.

The relationship of statin use to age-related macular degeneration (AMD) is unresolved. Several population-based studies (ARIC, MELBOURNE, Blue Mountains) have suggested that the use of statins is associated with a decreased risk of advanced AMD, whereas other studies (Beaver Dam) suggest there is no change in AMD risk with statin use. Other studies have suggested an increase in the risk of developing neovascular, or "wet," AMD in individuals who smoke or have other cardiac risk factors. All of these studies are limited by either small sample size or lack of randomized prospective data on the use of statins. Therefore, more data are required to assess the nature of this relationship. Corneal arcus, a nonreversible lipid deposit at the corneal limbus, is associated with age and hyperlipidemia. In the Blue Mountains Eye Study, the presence of arcus in persons aged 49 years and older was associated with higher total cholesterol and triglyceride levels.

Finally, statins do not appear to increase the risk of cataracts. In fact, some recent studies (eg, Blue Mountains) have suggested a protective effect.

American Academy of Ophthalmology website; www.aao.org.

American Heart Association website; www.americanheart.org.

CardioSource. American College of Cardiology website; www.acc.org.

European Society of Cardiology website; www.escardio.org.

Fong DS, Poon KY. Recent statin use and cataract surgery. *Am J Ophthalmol.* 2012; 153(2):222–228.e1.

Klein R, Knudtson MD, Klein BE. Statin use and the five-year incidence and progression of age-related macular degeneration. *Am J Ophthalmol.* 2007;144(1):1–6.

Müskens RP, Wolfs RC, Witteman JC, et al. Topical beta-blockers and mortality. *Ophthalmology.* 2008;115(11):2037–2043.

Song J, Deng PF, Stinnett SS, Epstein DL, Rao PV. Effects of cholesterol-lowering statins on the aqueous humor outflow pathway. *Invest Ophthalmol Vis Sci.* 2005;46(7):2424–2432.

Tan JS, Mitchell P, Rochtchina E, Wang JJ. Statin use and the long-term risk of incident cataract: The Blue Mountains Eye Study. *Am J Ophthalmol.* 2007;143(4):687–689.

CHAPTER 5

Acquired Heart Disease

Recent Developments

- Atherosclerotic *coronary artery disease (CAD)* remains by far the number-one killer in the United States and around the world.
- Primary prevention of CAD at a public health level requires lifestyle changes, including reduced intake of saturated fat and cholesterol, increased physical activity, and weight control.
- Smoking remains the number-one preventable risk factor for *cardiovascular disease (CVD)* worldwide.
- Markers of inflammation, such as high-sensitivity C-reactive protein (CRP), are strong risk factors for CAD.
- Randomized trials suggest that, regardless of cholesterol level, any patient at significant risk for vascular events should be given a statin.
- Primary *percutaneous coronary intervention (PCI)* performed by experienced operators is superior to thrombolysis for the treatment of acute *myocardial infarction (MI).*
- Stenting, using either a bare-metal stent or a drug-eluting stent, is useful in patients with acute MI and for prevention of MI in selected patients. It requires a postprocedure period of *dual antiplatelet therapy.*
- Prophylactic *implantable cardioverter-defibrillators (ICDs)* are indicated for patients who have survived a cardiac arrest or an episode of hemodynamically unstable ventricular tachycardia. ICDs are also indicated for severe left ventricular dysfunction after MI.

Ischemic Heart Disease

Atherosclerotic CAD is by far the number-one killer not only in the United States but also in the world. In the United States, it is estimated that every minute, 1 person dies because of CAD. The number of women who die from CVD is 10 times the number of women who die from breast cancer.

Pathophysiology

Abnormal cholesterol intake and metabolism are central factors in ischemic heart disease (IHD). The "fatty streak" is an accumulation of lipids and lipid-laden macrophages, called foam cells, under the endothelium of the coronary arteries. These cells organize in a plaque, and as the plaque becomes calcified, the lumen of the vessel narrows. The plaque can also become unstable and rupture. This rupture leads to turbulence and activation of the coagulation cascade, causing intravascular thrombosis. The result is partial or complete vessel occlusion, which causes the symptoms of unstable angina or MI.

Ischemia is defined as local, temporary oxygen deprivation associated with inadequate removal of metabolites caused by reduced tissue perfusion. IHD is typically caused by decreased perfusion of the myocardium secondary to stenotic or obstructed coronary arteries. The balance between arterial supply of and myocardial demand for oxygen determines whether ischemia occurs. Significant coronary stenosis, thrombosis, occlusion, reduced arterial pressure, hypoxemia, or severe anemia can impede the supply of oxygen to the myocardium. On the demand side, an increase in heart rate, ventricular contractility, or wall tension (which is determined by systolic arterial pressure, ventricular volume, and ventricular wall thickness) may increase utilization of oxygen. When the demand for oxygen exceeds the supply, ischemia occurs. If this ischemia becomes prolonged, infarction and myocardial necrosis result. The necrotic process begins in the subendocardium, usually after approximately 20 minutes of coronary obstruction, and progresses to transmural and complete infarction in 4–6 hours.

Risk Factors for Coronary Artery Disease

The majority of patients with CAD have some identifiable risk factors. These risk factors are evident in epidemiologic studies and include a positive family history, male sex, lipid abnormalities, diabetes mellitus, hypertension, physical inactivity, obesity, and smoking. Many of these risk factors may be modified and are discussed in more detail in Chapter 4. Markers of inflammation, particularly high-sensitivity CRP, may represent strong risk factors for CAD. CRP levels less than 1 mg/mL, between 1 and 3 mg/mL, and greater than 3 mg/mL identify patients at low, medium, and high risk, respectively, for future cardiovascular events.

CVD is the leading cause of death in women, accounting for one-third of all deaths, and kills more women than men each year. The average lifetime risk of CAD in women is very high, nearly 1 in 2. Compared with a man the same age, a 50-year-old woman with a single additional risk factor has a substantially higher lifetime risk for CAD. Fortunately, most CVD risk in women is modifiable with the recommendations previously discussed; optimizing modifiable risk is of crucial importance in women.

In addition, postmenopausal women are disproportionately affected by a stress-induced cardiomyopathy called takotsubo cardiomyopathy, or broken heart syndrome. This disorder may mimic an acute MI, but testing reveals no occlusive vascular disease. The etiology is unclear.

Clinical Syndromes

Clinical presentations of IHD include angina pectoris (ie, stable angina; variant, or Prinzmetal, angina), the acute coronary syndromes (ie, unstable angina, acute MI), congestive heart failure (CHF), sudden cardiac death, and asymptomatic IHD.

Angina pectoris

The cardinal symptom in patients with IHD is angina pectoris. It is usually manifested as precordial chest pain or tightness that is often triggered by physical exertion, emotional distress, or eating. Angina pectoris is usually due to atherosclerotic heart disease. Coronary vasospasm may occur at the site of a lesion or even in otherwise normal coronary arteries. Angina typically lasts 5–10 minutes and is usually relieved by rest, nitroglycerin, or both. Patients may present with pain radiating into other areas, including the jaw, arm, neck, shoulder, back, chest wall, or abdomen.

Often, angina is misinterpreted as indigestion or musculoskeletal pain. The level of physical activity that results in angina pectoris is clinically significant and is useful in determining the severity of CAD, treatment, and prognosis. Myocardial ischemia may be painless in diabetic patients and women, often delaying the diagnosis until the disease is more advanced. The pain associated with MI is similar to that of angina, but it is usually more severe and more prolonged.

Stable angina pectoris Angina is considered stable if it responds to rest or nitroglycerin and if the patterns of frequency, ease of onset, duration, and response to medication have not changed substantially over 3 months.

Variant (Prinzmetal) angina Variant angina occurs at rest and is not related to physical exertion. The ST segment is elevated on electrocardiography during the anginal episodes, which are caused by coronary artery spasm. Underlying atherosclerosis is present in 60%–80% of cases, and thrombosis and occlusion may result during the episodes of coronary artery spasm.

Acute coronary syndrome

Acute coronary syndrome (ACS) comprises the spectrum of unstable cardiac ischemia, from unstable angina to acute MI. Plaque rupture is considered the common underlying event. Unstable angina and acute MI should be considered closely related events, clinically differentiated by the presence or absence of markers of myocardial injury. In 2007, a task force representing groups from the United States and Europe established a definition of MI; it includes the detection of cardiac biomarkers (eg, troponin), ischemia symptoms, electrocardiogram (ECG) changes indicating new ischemia, pathologic Q waves on ECG, and evidence of loss of viable myocardium or wall-motion abnormalities on imaging.

If a coronary thrombus is occlusive and it persists, MI can result. The location and extent of the infarction depend on the anatomical distribution of the occluded vessel, the presence of additional stenotic lesions, and the adequacy of collateral circulation. If the patient has chest pain at rest, unstable angina is the diagnosis. If the ischemia is severe enough to cause myocardial necrosis, infarction results. *Acute MI* is further differentiated into *non–ST-segment elevation MI (NSTEMI)* and *ST-segment elevation MI (STEMI)*. Typical findings used to differentiate between these include

- *Unstable angina (chest pain at rest).* The ECG shows ST-segment depression and/or T-wave inversion. No cardiac biomarkers are detected, reflecting a lack of myocardial necrosis.

- *NSTEMI (subendocardial, nontransmural).* The ECG shows ST-segment depression and/or T-wave inversion. Cardiac biomarkers are detected. The MI may be considered incomplete; thus, patients may be more susceptible to reinfarction or extension. Aggressive workup and treatment are required to prevent progression to STEMI.
- *STEMI.* The ECG shows early ST-segment elevation and later Q waves. This condition involves full-thickness or nearly full-thickness necrosis of the ventricular wall; if the necrosis does not yet involve the full thickness of the ventricular wall, early reperfusion therapy is required to avoid progression to full-thickness necrosis.

Myocardial infarction may occur suddenly, without warning, in a previously asymptomatic patient or in a patient with stable or variant angina; MI may also follow a period of unstable angina. Patients commonly experience chest pain, nausea, vomiting, diaphoresis, weakness, anxiety, dyspnea, lightheadedness, and palpitations. Nearly 25% of myocardial infarcts are painless; painless MI is more common in persons with diabetes mellitus and with increasing age. These patients may present with CHF or syncope. Symptoms may begin during or after exertion or at rest.

The clinical findings in IHD vary and depend on the location and severity of myocardial ischemia or injury. Approximately half of all infarctions involve the inferior myocardial wall, and most of the remaining half involve the anterior regions. Examination may reveal pallor, coolness of the extremities, low-grade fever, signs of pulmonary congestion and increased central venous pressure (if left ventricular dysfunction is present), an S_3 or S_4 gallop, an apical systolic murmur (caused by papillary muscle dysfunction), hypertension, or hypotension. The ECG may demonstrate a variety of ST-segment and T-wave changes and arrhythmias.

Approximately 60% of patients who die of cardiac disease expire suddenly before reaching the hospital. However, the prognosis for those hospitalized with MI has become remarkably good. In some studies using thrombolytic therapy or PCI, the mortality rate has been in the range of 5%–8%. Mortality is affected by a wide variety of factors, such as the degree of heart failure, the extent of myocardial damage, the severity of the underlying atherosclerotic process, heart size, and previous ischemia.

Immediate coronary angiography and primary PCI (including stenting) of the infarct-related artery have been shown to be superior to thrombolysis when done promptly by experienced operators in high-volume centers. If the time from first medical contact to intervention ("door to balloon" time) is kept under 90 minutes, the outcome is improved and is superior to that of thrombolysis. This intervention, in conjunction with a platelet glycoprotein IIb/IIIa antagonist, is widely used in patients with acute MI.

The complications of MI depend on its severity and may include CHF, rupture of the ventricular wall, pericarditis, and arrhythmias. Regional and global ventricular contractile dysfunction may result in CHF or pulmonary edema. Mild to moderate heart failure occurs in nearly 50% of patients following MI. Some patients experience post-MI pericarditis, characterized by a pericardial friction rub 2–3 days after infarction. Injury along the conduction pathways of the atria or ventricles may result in bradycardia, heart block, supraventricular tachycardias, or ventricular arrhythmias. Arrhythmias often exacerbate ischemic injury by reducing the perfusion pressure in the coronary arteries. Most acute deaths from MI result from arrhythmia.

Congestive heart failure secondary to ischemic heart disease

Congestive heart failure is discussed later in this chapter.

Sudden cardiac death

Sudden cardiac death (SCD) is defined as unexpected nontraumatic death that occurs within 1 hour after onset of symptoms in clinically stable patients. A disproportionate number of SCDs occur in the early morning hours. SCD is usually caused by a severe arrhythmia, such as ventricular tachycardia, ventricular fibrillation, profound bradycardia, or asystole. SCD may result from MI, occur during an episode of angina, or occur without warning in a patient with frequent arrhythmias secondary to underlying IHD or ventricular dysfunction. Other causes of SCD are Wolff-Parkinson-White syndrome, long QT syndrome, torsades de pointes, atrioventricular block, aortic stenosis, myocarditis, cardiomyopathy, ruptured or dissecting aortic aneurysm, and pulmonary embolism. There is evidence that prophylactic ICDs are the optimal first-line therapy for patients who have survived a cardiac arrest or an episode of hemodynamically unstable ventricular tachycardia. Results from the Multicenter Automatic Defibrillator Implantation Trial II (MADIT II) demonstrate that ICDs are also the optimal first-line therapy for severe left ventricular dysfunction after MI.

Asymptomatic ischemic heart disease

Asymptomatic patients with IHD are at particular risk for unexpected MI, life-threatening arrhythmias, and SCD. Advanced CAD may develop in these patients and they may experience multiple infarcts before the correct diagnosis is made and appropriate treatment is initiated. Older adults, women, and individuals with diabetes mellitus are more likely to have painless ischemia. Approximately 25% of MIs are asymptomatic, but they may be detected on a subsequent ECG. A patient who has unexplained dyspnea, weakness, arrhythmias, or poor exercise tolerance requires cardiac testing to evaluate for the presence of undiagnosed IHD.

Noninvasive Cardiac Diagnostic Procedures

Noninvasive diagnostic testing in IHD includes electrocardiography, serum biomarker measurements, echocardiography, various types of stress testing, and imaging studies such as *cardiac computed tomography (CT)* and *cardiac magnetic resonance imaging (MRI).*

Electrocardiography

The ECG may appear normal between episodes of ischemia in patients with angina. During angina, the ST segments often become elevated or depressed by up to 5 mm. T waves may be inverted, they may become tall and peaked, or inverted T waves may normalize. These ECG findings, when associated with characteristic anginal pain, are virtually diagnostic of IHD. However, absence of ECG changes does not exclude, with certainty, myocardial ischemia.

During MI, QT-interval prolongation and peaked T waves may appear. The ST segments may be depressed or elevated. ST-segment elevation may persist for several days to weeks, then return to normal. T-wave inversion appears in the leads corresponding to the site of the infarct. Q waves or a reduction in the QRS amplitude appears with the onset of myocardial necrosis. Q waves are typically absent in a subendocardial (nontransmural) infarction. These findings usually occur in the ECG leads related to the site of the infarct and may be accompanied by reciprocal ST depression in the opposite leads. Tachycardia and ventricular arrhythmias are most common within the first few hours after the onset of infarction. Bradyarrhythmias, such as heart block, are more common with inferior infarction; ventricular tachycardia and fibrillation are more common with anteroseptal infarction.

Serum biomarker testing

Cardiac enzymes are released into the bloodstream when myocardial necrosis occurs and are therefore valuable in differentiating MI from unstable angina and noncardiac causes of chest pain. With the advent of assays for cardiac-specific troponins, serum biomarker testing has also proven useful in identifying patients with ACS who are at greatest risk for adverse outcomes.

Cardiac-specific troponins are accepted as the most sensitive and specific biochemical cardiac marker in ACS. Cardiac isoforms of troponins (troponins T and I) are important regulatory elements in myocardial cells and, unlike creatine kinase MB (CK-MB), are not normally present in the serum of healthy individuals. Troponins T and I have been shown to be more cardiac-specific and cardiac-sensitive than CK-MB, allowing for more accurate diagnosis of cardiac injury. Moreover, unlike CK-MB levels, levels of troponins T and I are not elevated in patients with skeletal muscle injury. Troponin levels remain elevated from 3 hours to 14 days after MI (long after CK-MB levels have normalized). Therefore, for patients who delay seeking medical attention for MI, troponin assays are the test of choice. The greater sensitivity of the cardiac troponin assay allows the detection of lesser amounts of myocardial damage. In fact, mildly elevated troponin levels may be found in patients with NSTEMI who otherwise would be considered to have unstable angina. However, troponin T is a less sensitive marker than is CK-MB in the early stages of infarction (6–12 hours), so the assay should be repeated 6–9 hours later.

In addition to being diagnostically valuable, troponin levels confer prognostic information. Patients with an ACS who present with normal CK-MB and elevated troponin T levels have an increased risk of death, risk of recurrent nonfatal infarction, and need for revascularization with PCI or *coronary artery bypass grafting (CABG).* Similarly, studies have shown that patients who have elevated troponin levels at the time of hospital admission are at increased risk of death, cardiogenic shock, or CHF. Finally, a quantitative relationship between the amount of troponin I measured and the risk of death in patients who present with ACS has been demonstrated. Patients who are at greatest risk for adverse outcomes can be identified in the emergency department, allowing for more appropriate medical decisions and therapeutic triage.

Serum myoglobin is the first marker to rise following myocardial damage, and levels can be elevated between 1 and 20 hours after infarction. Although myoglobin might appear to be ideal for early detection of MI, its performance is not consistent and its specificity for cardiac events is poor. Therefore, myoglobin should not be the only diagnostic marker used to identify patients with MI, but its early appearance with myocardial injury makes its absence useful in ruling out myocardial necrosis.

Echocardiography

Echocardiography employs 1- and 2-dimensional ultrasound and color flow Doppler techniques to image the ventricles and atria, the heart valves, left ventricular contraction and wall-motion abnormalities, left ventricular ejection fraction, and the pericardium. Patients with IHD, particularly following infarction, commonly have regional wall-motion abnormalities that correspond to the areas of myocardial injury. Other, less frequent complications of infarction, such as mitral regurgitation from papillary muscle injury, ventricular septal defect, ventricular aneurysm, ventricular thrombus, and pericardial effusion, can also be detected with echocardiography. Color flow Doppler imaging provides information on the flow of blood across abnormal valves, pressure differences within the chambers, intracardiac shunts, and cardiac output. Cardiac biomarkers are far more sensitive and specific than echocardiography in detecting cardiac injury.

Exercise echocardiography (stress echocardiography) is useful for imaging cardiac valve and wall-motion abnormalities and ventricular dysfunction induced by ischemia during exercise. Predischarge exercise stress echocardiography provides useful prognostic information following acute MI.

Exercise stress testing

Patients with angina may have normal findings on clinical examination, electrocardiography, and echocardiography between episodes of ischemia. Standardized exercise tests have been developed to induce myocardial ischemia under controlled conditions. The ECG, heart rate, blood pressure, and general physical status of the patient are monitored during the procedure. The endpoint in angina patients is a symptom or sign of cardiac ischemia, such as chest pain, dyspnea, ST-segment depression, arrhythmia, or hypotension. The level of exercise required to induce ischemia is inversely correlated with the likelihood of significant CAD. False-positive and false-negative results occur, and the sensitivity increases with the number of coronary arteries involved. A modified exercise stress test is also performed in patients with a recent MI to help determine functional status and prognosis.

Radionuclide scintigraphy and scans

The sensitivity of exercise testing can be increased via radionuclide techniques. Several agents are available for injection, including thallium-201, technetium-99m sestamibi, and technetium-99m tetrofosmin. Other techniques include thallium-201 myocardial and technetium-99 pyrophosphate scintigraphy, or blood pool isotope scans.

Thallium accumulates in normal myocardium and reveals a perfusion defect in areas of myocardial ischemia. Thallium scans have a high sensitivity and specificity for CAD. Reversible thallium or technetium-99m sestamibi defects are those that are present during exercise but resolve during rest. This correlates with myocardial ischemia. In contrast, a fixed thallium or sestamibi defect is present during both exercise and rest and represents a region of prior infarction or nonviable tissue. For patients unable to exercise vigorously enough to reach the required heart rates, a thallium scan or echocardiogram in conjunction with a pharmacologic stress test using intravenous adenosine, dipyridamole, or dobutamine may provide information similar to that of an exercise examination. Tomographic imaging of myocardial perfusion is possible with thallium-201 via a technique called *single-photon emission CT (SPECT),* which provides better imaging of infarcts, better detection of multivessel disease, and less severe artifacts.

A number of other imaging technologies are available and may add clinically useful information. *Positron emission tomography* can accurately differentiate metabolically active myocardium from scar tissue. *Coronary CT angiography* is useful in evaluating occlusive vascular disease and is most useful in ruling out atherosclerotic disease. *Electron beam CT* is useful in quantifying coronary artery calcification, which correlates with atherosclerosis and is highly sensitive but not specific. CT scanning can provide excellent resolution and may be an alternative to angiography in some patients; disadvantages include significant radiation exposure and the use of contrast media. Finally, *cardiac MRI* provides excellent imaging, and perfusion testing is possible with gadolinium. MRI may be contraindicated in some patients with ICDs or pacemakers but can be safely used in the presence of coronary stents. Cardiac CT and MRI are also useful in assessing congenital or acquired coronary abnormalities.

Invasive Cardiac Diagnostic Procedures

Coronary arteriography and *ventriculography* provide valuable information about the presence and severity of CAD and about ventricular function. These techniques can indicate the specific areas of coronary artery stenosis or occlusion, the number of involved vessels, the ventricular systolic and diastolic volumes, the ejection fraction, and regional wall-motion abnormalities. *Multiple gated acquisition (MUGA)* can also be performed for these purposes. This information helps the cardiologist and cardiac surgeon plan appropriate treatment for the patient. *Intravascular ultrasound imaging* is an evolving invasive modality for studying the intraluminal coronary anatomy and may be particularly useful in evaluating the effects of stents or angioplasty.

Coronary artery stenosis is hemodynamically significant when the arterial lumen diameter is narrowed by more than 50% or the cross-sectional area is reduced by more than 75%. Common indications for coronary arteriography are ACS, post-MI angina, stable angina unresponsive to medical therapy or revascularization, a markedly positive exercise stress test result, and a recent MI in a patient younger than 40 years. The technique may also be useful in evaluating valvular heart disease, ventricular septal defect, papillary muscle dysfunction, cardiomyopathy of unknown cause, or unexplained ventricular arrhythmias.

Management of Ischemic Heart Disease

The goals of management for the patient with CAD are to reduce the frequency of or eliminate angina, prevent myocardial damage, and prolong life. The first line of attack should include eliminating or reducing risk factors for atherosclerosis. Smoking cessation, dietary modification, weight loss, exercise, and improved control of diabetes mellitus and hypertension are critical steps. Fraker and colleagues have reported actual regression of atherosclerotic lesions following intensive lipid-lowering therapy, and statins should be considered for all CAD patients. Antiplatelet therapy with daily aspirin has also been advocated for all patients with CAD because it significantly reduces the risk of MI.

Aspirin appears to offer women and men equal benefit from reduction in primary MI risk, and it is of significant benefit in secondary prevention. Aspirin may also provide protection against stroke, but in low-risk patients, the risk of bleeding complications may outweigh the benefits. Aspirin use should be guided by an assessment of the patient's risk of stroke or MI. Hormone therapy, antioxidant vitamin supplementation, and folic acid therapy do not appear to provide any benefit in preventing CVD in women.

Fraker TD Jr, Fihn SD; 2002 Chronic Stable Angina Writing Committee, American College of Cardiology, American Heart Association, et al. 2007 chronic angina focused update of the ACC/AHA 2002 guidelines for the management of patients with chronic stable angina. *J Am Coll Cardiol.* 2007;50(23):2264–2274.

Treatment of stable angina pectoris

Medical management of angina pectoris is designed to deliver as much oxygen as possible to the potentially ischemic myocardium, to reduce the oxygen demand to a level at which symptoms are eliminated or reduced to a comfortable level, or both.

Therapeutic agents include

- *β-Adrenergic blockers.* These represent the first line of treatment. They reduce heart rate and contractility (decreasing oxygen demand) and are demonstrated to prolong life in CAD patients. They should be used with caution when left ventricular dysfunction is present.
- *Nitrates and nitroglycerin.* These agents increase oxygen delivery through coronary vasodilation. Systemic effects (eg, venous dilation, decrease in blood pressure) decrease oxygen demand. They should be used with caution in patients taking erectile dysfunction drugs.
- *Slow calcium channel blockers.* These agents are good for long-term angina treatment. They should be used with caution when left ventricular dysfunction is present.
- *Aspirin with or without clopidogrel, prasugrel, or ticagrelor.* These drugs can be used for anticoagulation.

Improving the oxygen-carrying capacity of the blood by treating anemia or coexisting pulmonary disease provides some additional benefit. Patients in whom medical therapy is unsuccessful may be candidates for revascularization with either PCI or CABG.

Revascularization may improve coronary blood flow, control angina, and increase exercise tolerance. In high-risk patients, the risk of infarction is reduced and long-term survival is enhanced. Revascularization is indicated in otherwise healthy patients with advanced left main CAD, left ventricular dysfunction with 3-vessel disease, or angina that is unresponsive to medical treatment and in patients on medical therapy who have ischemia on exercise testing. Revascularization procedures include PCI with or without stenting and CABG.

PCI was developed as an alternative to surgical revascularization. Angioplasty, one PCI technique, involves passing a balloon catheter into a stenosed vessel and inflating the balloon at the site of the narrowing to widen the lumen. Although 85%–90% of vessels can be opened with PCI, the rate of restenosis is approximately 25%–40% at 6 months. The insertion of a wire-mesh *stent* at the time of PCI improves patency and reduces the risk of restenosis by nearly 50%. Drug-eluting stents are superior to bare-metal stents in preventing restenosis but are also more likely to lead to late stent thrombosis. Stent thrombosis may result in MI or death, so patients receiving stents should receive a platelet IIb/IIIa receptor antagonist (abciximab, eptifibatide, or tirofiban) along with heparin, aspirin, and clopidogrel at the time of stenting (Table 5-1). European guidelines are similar but recommend prasugrel or ticagrelor over clopidogrel following PCI. Dual antiplatelet therapy (DAT; aspirin plus clopidogrel, prasugrel, or ticagrelor) should continue for at least 1 month poststenting for a bare-metal stent and at least 1 year for a drug-eluting stent. DAT should not be stopped during this period, and elective surgery should be postponed unless the patient can continue on DAT. Patients intolerant of aspirin may use clopidogrel alone. Prasugrel appears to have a better anticoagulant effect than clopidogrel but may pose a higher risk of serious bleeding.

Table 5-1 Summary of ACC/AHA Guideline Recommendations for Medical Management of ACS and Acute MI*

Medication	Acute Therapies for ACS	Acute Therapies for Acute MI	Discharge Therapies
Aspirin	IA	IA	IA
Clopidogrel in patients allergic to aspirin	IA	IC	IA
Clopidogrel, intended medical management	IA	—	IA
Clopidogrel, early catheterization/PCI	IA (prior to or at time of PCI)	IB	IA
Prasugrel (as an alternative to clopidogrel), for unstable angina/non-STEMI patients undergoing PCI and for primary PCI	IB†	IB†	IB†
Ticagrelor (as an alternative to clopidogrel)	IB	IB	IB
Clopidogrel and glycoprotein IIb/IIIa inhibitor, up front (prior to catheterization)	IIaB	—	—
Heparin (unfractionated or low-molecular-weight)	IA	IC‡	—
Fondaparinux	IB	IC	—
Bivalirudin	IB	IB§	—
Bivalirudin for early invasive strategy (without glycoprotein IIb/IIIa inhibitor), if clopidogrel at least 300 mg was administered 6 hours before planned catheterization or PCI	IIaB	—	—

Table 5-1 *(continued)*

β-Blockers (oral)	IB	IA	IB
β-Blockers (intravenous)[‖]	IIaB[‖]	IIaB[‖]	—
ACE inhibitors	IB[‖]	IA/IIaB[#]	IA/IIaB[**]
Glycoprotein IIb/IIIa inhibitors for intended early catheterization/PCI:			
Eptifibatide/tirofiban	IA	IIaB	—
Abciximab	IA	IIaA	—
Glycoprotein IIb/IIIa inhibitors in addition to clopidogrel for high-risk patients without intended early catheterization/PCI:			
Eptifibatide and or tirofiban	IIbB	—	—
Abciximab	IIIA	—	—
Lipid-lowering agent[††]	—	—	IA
Smoking cessation counseling	—	—	IB
Nonsteroidal anti-inflammatory agents (other than aspirin)	IIIC	IIIC	—

ACC = American College of Cardiology; ACE = angiotensin-converting enzyme; ACS = acute coronary syndrome; AHA = American Heart Association; MI = myocardial infarction; NSTEMI = non–ST-segment elevation myocardial infarction; PCI = percutaneous coronary intervention; STEMI = ST-segment elevation MI.

*Class I indicates that treatment is useful and effective, class IIa indicates that the weight of the evidence is in favor of usefulness and efficacy, class IIb indicates that the weight of the evidence is less well established, and class III indicates that the intervention is not useful or not effective and may be harmful. Type A recommendations are based on data derived from multiple randomized clinical trials or meta-analyses, type B recommendations are based on data derived from a single randomized clinical trial or large nonrandomized studies, and type C recommendations are based on consensus of expert opinion or on data derived from small studies, retrospective studies, or registries.

†In STEMI patients with a prior history of stroke and transient ischemic attack for whom primary PCI is planned, prasugrel is not recommended for use in dual antiplatelet therapy (IIIC).

‡Use of unfractionated heparin, enoxaparin, or fondaparinux has established efficacy and should be continued (IC) for a minimum of 48 hours and preferably for the duration of the hospitalization, up to 8 days. Enoxaparin or fondaparinux is preferred if therapy is given for more than 48 hours because of the risk of heparin-induced thrombocytopenia (IA). Because of the risk of catheter thrombosis, fondaparinux should not be used as the sole anticoagulant to support PCI.

§With primary PCI, with or without prior heparin bolus.

‖For patients with hypertension and no heart failure, low-output state, increased risk of shock, or other contraindications to β-blockers.

#For patients with persistent hypertension despite treatment, diabetes mellitus, heart failure, or any left ventricular dysfunction.

**Class IA for patients with heart failure or ejection fraction <0.40, class IIaB for others, in the absence of hypotension (systolic blood pressure <100 mm Hg). Angiotensin receptor blocker (valsartan or candesartan) for patients with ACE inhibitor intolerance.

††For patients with a low-density-lipoprotein cholesterol level >70 mg/dL.

Modified with permission from Bashore TM, Granger CB, Hranitzky P, Patel MR. Heart disease. In: Papadakis M, McPhee SJ, Rabow MW, eds. *Current Medical Diagnosis and Treatment 2013.* 48th ed. Lange Current Series. New York: McGraw-Hill; 2013:eTable 10-9.1.

PCI is recommended for patients with lesions amenable to passing a catheter, patients with a 1-vessel or 2-vessel disease but without complex disease of the left anterior descending coronary artery, and nondiabetic patients with a good ejection fraction with multivessel disease. Diabetic patients do well with PCI if the procedure is paired with a stent and a glycoprotein IIb/IIIa agent. PCI and CABG have similar mortality rates, but patients undergoing PCI are more likely to require a second procedure.

When angioplasty is inappropriate or ineffective and medical therapy has failed to control symptoms in severe multivessel disease, CABG may be considered. CABG may be indicated in patients with high-risk disease, including those with significant left main, proximal left anterior descending, or 3-vessel disease, especially if accompanied by left ventricular dysfunction. In many other situations, medical therapy may be superior to CABG in prolonging survival. During CABG, a shunt is installed from the aorta to the diseased coronary artery. It bypasses the area of obstruction and increases blood flow, thereby eliminating angina and often reducing the risk of infarction and cardiac death. CABG has also been shown to increase left ventricular function, improve quality of life, and relieve angina. Previously, saphenous veins were most commonly used as the bypass material, but use of the internal mammary artery has become the standard for the left anterior descending artery because of its improved long-term patency rate. Some patients now receive "off-pump bypass surgery," in which the grafts are sewn onto the beating heart. This technique could avoid the adverse effects of cardiopulmonary bypass, which include memory, cognitive, and other neurologic deficits.

Although revascularization may produce good outcomes, the underlying disease process must continue to be managed. The Bypass Angioplasty Revascularization Investigation has demonstrated that even after revascularization procedures (ie, PCI, CABG), arterial disease will continue to progress unless cardiac risk factors are reduced.

Alderman EL, Kip KE, Whitlow PL, et al; Bypass Angioplasty Revascularization Investigation. Native coronary disease progression exceeds failed revascularization as cause of angina after five years in the Bypass Angioplasty Revascularization Investigation (BARI). *J Am Coll Cardiol.* 2004;44(4):766–774.

O'Gara PT, Kushner FG, Ascheim DD, et al; American College of Cardiology Foundation/American Heart Association Task Force on Practice Guidelines. 2013 ACCF/AHA guideline for the management of ST-elevation myocardial infarction: a report of the American College of Cardiology Foundation/American Heart Association Task Force on Practice Guidelines. *Circulation.* 2013;127(4):e362–e425. Epub 2012 Dec 17.

Task Force on the Management of ST-segment Elevation Acute Myocardial Infarction of the European Society of Cardiology; Steg PG, James SK, Atar D, et al. ESC guidelines for the management of acute myocardial infarction in patients presenting with ST-segment elevation. *Eur Heart J.* 2012;33(20):2569–2619. Epub 2012 Aug 24.

Thygesen K, Alpert JS, White HD; Joint ESC/ACCF/AHA/WHF Task Force for the Redefinition of Myocardial Infarction. Universal definition of myocardial infarction. *Circulation.* 2007;116(22):2634–2653. Epub 2007 Oct 19.

Yusuf S, Hawken S, Ounpuu S, et al; INTERHEART Study Investigators. Effect of potentially modifiable risk factors associated with myocardial infarction in 52 countries (the INTERHEART study): case-control study. *Lancet.* 2004;364(9438):937–952.

Treatment of acute coronary syndromes

Patients with an ACS are admitted to a hospital or a chest pain observation unit for monitoring and treatment. They are initially treated aggressively with anti-ischemic pharmacotherapy. Once these initial measures are instituted, further management and triage of patients with an ACS is based on the presence or absence of ST-segment elevation. Patients with ST-segment elevation ACS undergo reperfusion therapy with either thrombolysis or catheter-based interventions; patients with non–ST-segment elevation ACS may be appropriately followed up with either medical treatment alone or a more aggressive interventional approach. The use of a risk calculator (eg, TIMI, GRACE, PURSUIT) may help identify high-risk patients and determine subsequent management; the TIMI and GRACE risk calculators are available at www.timi.org and www.mdcalc.com/grace-acs-risk-and-mortality-calculator, respectively. Therapy for ACS and MI, as well as recommended therapy at the time of discharge, is summarized in Table 5-1.

Management of non–ST-segment elevation ACS In general, myocardial oxygen demands are managed with medications and supplemental oxygen. β-Blocker therapy reduces myocardial oxygen demands and should be considered for all patients with evolving MI if no contraindication exists. For patients not receiving reperfusion therapy, β-blocker therapy provides a survival benefit, particularly for high-risk patients (older patients and those with previous MI and mild pulmonary venous congestion). Medical therapy for NSTEMI includes

- β-adrenergic blockers
- angiotensin-converting enzyme (ACE) inhibitors (eg, captopril, enalapril, lisinopril, ramipril)
- nitrates and/or nitroglycerin
- DAT (aspirin plus clopidogrel, prasugrel, or ticagrelor)
- antithrombin therapy

CHF and pulmonary edema should be treated if present. If β-blockers cannot be used, the clinician may consider verapamil or diltiazem. ACE inhibitors decrease the risk of death if given within 24 hours of MI, but they should be avoided if hypotension or renal insufficiency is present.

Antithrombin therapy is beneficial in ACS. It involves a variety of agents, including unfractionated heparin (UFH); low-molecular-weight heparins, including enoxaparin; the direct thrombin inhibitors (hirudin and bivalirudin); and the factor Xa inhibitor fondaparinux. Controlled studies have yet to determine the optimal regimen, but fondaparinux and enoxaparin appear slightly better than UFH. Fondaparinux appears to cause fewer bleeding complications than the other agents, but the anticoagulation is more difficult to reverse because the half-life is longer; thus, UFH may be superior if surgery is anticipated within 24 hours.

Glycoprotein IIb/IIIa inhibitors (eg, tirofiban, abciximab, eptifibatide) have been shown to reduce the risk of death and MI in patients with non–ST-segment elevation ACS, as well as after coronary angioplasty and stenting. The glycoprotein IIb/IIIa receptor is present on the surface of platelets. When platelets are activated, this receptor increases its affinity for fibrinogen and other ligands, resulting in platelet aggregation. This mechanism constitutes the final and obligatory pathway for platelet aggregation. The platelet glycoprotein IIb/IIIa receptor antagonists act by preventing fibrinogen binding and thereby preventing platelet aggregation. Platelets are involved in the development of both ACS and complications after PCI. The benefits of glycoprotein IIb/IIIa inhibitors are less demonstrated with the use of new antiplatelet agents (eg, prasugrel, ticagrelor).

Once unstable angina and NSTEMI have been managed as described, patients may be evaluated with either a conservative noninvasive approach or an early invasive (angiographic) strategy, depending on their level of risk for adverse outcomes. Controlled trials have shown the superiority of an invasive approach in managing ACS patients, particularly patients with refractory angina or hemodynamic instability and patients at elevated risk as measured by bedside risk stratification tools (eg, TIMI, GRACE). The decision to proceed from diagnostic angiography to revascularization is influenced not only by the coronary anatomy but by a number of additional factors, including anticipated life expectancy, ventricular function, comorbidity, functional capacity, severity of symptoms, and quantity of viable myocardium at risk.

Patients should also have a serum lipid profile drawn and be discharged on a statin agent.

Management of ST-segment elevation ACS Modern therapy for evolving Q-wave MI involves rapid and effective reperfusion, because necrosis is a time-dependent process. Optimal myocardial salvage requires that nearly complete reperfusion be achieved as soon as possible: reperfusion within 1 hour of symptom onset yields maximal benefit; within 6 hours of symptom onset, significant benefit; 6–12 hours after symptom onset, some benefit. The benefit of reperfusion therapy after 12 hours of symptom onset has not been established.

Methods of reperfusion include thrombolysis and catheter-based PCIs (balloon angioplasty with or without stent placement). Initial medical management before and after reperfusion therapy should include aspirin, clopidogrel, morphine (for pain), and β-blockers if no contraindications exist. Nonsteroidal agents besides aspirin should not be used acutely or during hospitalization, as they increase the risk of CHF and death. Other adjuncts to therapy may include low-molecular-weight heparins and glycoprotein IIb/IIIa inhibitors.

Numerous clinical trials have shown the superiority of early PCI over thrombolysis, particularly if performed in the first 90 minutes following medical contact. Hospitals without PCI capability should transfer the patient to a facility that can perform PCI if the procedure can be done within 90 minutes. Otherwise, thrombolytic therapy should be started within 30 minutes of first medical contact. PCI following full-dose thrombolytics carries significant risks but may be done in high-risk patients or if thrombolytic therapy has failed ("rescue PCI"). Totally occluded arteries generally do not benefit from PCI.

Thrombolysis Patients with a STEMI treated with thrombolytics in the first 3 hours show a 50% reduction in mortality; those treated at 12 hours show a 10% reduction. Thrombolytic agents lyse coronary thrombi and restore coronary blood flow in most patients; several such agents are available. *Tissue plasminogen activators (tPAs),* including alteplase, reteplase, and tenecteplase, are the most commonly used thrombolytics because they are more effective in opening arteries and reducing mortality than is streptokinase. When any tPA is used, intravenous heparin should be administered concurrently.

Major bleeding complications occur in up to 5% of patients undergoing thrombolytic therapy. Contraindications to thrombolysis include known sites of potential bleeding, a history of cerebrovascular accident, recent surgery, and prolonged cardiopulmonary resuscitation efforts. Thrombolysis should not be used in the treatment of NSTEMI due to decreased benefits and, possibly, increased hemorrhagic risks.

Congestive Heart Failure

The epidemiologic magnitude of CHF is staggering. Approximately 5 million patients in the United States have CHF, and there are 500,000 new cases per year. It is estimated that CHF will develop in 20% of the population older than 40 years. Many of the patients consulting an ophthalmologist belong to the older population, a group especially prone to this condition. If the heart cannot meet the metabolic demands of the tissues, heart failure is the diagnosis. The cardiac pump may be in failure, or it may be near normal but unable to keep up with demand. The direct result of heart failure is circulatory failure.

Symptoms and signs of CHF may occur when the heart is not able to pump enough blood over a prolonged period to meet the body's requirements. *Compensated CHF* refers to situations in which the clinical manifestations of CHF have been controlled by treatment. *Decompensated CHF* represents heart failure with symptoms that are not under control. *Refractory CHF* exists when previous therapeutic measures have failed to control the clinical manifestations of the syndrome. Pulmonary edema usually results from severe left ventricular failure with increased pulmonary capillary pressure, causing parenchymal and intra-alveolar fluid accumulation in the lung. Heart failure is often preventable with early detection and intervention, and this is emphasized by guidelines and classifications that recognize 4 stages of heart failure, including stages for those at risk and those with no current signs of CHF. Figure 5-1 illustrates the stages and recommended therapy at each stage. The New York Heart Association has also developed a classification for heart failure symptoms, ranging from class I (no symptoms) to class IV (symptoms at rest).

Symptoms

Heart failure causes a variety of symptoms, depending on the severity of ventricular dysfunction. Symptoms may result from inadequate tissue perfusion caused by pump failure or from the failing heart's inability to empty adequately, leading to edema and fluid accumulation in the lungs, extremities, and other sites. The most frequent symptoms of left ventricular failure are dyspnea with exertion or at rest, orthopnea, paroxysmal nocturnal dyspnea, diaphoresis, generalized weakness, fatigue, anxiety, and lightheadedness. With more severe CHF, the patient may also experience a productive cough; copious pink, frothy sputum; and confusion. Angina may also occur if the CHF results from IHD. Right-sided heart failure may occur separately from or secondary to chronic left-sided heart failure. Peripheral edema typically develops in patients with right-sided heart failure.

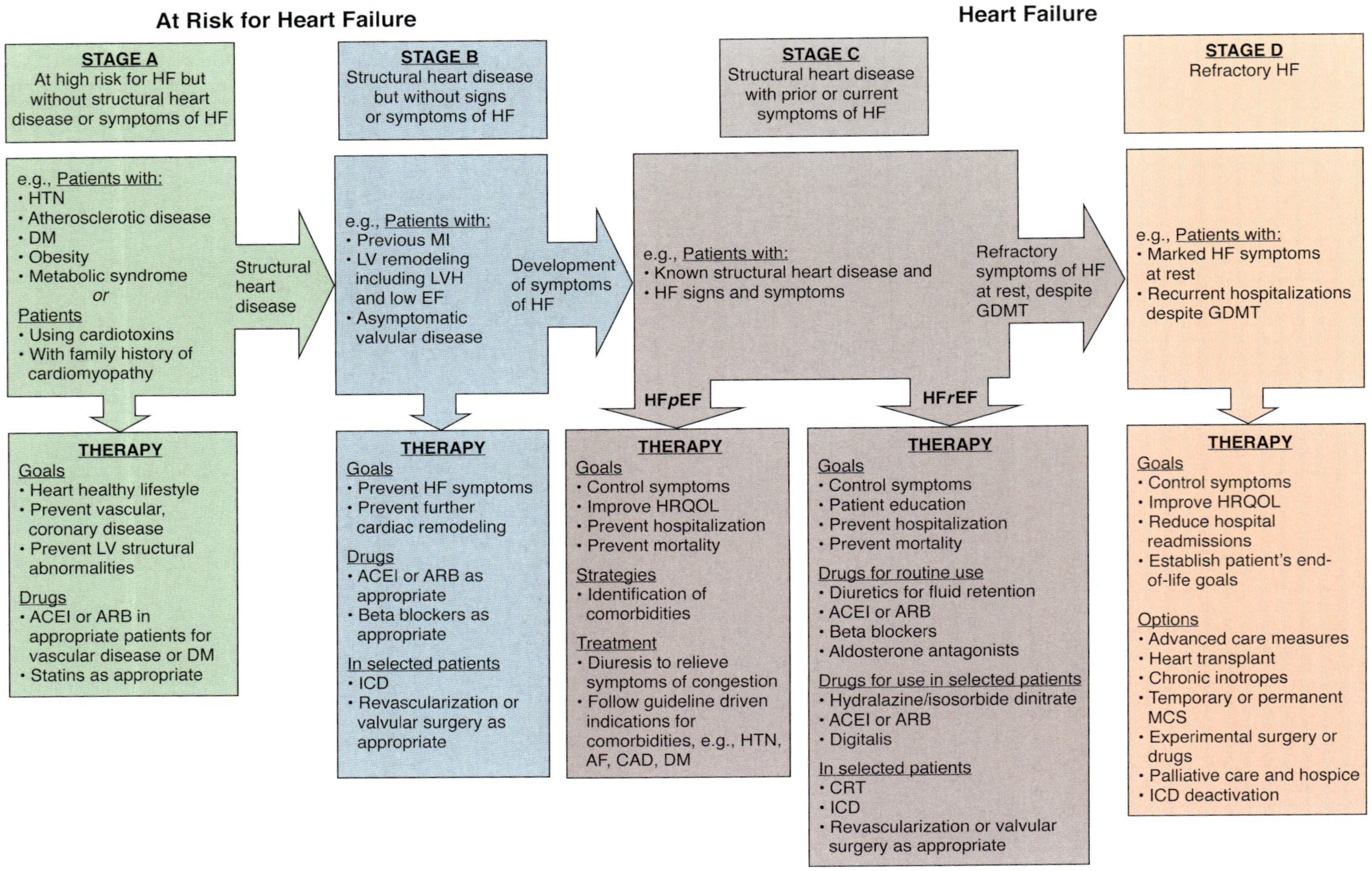

Figure 5-1 Stages in the development of heart failure. ACEI = ACE inhibitors; AF = atrial fibrillation; ARB = angiotensin II receptor blocker; CAD = coronary artery disease; CRT = cardiac resynchronization therapy; DM = diabetes mellitus; EF = ejection fraction; GDMT = guideline-directed medical therapy; HF = heart failure; HF*p*EF = heart failure with preserved ejection fraction; HF*r*EF = heart failure with reduced ejection fraction; HRQOL = health-related quality of life; HTN = hypertension; ICD = implantable cardioverter-defibrillator; LV = left ventricular; LVH = left ventricular hypertrophy; MCS = mechanical circulatory support; MI = myocardial infarction. *(Reproduced with permission from Yancy CW,*

Clinical Signs

Examination findings in acute left ventricular failure may include respiratory distress, use of the respiratory accessory muscles, pinkish sputum or frank hemoptysis, coarse rales on pulmonary auscultation, expiratory wheezes, a rapid heart rate, an S gallop, diaphoresis, and deterioration in mental status. Blood pressure is often markedly elevated but may be reduced during MI. Long-standing cases of CHF show signs of right ventricular failure, especially elevated central venous pressure, pedal edema, hepatomegaly, and cyanosis. In some patients, pleural effusion or ascites may be detected.

Diagnostic Evaluation

The history and clinical examination are the most important components in the diagnostic assessment of CHF. Diagnostic studies that are helpful in evaluating CHF and its underlying causes include chest radiography, electrocardiography, blood gas analysis, complete blood counts, serum electrolyte tests, blood urea nitrogen and creatinine tests, liver function tests, and urinalysis. Measurement of serum B-type natriuretic peptide (BNP), a peptide associated with reduced left ventricular ejection fraction and increased left ventricular filling pressure, may be helpful in determining the underlying cause, assessing disease severity and prognosis, and guiding the treatment of CHF. If the primary mechanism of heart failure is unclear, additional tests may prove useful in selected patients. Such tests may include echocardiography, exercise stress testing, cardiac nuclear imaging studies, coronary arteriography, right-sided and/or left-sided heart catheterization, Holter monitoring, pulmonary function tests, HIV testing, and thyroid function tests.

The ECG may reveal acute ischemic changes, acute or previous ventricular hypertrophy, chamber enlargement, and atrial fibrillation or other arrhythmias. Typical chest radiograph findings are prominent pulmonary vessels, interstitial or alveolar pulmonary edema, cardiomegaly, and pleural effusions. Patients with severe pump failure may have abnormal serum electrolyte levels owing to poor renal perfusion. Abnormalities in the blood or urine may help detect severe anemia or renal failure as a precipitating factor in CHF. Abnormal liver enzyme levels are common if venous congestion is present as a result of right ventricular failure.

Echocardiography and other cardiac studies can help differentiate the many cardiac causes of CHF, including IHD, valvular heart disease, cardiomyopathies, and cardiac arrhythmias. Coronary angiography can be helpful in identifying patients with cardiac ischemia and CHF, for which revascularization may lead to symptomatic improvement.

Ejection fraction (EF) is the calculated proportion of blood ejected by the ventricle during a single or average contraction. In patients without CHF, the EF is more than 0.50. An EF of 0.40–0.50 indicates mild impairment; 0.25–0.39, moderate impairment; and less than 0.25, severe impairment. Ejection fraction can be measured using echocardiography, radionuclide ventriculography, or contrast ventriculography. Echocardiography is the most useful and least invasive method of determining and sequentially following EF and the systolic state of the ventricles.

Etiology

As was noted previously, IHD is the most common cause of CHF. Cumulative injury to the ventricular myocardium from ischemia and infarction can lead to impaired ventricular systolic and diastolic function and, ultimately, pump failure. Additional causes of systolic dysfunction to be considered include

- valvular heart disease (aortic stenosis and aortic or mitral regurgitation)
- cardiomyopathies (idiopathic, metabolic, infectious, toxic, or connective tissue disease)
- myocarditis (secondary to viral or inflammatory diseases)
- infiltrative diseases (amyloidosis, sarcoidosis, and metastatic disease)
- left ventricular hypertrophy

Systolic dysfunction and diastolic dysfunction often occur simultaneously in the common causes of CHF—namely, IHD, valvular disease, and the congestive cardiomyopathies. Some of the causes of high-cardiac-output heart failure are severe anemia, hyperthyroidism, arteriovenous fistulas, beriberi, and Paget disease.

In high-output failure, the demand for oxygen is so great that the heart eventually fails because it cannot maintain the excessive cardiac output indefinitely. In some patients, heart failure may be more complex—for example, CHF may develop in a patient with IHD who has become severely anemic. Pure right ventricular failure may result from chronic obstructive pulmonary disease, pulmonary hypertension, tricuspid or pulmonary valve disease, right ventricular infarction, or constrictive pericarditis.

Pathophysiology and Clinical Course

The left and right ventricles function as pumping chambers, and their action can be subdivided into a *systolic,* or contraction, phase and a *diastolic,* or relaxation, phase. During systole, the ventricular muscle actively contracts, developing pressure and ejecting blood into the aorta or pulmonary artery for forward perfusion. During diastole, the ventricular muscle actively and passively relaxes and allows refilling of the ventricle from the corresponding atrium. Either or both of these phases may become impaired. Some of the symptoms and clinical signs of CHF can be distinguished as being attributable to systolic or diastolic impairment. Treatment varies, depending on which type of dysfunction predominates.

Systolic dysfunction

The ability of the heart to contract and eject blood is determined by preload, afterload, and contractility. *Preload* refers to the amount of stretch to which muscle fibers are subjected at the end of diastole, or refilling. Preload is determined by blood volume and venous return. Excessive preload is often called *volume overload.* Up to a point, as the preload increases, the force of contraction also increases, allowing adequate emptying of the ventricle.

Afterload is the amount of tension or force in the ventricular muscle mass just after onset of contraction, as the ventricle begins emptying. Clinically, afterload represents the pressure that the ventricle must withstand during contraction. Thus, the aortic pressure determines afterload for the left ventricle, whereas the pulmonary artery pressure determines afterload for the right. Even a normal ventricle may fail with extremely high preload or afterload.

Contractility refers to the intrinsic ability of the myocardial fibers to contract, independent of the preload or afterload conditions. Contractility can be adversely affected by metabolic, ischemic, or other structural derangement of the myocardial cells. Abnormal intracellular modulation of calcium ions is a key component in heart failure. Clinical disorders that affect preload, afterload, or contractility result in systolic dysfunction—and therapy directed toward improving these parameters can be used to treat systolic dysfunction.

Diastolic dysfunction

Several of the disorders that impair the diastolic, or relaxation, properties of the ventricle were listed previously among the causes of CHF. Diastolic dysfunction causes elevated filling pressures in the ventricles and atria. In the left ventricle, diastolic dysfunction causes pulmonary venous hypertension and its clinical manifestations, such as dyspnea on exertion, orthopnea, and paroxysmal nocturnal dyspnea. Clinical signs of diastolic dysfunction are pulmonary edema with rales, lung congestion visible on chest radiograph, and hypoxemia.

The clinical course of CHF may follow a downward spiral of left ventricular systolic and diastolic dysfunction, ventricular dilation, and a decline in the EF, followed by right-sided heart failure. A continuous reduction in cardiac output and tissue perfusion may be accompanied by increasing pulmonary and systemic venous congestion. Appropriate treatment may slow or even halt progression in some patients. BNP, which is synthesized in the cardiac ventricles and whose release is directly proportional to ventricular volume expansion and pressure overload, may indicate the course of CHF. Levels of BNP correlate with left ventricular pressure, the amount of dyspnea, and the state of neurohumoral modulation. In addition, BNP levels correlate well with the New York Heart Association CHF classification.

Medical and Nonsurgical Management

Appropriate treatment at each stage of CHF is summarized in Figure 5-1. In general, most symptomatic patients should be treated with a combination of a diuretic and an ACE inhibitor. Diuretics, whether oral thiazide-type or loop diuretics, reduce the blood volume and thus preload. More severely affected CHF patients should receive a loop diuretic (eg, furosemide, bumetanide, torsemide) either orally or intravenously. Hypokalemia may result from the use of these agents, requiring the use of potassium-sparing agents (eg, spironolactone, triamterene, amiloride), but these potassium-sparing agents tend to be less potent diuretics.

Management of systolic dysfunction

Reducing afterload is the most effective way to manage systolic dysfunction in most clinical situations. Reducing vascular resistance and lowering arterial blood pressure decrease the burden on the left ventricle and enhance contraction and ejection. Regardless of the baseline values, lowering blood pressure (while maintaining adequate tissue perfusion) is the mainstay of treatment of systolic dysfunction. Therapeutic options include

- *ACE inhibitors.* ACE inhibitors—which include captopril, enalapril, lisinopril, and ramipril—are the agents that decrease afterload most effectively. They decrease clinical signs of CHF and morbidity and mortality rates.
- *β-Blockers.* These include carvedilol, bisoprolol, and metoprolol. They decrease mortality and hospitalization rates. If not contraindicated, they should be used in almost all CHF patients.
- *Angiotensin II receptor blockers.* These include candesartan and valsartan. They may be used when hypotension from ACE inhibitors would not be tolerated.
- *Amlodipine.* Other calcium channel blockers should be avoided in CHF.
- *Other afterload-reducing agents.* These include hydralazine, clonidine, and, for patients intolerant of ACE inhibitors due to renal disease, α-adrenergic blockers (eg, prazosin, doxazosin).

For patients with systolic dysfunction, the contractility of the left ventricle can be enhanced with inotropic agents. *Digoxin,* or *digitalis,* is a time-honored drug for increasing contractility and was once a mainstay of treatment, but it raises safety and toxicity concerns. Thus, digoxin is now reserved largely for patients who remain symptomatic despite the use of diuretics and ACE inhibitors and for patients with CHF and atrial fibrillation requiring rate control. With the exception of digoxin, oral inotropic agents have not proven safe or effective in patients with chronic CHF; however, intravenous inotropic agents play a key role in treating patients hospitalized for worsening heart failure.

Management of diastolic dysfunction

Diastolic function can be improved by reducing preload, which in turn lowers filling pressures in the ventricle. Preload can be reduced by reducing circulating blood volume, by increasing the capacitance of the venous bed, and by improving systolic function to more effectively empty the ventricle. Diuretics are the most effective agents for reducing blood volume. Oral thiazide-type and loop diuretics are effective for long-term diuresis, but, as noted earlier, intravenous loop diuretics such as furosemide and bumetanide are more effective in the treatment of severe CHF or pulmonary edema. Venous capacitance can be increased by administering venous dilators, particularly the nitrates. Intravenous furosemide and morphine also have some venodilation effects, partially explaining their effectiveness in treating pulmonary edema. Any of the measures previously discussed that improve systolic function also indirectly enhance diastolic function by reducing the residual blood volume in the ventricle following contraction.

Other approaches to CHF

Other strategies for managing CHF include seeking underlying causes and/or contributing factors responsible for the failure and correcting them, if possible. Precipitating factors can include excessive salt or fluid intake, poor medication adherence, excessive activity, obesity, pulmonary infection or embolism, MI, renal disease, anemia, thyrotoxicosis, and arrhythmias.

Intermittent arrhythmias may seriously compromise ventricular function. Tachyarrhythmias may aggravate ischemia; bradyarrhythmias may decrease cardiac output and blood pressure further. As previously discussed, β-blockers should be considered for these patients and all patients with CHF for their effects on overall prognosis and particularly SCD. Amiodarone was not beneficial in the Sudden Cardiac Death in Heart Failure Trial (SCD-HeFT), and most other antiarrhythmic agents are contraindicated in CHF because they may decrease cardiac function and be paradoxically proarrhythmic. ICDs can be useful adjuncts to medical therapy in patients with CHF, cardiomyopathy, and an EF of 0.35 or less, and they improved mortality in both the MADIT II and SCD-HeFT trials. Biventricular pacing also improves mortality rates and decreases rehospitalization rates in patients with CHF and a wide QRS complex by improving contraction efficiency. Patients with heart block or other severe bradyarrhythmias may also require cardiac pacing.

Patients with a dilated cardiomyopathy and atrial fibrillation should receive anticoagulation therapy unless contraindications exist. Many physicians also prescribe anticoagulation for patients with a dilated cardiomyopathy, low EF, and normal sinus rhythm, if no contraindications exist. Options include warfarin, DAT, and newer agents such as dabigatran, apixaban, and rivaroxaban. Risk factors, cost, tolerability, and potential drug interactions should all be considered during agent selection.

Other measures that can help in managing CHF are restricting dietary sodium, avoiding fluid overload by carefully monitoring oral and intravenous fluid intake, controlling pain and anxiety, treating concomitant metabolic and pulmonary diseases, and providing supplemental oxygen to hypoxemic patients. Finally, all patients with CHF should receive an influenza vaccination and the pneumococcal vaccine.

Bardy GH, Lee KL, Mark DB, et al; Sudden Cardiac Death in Heart Failure Trial (SCD-HeFT) Investigators. Amiodarone or an implantable cardioverter-defibrillator for congestive heart failure. *N Engl J Med.* 2005;352(3):225–237.

Invasive or Surgical Management

Depending on the underlying causes, other surgical procedures that may benefit patients with CHF include percutaneous balloon valvuloplasty, mitral commissurotomy, mitral or aortic valve replacement, left ventricular aneurysmectomy, and pericardiectomy. Patients with CAD, the leading cause of CHF, may benefit from coronary revascularization by either CABG or PCI. Cardiac transplantation has become an effective surgical treatment for patients with refractory CHF. Many transplant centers have achieved a 5-year survival rate that exceeds 75%. The use of corticosteroids and immunosuppressive agents, such as cyclosporine, tacrolimus, sirolimus, azathioprine, and mycophenolate, has reduced transplant rejection and mortality. Implantable ventricular assist devices may help to maintain patients awaiting cardiac transplantation.

Finally, as many of these patients are older and have multiple comorbidities, palliative care directed only at symptomatic improvement should also be considered.

Hunt SA, Abraham WT, Chin MH, et al; American College of Cardiology Foundation, American Heart Association. 2009 focused update incorporated into the ACC/AHA 2005 guidelines for the diagnosis and management of heart failure in adults: a report of the

American College of Cardiology Foundation/American Heart Association Task Force on Practice Guidelines developed in collaboration with the International Society for Heart and Lung Transplantation. *J Am Coll Cardiol.* 2009;53(15):e1–e90.

McMurray JJ, Adamopoulos S, Anker SD, et al; ESC Committee for Practice Guidelines. ESC guidelines for the diagnosis and treatment of acute and chronic heart failure 2012: the Task Force for the Diagnosis and Treatment of Acute and Chronic Heart Failure 2012 of the European Society of Cardiology. Developed in collaboration with the Heart Failure Association (HFA) of the ESC. *Eur Heart J.* 2012;33(14):1787–1847.

Yancy CW, Jessup M, Bozkurt B, et al. 2013 ACCF/AHA guideline for the management of heart failure: executive summary: a report of the American College of Cardiology Foundation/American Heart Association Task Force on Practice Guidelines. *Circulation.* 2013;128(16):1810–1852. Epub 2013 Jun 5.

Disorders of Cardiac Rhythm

Abnormalities of cardiac rhythm can vary widely, from asymptomatic premature atrial complexes and mild sinus bradycardia to life-threatening ventricular tachycardia and fibrillation. Disorders of cardiac rhythm can be categorized into several groups, including bradyarrhythmias and conduction disturbances, ectopic or premature contractions, and tachyarrhythmias.

Although many rhythm and conduction disturbances are caused by underlying IHD, they are also attributable to valvular heart disease, myocarditis, cardiomyopathy, congenital aberrant conduction pathways, pulmonary disease, toxic or metabolic disorders, neurogenic causes, and cardiac trauma.

The electrical impulse that initiates each heartbeat normally begins in the *sinoatrial (SA) node* and is conducted down through the atria and ventricles, resulting in a coordinated series of contractions of these chambers. The SA node is the primary pacemaker of the heart. It controls the heart rate and is influenced by neural, biochemical, and pharmacologic factors. If the SA node function is depressed or absent, secondary pacemakers in the *atrioventricular (AV) junction,* the *bundle of His,* or the *ventricular muscle* can generate stimuli and maintain the heartbeat. Normally, stimulus formation in these secondary pacemaker sites is slower than stimulus formation in the SA node. However, abnormal stimuli can also be generated at any of these sites at a rapid pace, resulting in tachycardia.

Bradyarrhythmias and Conduction Disturbances

A *bradyarrhythmia* is any rhythm resulting in a ventricular rate of less than 60 beats per minute (bpm). Bradyarrhythmias and conduction blocks are generally asymptomatic, although they may cause lightheadedness or syncope in rare cases. In some cases, simply discontinuing the inciting medication leads to resolution of the bradycardia. Treatment is generally not necessary except in cases of syncope or hemodynamic instability. In those cases, the placement of a cardiac pacemaker is usually the definitive treatment.

Premature Contractions

The principal types of premature contractions are *premature atrial complexes (PACs), premature junctional complexes (PJCs),* and *premature ventricular complexes (PVCs).* These complexes result from ectopic premature depolarization arising from the atria (PAC), the AV node or proximal His-Purkinje system (PJC), or the ventricles (PVC). Patients often experience no symptoms or may have a sensation of "skipped beats." Often, no treatment is necessary, but β-blockers or calcium channel blockers can be helpful in symptomatic patients. The correction of underlying abnormalities (eg, drug toxicity, electrolyte imbalance, hyperthyroidism) is often curative.

Premature ventricular complexes typically require no therapy. However, frequent or complex PVCs in the presence of cardiac disease are markers of an increased risk of SCD. Symptomatic patients requiring treatment are best treated with class II drugs (β-blockers) because class I and III drugs appear to worsen the arrhythmia in 5%–20% of patients. While clinically useful, the Vaughan Williams classification of antiarrhythmic drugs (Table 5-2) represents an oversimplification, since many of these medications appear to have multiple mechanisms of action.

Tachyarrhythmias

Tachyarrhythmia is defined as a heart rate in excess of 100 bpm. Tachycardias are classified as supraventricular or ventricular, depending on the mechanism and site of origin. *Narrow complex tachycardias* are almost exclusively supraventricular in origin; *wide complex tachycardias* may be either supraventricular or ventricular in origin. Correct identification of the origin and mechanisms of the tachycardia is critical to selecting appropriate treatment. The patient with a supraventricular tachycardia often describes palpitations and in some cases is syncopal. Symptoms often correlate with a higher ventricular rate.

Table 5-2 Vaughan Williams Classification of Antiarrhythmic Drugs

Class	Drugs	Mechanism of Action	Indications for Use
Class Ia	Disopyramide, procainamide, quinidine	Sodium channel blockers slow conduction velocity, prolong APD	SVT and VT, prevent VF, symptomatic PVCs
Class Ib	Lidocaine, mexiletine, phenytoin	Shorten APD, no effect on conduction velocity	VT, symptomatic PVCs, prevent VF
Class Ic	Flecainide, propafenone	Slow conduction velocity, may mildly prolong APD	Refractory SVT, VT, or VF
Class II	Carvedilol, esmolol, metoprolol, propranolol	β-Blockers block β-adrenergic receptors	SVT, prevent VF, prevent recurrent AF
Class III	Amiodarone, dofetilide, dronedarone, ibutilide, sotalol	Prolong APD, no effect on conduction	Amiodarone: VT, VF, SVT, AF Dofetilide, dronedarone, or ibutilide: AF, atrial flutter Sotalol: VT, AF
Class IV	Diltiazem, verapamil	Nondihydropyridine slow calcium channel blockers	SVT

AF = atrial fibrillation; APD = action potential duration; PVC = premature ventricular contraction; SVT = supraventricular tachycardia; VF = ventricular fibrillation; VT = ventricular tachycardia.

Data from Makielski JC. Myocardial action potential and action of antiarrhythmic drugs. In: *UpToDate*, Downey BC (ed), Waltham, MA. Available at www.uptodate.com. Accessed July 23, 2014.

The category of supraventricular tachycardias includes paroxysmal atrial tachycardia, AV junctional tachycardia, atrial flutter, and atrial fibrillation. The exact site of the pacing focus may be difficult to determine when the heart rate is very rapid. The prognosis for supraventricular tachycardias is usually better than that associated with ventricular tachycardia. Supraventricular tachycardias may be paroxysmal or chronic, as with chronic atrial fibrillation. Causes include emotional stress; caffeine, alcohol, or drug use; thyrotoxicosis; lung disease; and cardiac disease. β-Blockers are often useful in the management of these disorders, and catheter-guided radiofrequency ablation may be curative in patients with refractory supraventricular tachycardia.

Atrial fibrillation

Atrial fibrillation is caused by multiple simultaneous wavelets occurring in both the right and the left atria, resulting in a chaotic electrical rhythm with ineffective atrial contraction. Cardiac output can be reduced markedly when the ventricular rate is very rapid, possibly resulting in CHF. Atrial thrombi may accumulate from stagnation of blood in the atrial appendages. These thrombi may embolize to the lungs, brain, or other organs. Anticoagulation therapy is indicated for patients with chronic atrial fibrillation and chronic atrial flutter associated with valvular disease, cardiomyopathy, or cardiomegaly and before conversion to sinus rhythm is attempted. Several risk stratification tools (eg, CHADS2) have been devised to weigh the risk of embolism versus the risk of bleeding in these patients. Warfarin appears to be superior to aspirin for anticoagulation in this situation. Other classes of anticoagulants (eg, direct thrombin inhibitors, factor Xa inhibitors) may also be useful, but risk factors, cost, tolerability, patient preference, and potential drug interactions should all be considered.

Conversion of atrial fibrillation can be attempted with quinidine, procainamide, ibutilide, or direct-current (DC) cardioversion. In many patients with chronic atrial fibrillation, maintenance therapy is directed toward controlling the ventricular rate, which can usually be accomplished with digoxin, verapamil, or β-blockers.

Other curative approaches have been developed for both atrial fibrillation and atrial flutter. These treatments include radiofrequency catheter ablation and the surgical maze procedure. The maze procedure interrupts all possible reentry circuits to the atrium with multiple incisions. A single uninterrupted pathway is left intact to allow normal conduction from the SA node to the AV node.

Calkins H, Brugada J, Packer DL, et al; European Heart Rhythm Association, European Cardiac Arrhythmia Society, American College of Cardiology, American Heart Association, Society of Thoracic Surgeons. HRS/EHRA/ECAS expert consensus statement on catheter and surgical ablation of atrial fibrillation: recommendations for personnel, policy, procedures and follow-up. A report of the Heart Rhythm Society (HRS) Task Force on Catheter and Surgical Ablation of Atrial Fibrillation. *Heart Rhythm.* 2007;4(6):816–861.

Ventricular tachyarrhythmias

Ventricular tachycardia The ventricular tachyarrhythmias include ventricular tachycardia (VT), torsades de pointes (a variant of VT), ventricular flutter, and ventricular fibrillation. These arrhythmias may present with palpitations, heart failure, or syncope or may progress rapidly to SCD. VT occurs infrequently in young patients with no organic heart disease. Brief episodes of VT cause palpitations; prolonged attacks in patients with organic cardiac disease can lead to heart failure or cardiac shock. If the rate is not very high and there is no significant underlying heart disease, VT may be well tolerated; however, it may degenerate into ventricular fibrillation, resulting in hemodynamic collapse and death.

Treatment with immediate synchronized DC cardioversion is indicated for sustained VT associated with hemodynamic compromise, severe CHF, or ongoing ischemia or infarction. Pharmacologic cardioversion with intravenous procainamide or lidocaine and amiodarone may be attempted in patients with clinically stable VT. Amiodarone is probably the agent of choice for recurrent VT if its adverse effects are tolerated.

Electrophysiologic testing is often performed on patients with suspected or documented ventricular arrhythmias. In this procedure, direct transcatheter electrical stimulation of various sites in the ventricle induces arrhythmias. Given the efficacy and low risk associated with implantation, ICDs, in conjunction with antiarrhythmic drugs, have become the treatment of choice for patients with life-threatening ventricular arrhythmias. Less common therapies include ventricular aneurysmectomy, ventricular electrical mapping and resection of the arrhythmogenic focus, and radiofrequency catheter ablation.

Ventricular fibrillation Ventricular fibrillation (VF) is the most ominous of all the cardiac arrhythmias because it is fatal when untreated or when refractory to treatment. It is a major cause of SCD outside the hospital. The ventricular contractions are rapid and uncoordinated, resulting in ineffective ventricular pumping that soon leads to syncope, convulsions, and death if the VF is not interrupted. The prognosis is generally poor because each episode can be fatal.

Cardiopulmonary resuscitation efforts must be initiated emergently. Immediate unsynchronized DC cardioversion is the primary therapy. After successful cardioversion, continuous intravenous infusion of effective antiarrhythmic therapy should be maintained until any reversible causes have been corrected. The choice of long-term antiarrhythmic therapy depends on the conditions responsible for the initial VF episode. Primary VF occurring within the first 72 hours of an acute MI is not associated with an elevated risk of recurrence and does not require long-term antiarrhythmic therapy. However, VF without an identifiable and reversible cause requires long-term therapy in the form of either prophylactic antiarrhythmic drug therapy (eg, amiodarone, sotalol) or implantation of an automatic defibrillator.

Implantable cardioverter-defibrillators ICDs monitor the heart rhythm and, when a tachyarrhythmia is identified, deliver therapy. Their evolution has been impressive. Initially, a thoracotomy was necessary to implant an epicardial patch or patches. The overwhelming majority of patients now receive a transvenous system, which significantly reduces the morbidity and mortality associated with the implantation of these devices. Current-generation ICDs are generally implanted in the prepectoral region (similar to pacemaker implantation). Although first-generation ICDs delivered only high-energy "defibrillating" shocks, current-generation devices provide tiered therapy, including pacing algorithms for tachycardia, low-energy cardioversion for stable VT, high-energy cardioversion for VT or VF, single-chamber or dual-chamber pacing support for bradycardia, and stored diagnostic information for rhythm discrimination.

ICDs treat arrhythmias when they occur and do not prevent them. Most patients require concomitant antiarrhythmic therapy to reduce the frequency of device discharges or facilitate antitachycardia pacing by slowing the ventricular rate. The development of an effective and safe antiarrhythmic prescription may be complex and requires the skills of a trained electrophysiologist. Generally, the acute management of life-threatening ventricular arrhythmias in these patients does not differ from that of other patients with similar rhythm disturbances. If the device fails to terminate an arrhythmia, cardiopulmonary resuscitation and external defibrillation should proceed normally. Three randomized prospective studies have demonstrated that automated ICDs are the preferred first-line therapy for patients who have survived a cardiac arrest or an episode of hemodynamically unstable VT. At 2-year follow-up, the automated ICD was associated with a 20%–30% relative reduction in the risk of death. The MUSTT (Multicenter Unsustained Tachycardia Trial) and MADIT trials have also proven the benefit of ICDs used for primary prevention of sudden death in patients with CAD, reduced EFs, nonsustained VT, or inducible ventricular arrhythmias during electrophysiologic testing. Following an MI, ICDs appear to be the best available therapy for preventing SCD. An ICD should be considered for patients on optimal medical therapy who have left ventricular dysfunction from an MI at least 40 days previously and an expected survival with good functional status of at least 1 year. Ongoing trials may expand the role of ICDs in the primary prevention of sudden death.

Camm AJ, Lip GY, De Caterina R, et al; ESC Committee for Practice Guidelines. 2012 focused update of the ESC guidelines for the management of atrial fibrillation: an update of the 2010 ESC guidelines for the management of atrial fibrillation. Developed with the special contribution of the European Heart Rhythm Association. *Eur Heart J.* 2012;33(21): 2719–2747.

Epstein AE, DiMarco JP, Ellenbogen KA, et al; American College of Cardiology/American Heart Association Task Force on Practice Guidelines (Writing Committee to Revise the ACC/AHA/NASPE 2002 Guideline Update for Implantation of Cardiac Pacemakers and Antiarrhythmia Devices), American Association for Thoracic Surgery, Society of Thoracic Surgeons. ACC/AHA/HRS 2008 guidelines for device-based therapy of cardiac rhythm abnormalities: a report of the American College of Cardiology/American Heart Association Task Force on Practice Guidelines. *Circulation.* 2008;117(21):e350–e408.

Ophthalmic considerations Many of the adult patients seen and treated by ophthalmologists are in the age group at risk for IHD and its many complications. They often undergo stressful eye surgery under local or general anesthesia, and ophthalmologists need to be cognizant of these patients' risks of myocardial ischemia, MI, CHF, and arrhythmias. Similarly, ophthalmologists need to be aware of the association between proliferative diabetic retinopathy and IHD. This information should be given to the primary medical care provider of patients with proliferative diabetic retinopathy but no diagnosis of IHD so that appropriate screening tests can be considered.

Cardiac complications of noncardiac surgery are a major cause of perioperative morbidity and mortality, MI being the most significant. Older age, preexisting CAD, and CHF are the principal risk factors for development of these complications.

ICDs are increasingly used for the management of cardiac arrhythmias. While no cases of discharge of an ICD during ocular surgery have been reported, the ophthalmologist should discuss the status and possible perioperative disabling of the ICD with the cardiologist before ocular surgery to avoid surgical complications.

Finally, ophthalmologists should be aware of the potential ocular adverse effects associated with medications commonly used in treating CVD. Following are the medications of clinical relevance:

- *Amiodarone.* Corneal microdeposits probably occur in nearly all patients who use amiodarone for a long time. The corneal epithelial whorl-like deposition is indistinguishable from that due to chloroquine. Visual changes are unusual; patients most often report hazy vision or colored halos around lights. Occasionally, a patient may report that bright lights, especially headlights at night, cause a significant glare problem. An adverse effect that has been seen secondary to photosensitivity reactions is discoloration (usually slate-gray or blue) of periocular skin. A rare adverse effect is amiodarone optic neuropathy, which is characterized by an insidious onset, slow progression, bilateral vision loss, and protracted disc swelling that tends to stabilize within several months of discontinuing the medication. Patients on long-term amiodarone therapy should have a baseline ophthalmic examination, follow-up examinations every 6–12 months, and immediate evaluation of any new visual disturbances. Due to this drug's photosensitizing effects, UV-blocking spectacle lenses should be considered in selected cases of chronic eyelid disease or macular disease.
- *β-Blockers.* As with other β-adrenergic blocking agents, use of β-blockers can lead to a keratoconjunctivitis sicca–like syndrome, probably due to decreased lacrimation. Some β-blockers may decrease tear secretion, may possibly enhance migraine ocular scotomata, and may decrease intraocular pressure (IOP). Topical β-blockers, particularly timolol, may be less effective in lowering IOP in patients taking systemic β-blockers. Visual disturbances and vivid visual hallucinations may also be associated with the systemic use of β-blockers.
- *Digoxin.* Glare and disturbances of color vision are the most striking and the most common ocular adverse effects. They include decreased vision and problems with color vision, such as blue-yellow pattern defects; a yellow, green, blue, or red tinge to objects; and colored halos (mainly blue) around lights. Patients on digoxin may also describe yellow or green flickering vision, colored borders around objects, glare phenomena, light flashes, scintillating scotomata, a frosted appearance to objects, and formed visual hallucinations.

- *ACE inhibitors.* These agents may cause angioedema involving the eye and orbit. The presumed mechanism is the disruption of bradykinin metabolism.

Agency for Healthcare Research and Quality, US Department of Health and Human Services. [US and international guidelines]; www.guideline.gov.

American Academy of Ophthalmology website; www.aao.org.

American College of Cardiology website; www.cardiosource.org.

American Heart Association website; www.heart.org.

European Society of Cardiology website; www.escardio.org.

Johnson LN, Krohel GB, Thomas ER. The clinical spectrum of amiodarone-associated optic neuropathy. *J Natl Med Assoc.* 2004;96(11):1477–1491.

Stoller GL. Ophthalmic surgery and the implantable cardioverter defibrillator. *Arch Ophthalmol.* 2006;124(1):123–125.

UpToDate; www.uptodate.com.

CHAPTER 6

Cerebrovascular Disease

Recent Developments

- Intravenous recombinant tissue plasminogen activator (rtPA) is strongly recommended for carefully selected patients who meet additional exclusion criteria and who can be treated within 4½ hours of onset of ischemic stroke.
- Carotid endarterectomy (CEA) is beneficial for symptomatic patients with recent nondisabling carotid artery ischemic events and ipsilateral carotid artery stenosis of 70%–99%. CEA is not beneficial for symptomatic patients with 0%–29% or 100% stenosis.
- Newer oral anticoagulants, which include direct thrombin inhibitors and factor Xa inhibitors, should be considered for carefully selected patients with nonvalvular atrial fibrillation.
- Patients with acute ischemic stroke presenting within 48 hours of symptom onset should be given aspirin (160–325 mg/day) to prevent recurrent stroke, reduce stroke mortality, and decrease morbidity, provided contraindications such as allergy and gastrointestinal bleeding are absent and rtPA was not or will not be used as treatment. Patients who are not tPA candidates may be considered for intra-arterial (IA) therapies.
- Statin use reduces the risk of stroke and coronary events in patients with coronary artery disease and in those who have had an ischemic stroke of atherosclerotic origin.

Introduction

Stroke is the third leading cause of death in developed countries, ranking behind heart disease and cancer. From 2000 to 2010, the relative rate of stroke death decreased by 35.8% in the United States, and the actual number of US stroke deaths declined by 22.8%; yet the number of strokes occurring annually in the United States remains approximately 795,000, of which 610,000 are first attacks. Better control of hypertension, cholesterol levels, and diabetes mellitus, as well as increases in smoking cessation, have contributed to this drop in stroke mortality. The annual incidence of ischemic stroke has increased in Eastern Europe, China, and other nations where the widespread adoption of unhealthful lifestyles has accompanied improved economic status. Stroke is the leading cause of long-term disability in the United States today.

There are 2 primary types of stroke: ischemic stroke and hemorrhagic stroke. For extensive discussion of the ophthalmic manifestations of cerebrovascular disease, see BCSC Section 5, *Neuro-Ophthalmology.*

Cerebral Ischemia

Cerebral ischemia results from interference with circulation to the brain. Usually, cerebral circulation is maintained by a very efficient collateral arterial system that includes the 2 carotid and the 2 vertebral arteries, anastomoses in the circle of Willis, and collateral circulation in the cerebral hemispheres. However, atheromas and congenital arteriovenous malformations can lead to a reduction in cerebral blood flow. This reduction may be generalized or localized. Interruptions in cerebral blood flow can result in permanent neurologic deficits, depending on the extent and duration of the cerebral ischemia.

There are varying degrees of ischemia, which may be classified by severity and duration. A *transient ischemic attack (TIA)* is a focal loss of neurologic function of sudden onset, persisting for less than 24 hours and clearing without residual signs. Most TIAs last only a few minutes, and the symptoms are primarily associated with insufficiency of the internal carotid, middle cerebral, or vertebrobasilar arterial territories. A *completed stroke* is an ischemic event that produces a stable, permanent neurologic disability. Most ischemic strokes consist of small regions of complete ischemia in conjunction with a larger area of incomplete ischemia. This ischemic but not infarcted area has been termed the *penumbra.* The penumbra is dynamic, resulting in changes to the once passive approach to treating patients with acute cerebral ischemia. Clinical manifestations of cerebral ischemia reflect the functions associated with the area of ischemia and include paresis, paresthesia, vision loss, language disturbances, vertigo, diplopia, ataxia, dysarthria, headache, nausea, and vomiting.

Emboli or thrombi caused by atherosclerosis, hypertension, or diabetes mellitus and located in large, medium, and small arteries account for most strokes. Strokes caused by emboli of cardiac origin account for 20% of the total ischemic stroke incidence. Atrial fibrillation is the most common cause of cardioembolic strokes, occurring in up to 20% of such patients. Mural thrombi forming on the endocardium in conjunction with myocardial infarction (MI) account for 8%–10% of the total stroke incidence worldwide. Mitral stenosis and atrial myxoma are other cardiac conditions associated with intracranial embolism. Cerebral autosomal dominant arteriopathy with subcortical infarcts and leukoencephalopathy (CADASIL), a rare genetic small-vessel vasculopathy, can mimic multiple sclerosis and cause ischemic stroke.

Nonarteriosclerotic causes of thrombotic occlusion leading to TIA and stroke include internal carotid dissection (causing the classic triad of Horner sign, neck pain/headache, and neurologic signs and symptoms) and inflammatory arteritis (eg, collagen vascular disease, giant cell arteritis, meningovascular syphilis, acute and chronic meningitis, and moyamoya disease).

Another cause of cerebral ischemia is increased viscosity of the blood due to pregnancy and the postpartum period, use of oral contraceptives, postoperative and posttraumatic states, hyperviscosity syndromes, polycythemia, and sickle cell disease. Also, stroke may occur as a result of hypoxemia caused by conditions such as carbon monoxide poisoning, chronic obstructive pulmonary disease, profound anemia, and pulmonary emboli, in which there is decreased oxygenation and oxygen-carrying capacity of the blood.

Diagnosis and Management

The diagnosis of ischemic stroke and TIAs should be differentiated from the diagnosis of diabetic and convulsive seizures, migraine, vertigo, and neoplasms. Although the presentation of stroke is usually characteristic, the diagnosis should be differentiated from that of other conditions that may mimic strokes, such as multiple sclerosis, subdural hematoma, cranial nerve palsy, encephalitis, hypoglycemia, seizures, brain tumor, hypertensive encephalopathy, syncope, migraine, and functional disorder.

A detailed history, including the time and duration of onset, is important. Also, an assessment of risk factors is critical for treating a patient with suspected stroke. Nonmodifiable risk factors include age older than 60 years, male sex, and family history or prior history of stroke or TIAs. Modifiable risk factors include diabetes mellitus, hypertension, hyperlipidemia, cardiac arrhythmias, smoking, alcohol use, illicit drug use, migraine, and hypercoagulable states.

The clinical severity of a stroke can be determined using the US National Institutes of Health Stroke Scale, which assesses level of consciousness, gaze, visual fields, facial strength, motor function of the arms and legs, ataxia, sensation, language, dysarthria, and inattention, giving a specified number of points to each impairment uncovered. A scale of 0–42 is used for the assessment, with *0* being normal function and *42* being the most severe functional impairment. More information on this scale, as well as training in its use and certification, is available at www.strokeassociation.org.

Diagnostic studies

For practical purposes, diagnostic studies may be separated into those done in an acute care setting, such as in the emergency department, and those done in a more subacute setting, such as in a stable inpatient or stable outpatient setting. Emergent testing assesses the patient's clinical stability and the possibility of stroke mimics or conditions that could contribute to stroke; the tests should include blood glucose, complete blood count, blood chemistry, coagulation studies such as PT/aPTT (prothrombin time/activated partial thromboplastin time), international normalized ratio, troponins, and electrocardiogram. Ideally, all suspected cases of stroke and TIA should receive urgent *computed tomography (CT)* of the brain. The scan should be completed without contrast because contrast and blood appear similar on CT, and this similarity can result in misinterpretation of the image. CT is very sensitive for the presence of intracranial hemorrhage.

Once the urgent investigations are complete, imaging studies such as *magnetic resonance imaging (MRI)*, *magnetic resonance cerebral angiography*, *CT angiography*, and *conventional catheter angiography* can be considered. MRI is often more sensitive than CT in detecting an evolving stroke within hours of its onset, whereas CT results may be negative for up to several days after an acute cerebral infarct. These techniques can distinguish between acute and chronic infarction and help date hemorrhagic infarction; they can also evaluate for unsuspected space-occupying lesions. MRI, CT, or catheter angiography may be necessary to examine the intracranial and extracranial vessels for stenoses or to identify an aneurysm. Carotid duplex ultrasonography may be used to evaluate the patency of the extracranial carotid arteries; transcranial Doppler ultrasonography can evaluate the intracranial arteries. *Diffusion-weighted MRI, apparent diffusion coefficient (ADC) mapping,* and *CT perfusion imaging* are useful in the evaluation of early cerebral ischemia and regional blood flow. Early detection of these conditions by such techniques may allow for early treatment, which may be beneficial in salvaging tissue at risk. *Cerebral arteriography* is usually required only if the cause is unclear or if intra-arterial thrombolysis or surgical intervention is being strongly considered.

Investigation of the systemic arteries and the heart is essential in determining the cause of cerebral ischemia. Differences between upper limb pulse rates and blood pressure (BP) may indicate serious subclavian disease. Multiple bruits may suggest widespread arterial disease but may be present without significant occlusion. Evidence of a cardioembolic source should be pursued aggressively, especially in younger normotensive persons with cerebral ischemia and in older patients, for whom atrial fibrillation is included in the differential diagnosis. Electrocardiography and telemetry or Holter monitoring should be routine to exclude cardiac dysrhythmia and occult MI. Echocardiography is often helpful in excluding intracardiac emboli; transesophageal Doppler echocardiography is most sensitive in this regard. Lumbar puncture is rarely required in the evaluation of stroke or TIA, unless meningovascular syphilis, meningitis, or subarachnoid hemorrhage is a serious consideration.

Treatment

The goals of treating ischemic stroke are to restore blood flow to the brain and to salvage ischemic brain tissue that has not already infarcted. Achieving these goals involves ensuring the patient's medical stability and determining whether the patient is eligible for thrombolytic therapy. There is a narrow window in which to accomplish these objectives, typically within 4½ hours of the onset of symptoms.

Thrombolytic and antithrombotic agents are the primary drugs used in the treatment of ischemic stroke. One such drug is recombinant tissue plasminogen activator (rtPA), a fibrinolytic agent that converts plasminogen into plasmin in the presence of fibrin. This initiates fibrinolysis at the thrombus site, thereby improving blood flow to ischemic areas not yet infarcted (ischemic penumbra). In the US National Institute of Neurological Diseases and Stroke (NINDS) rtPA Stroke Study, the administration of rtPA within 3 hours of acute ischemic stroke was associated with improved function at 3 months but not with earlier neurologic improvement or lower mortality. The European Cooperative Acute Stroke Study III (ECASS III) showed a benefit of rtPA initiated up to 4½ hours after the onset of stroke. However, the exclusion criteria for patients treated 3–4½ hours from symptom onset (age >80 years, severe stroke, diabetes mellitus with a previous infarct, and any anticoagulant use) were more restrictive than for those treated at 3 hours or less. Most studies indicate that the sooner rtPA is initiated, the more likely it is to be beneficial.

The most serious complication of administering rtPA is symptomatic intracranial hemorrhage, which occurs in 6.4% of treated patients and has a mortality rate of 50%. Recently, stroke centers have used intra-arterial catheter-directed treatment for delivering thrombolytic agents directly to the site of the vascular occlusion. This has been shown to improve recanalization rates and clinical outcomes and is recommended for middle cerebral artery infarctions up to 6 hours after stroke onset.

Patients with a large cerebral artery occlusion are less likely to benefit from rtPA; endovascular clot removal is often performed in these patients after treatment with rtPA. Clot removal or thrombectomy can be performed within 8 hours of stroke onset and is a reasonable alternative for those patients who cannot receive rtPA. In the Solitaire With the Intention for Thrombectomy (SWIFT) trial, which compared the Solitaire Flow Restoration device (Covidien, Dublin, Ireland) and the Merci Retriever (University of California, Los Angeles) in the treatment of patients with acute ischemic stroke, the Solitaire device achieved better safety, angiographic, and clinical outcomes than did the Merci Retriever.

In addition to thrombolytic drugs, 2 major classes of antithrombotic agents can be used to treat ischemic stroke: antiplatelets and anticoagulants. Although aspirin, clopidogrel, and aspirin/extended-release dipyridamole combination are acceptable drug choices for secondary stroke prevention, aspirin is the only antiplatelet agent that is effective in the early treatment of ischemic stroke. Two large clinical trials showed a benefit of treatment with aspirin over placebo in short-term mortality and recurrent stroke risk when aspirin is initiated within 48 hours of ischemic stroke onset. Early use of combination antiplatelet agents such as aspirin with clopidogrel for acute ischemic stroke may be beneficial, but the available evidence is not consistent and is limited to the specific populations studied. Heparin and related agents are not effective in reduction of mortality or recurrent stroke in patients with cardioembolic or noncardioembolic stroke. In fact, these agents are associated with higher mortality and a worse outcome. Use of heparin may be considered in the acute care setting for stroke due to postoperative atrial fibrillation in patients with mechanical heart valves or in those with cervicocephalic arterial dissections.

A cornerstone of stroke management is to prevent future events, especially because most stroke patients do not receive the acute care treatment previously discussed. Hypertension is the most important risk factor for stroke; thus, patients with hypertension after a stroke should be treated even in the absence of a history of high blood pressure. Hyperlipidemia is also an important and modifiable risk factor for stroke recurrence. There is evidence that the use of high-dose statins in patients with a low-density lipoprotein (LDL) cholesterol level greater than 100 mg/dL (2.59 mmol/L) may be beneficial in preventing future ischemic strokes.

Adams H, Adams R, Del Zoppo G, Goldstein LB; Stroke Council of the American Heart Association; American Stroke Association. Guidelines for the early management of patients with ischemic stroke: 2005 guidelines update a scientific statement from the Stroke Council of the American Heart Association/American Stroke Association. *Stroke.* 2005;36(4): 916–923.

Brott T, Bogousslavsky J. Treatment of acute ischemic stroke. *N Engl J Med.* 2000;343(10): 710–722.

Carotid Occlusive Disease

Carotid atherosclerosis occurs most frequently in the proximal internal carotid artery (origin) and at the carotid bifurcation. The progression of luminal narrowing and ulceration leads to ischemic stroke or TIA from embolization, thrombosis, or hemodynamic compromise. Carotid atherosclerosis can be asymptomatic or symptomatic. This is an important distinction, as the management recommendations for these 2 conditions differ.

Asymptomatic carotid bruits occur in 4% of the population older than 40 years, and the annual stroke rate in these individuals is 1.5%. This same population has an annual mortality rate of 4%, primarily from complications of heart disease. The presence of a carotid bruit is a better predictor of arteriosclerotic disease than of stroke. Patients with asymptomatic carotid artery stenosis should be screened for modifiable risk factors for stroke, with lifestyle changes suggested and medical therapy such as antihypertensive and cholesterol-lowering medications prescribed as necessary. The physician should assess life expectancy and comorbid conditions before considering the patient for carotid revascularization, and the patient should be aware of the risks and benefits of the procedure. The use of aspirin in conjunction with CEA is recommended unless contraindicated. In carefully selected patients at high risk for stroke with asymptomatic carotid stenosis (minimum of 60% stenosis confirmed by angiography and 70% by Doppler ultrasonography), prophylactic CEA, performed in a medical center with less than 3% morbidity and mortality, is beneficial. Prophylactic carotid artery stenting (CAS) may be considered in carefully selected patients (stenosis ≥60% on angiography, ≥70% on Doppler ultrasonography, or ≥80% on CT angiography/MR angiography) if the stenosis was 50%–69% on ultrasonography. However, the advantage of CEA over medical therapy is currently not well established. The usefulness of CAS compared to CEA in this asymptomatic population, which is at high risk for surgery, is uncertain.

Patients with TIA or previous stroke in the territory of carotid stenosis are considered symptomatic. The risk of stroke within a year of onset of symptoms is 8% in patients with TIA; the risk thereafter is approximately 6% per year, with a 5-year risk of 35%–50%.

For patients with recent (within the past 6 months) TIA or ischemic stroke and severe (70%–99%) ipsilateral carotid artery stenosis, CEA is recommended if the perioperative morbidity and mortality risk is less than 6%. For patients with recent events and moderate ipsilateral stenosis (50%–69%), CEA is recommended depending on patient-specific factors such as age, sex, and comorbidities and depending on whether the perioperative risk is less than 6%. There is no benefit of CEA or CAS for stenosis of less than 50%. As there is no contraindication to early revascularization with CEA, surgery can be performed within 2 weeks of a TIA or stroke. CAS is considered as an alternative to CEA in symptomatic patients when the patient is at low risk for endovascular intervention *and* the residual lumen diameter indicates internal carotid artery stenosis of greater than 70% by noninvasive imaging or greater than 50% by catheter angiography. CAS may also be considered in patients with severe stenosis that is difficult to assess surgically; in those with medical comorbidities that greatly increase surgical risk; or in other specific conditions, such as radiation-induced stenosis or restenosis after CEA. It is important to note that CAS is a treatment option for symptomatic patients only when the interventionist's morbidity and mortality rates are 4%–6%.

The Carotid Revascularization Endarterectomy Versus Stenting Trial (CREST) randomly assigned patients with asymptomatic or symptomatic carotid disease to CEA or CAS. The primary endpoint of the trial—a composite of any stroke, MI, or death within 30 days of the procedure and ipsilateral stroke during long-term follow-up—was similar in both groups, including the rate of ipsilateral stroke at 31 days to 4 years after the procedure. Interestingly, the study showed that endarterectomy had a greater benefit in older patients (≥70 years), whereas stenting was more beneficial in younger age groups. There was a greater incidence of stroke at 30 days in the stenting group versus the endarterectomy group, but the incidence of MI was significantly lower in the CAS group. A CREST substudy found that at 1 year, despite the higher rate of stroke with stenting, there were no significant differences in any quality of life measure between the CEA and CAS groups.

In addition to cerebral conditions, ocular conditions such as transient monocular visual loss (TMVL) and retinal TIAs can be associated with carotid stenosis. The ophthalmologist is often the first physician to see a patient with TMVL, which is usually embolic, having either a carotid or a cardiac source. The annual stroke rate among patients with isolated TMVL, retinal infarcts, or TIAs is approximately 2%, 3%, and 8%, respectively. Untreated patients with TMVL, retinal infarcts, or TIAs have a 30% risk of MI and an 18% risk of death over a 5-year period. A cardiac source of embolization should be excluded for all patients presenting with isolated TMVL. Transthoracic echocardiography can identify multiple potential cardiac causes for embolism and, as expected, the yield is highest if the clinical history and physical examination suggest a cardiac source such as atrial fibrillation, rheumatic mitral stenosis, diffuse atherosclerosis, left ventricular aneurysm, or clinical endocarditis. Transesophageal echocardiography is superior to transthoracic echocardiography in diagnosing a cardiac source, but despite this improved diagnostic yield, the efficacy of transesophageal echocardiography in cryptogenic stroke or TIA is controversial. Other modalities that are being used in the diagnosis of cardioembolic sources of stroke include inpatient telemetry, ambulatory Holter monitoring, loop recorders, and surgically implantable cardiac monitors.

If evidence suggests that a carotid lesion is the cause of the TMVL, or if venous stasis retinopathy is present, duplex ultrasonography should be performed to determine the presence of vessel wall disease or carotid stenosis.

The following approach should be considered for a patient presenting with a cerebral or retinal TIA:

- emergency department or urgent outpatient evaluation or hospital admission if the event occurred within the previous 48 hours
- patient evaluation for the presence of risk factors associated with atherogenesis: hypertension, diabetes mellitus, obesity, hyperlipidemia, and smoking
- institution of appropriate medical therapy
- evaluation by appropriate testing for the presence of a cardiac source of emboli
- determination using duplex ultrasonography of the possibility of carotid stenosis

If ipsilateral carotid stenosis exceeds 70%, if bilateral carotid stenosis greater than 50% is present, or if long-term evidence indicates progressive disease, CEA should be considered—but only if the surgeon's perioperative stroke and death rate is less than 6%. Otherwise, antiplatelet therapy with aspirin (325 mg/day), aspirin/extended-release dipyridamole combination, or clopidogrel should be initiated. A patient presenting with TIA symptoms who has previously undergone CEA should be evaluated and treated similarly. Special attention should be paid to evaluating early restenosis and thrombosis.

Intracranial Hemorrhage

Intracranial hemorrhage constitutes approximately 15% of acute cerebrovascular disorders. Bleeding from aneurysms of the arteries composing the circle of Willis, bleeding from arterioles damaged by hypertension or arteriosclerosis, and trauma are the most common causes of intracranial hemorrhage. Although there are many causes of intracranial hemorrhage, the anatomical location of the bleeding greatly influences the clinical picture. By location, hemorrhages can be broadly categorized as follows:

- subarachnoid hemorrhage
- intracerebral hemorrhage
- intraventricular hemorrhage

A variety of vascular malformations within and on the surface of the brain parenchyma may present with seizures and headaches. Arteriovenous malformations (AVMs) produce symptoms more commonly than do other types of cerebrovascular malformations.

Approximately 85% of congenital saccular, or "berry," aneurysms develop in the anterior part of the circle of Willis derived from the internal carotid artery in its major branches. The most common site is at the origin of the posterior communicating artery from the internal carotid artery. Such an aneurysm typically presents with headache and third nerve palsy involving the pupil. Vascular malformations within and on the surface of the brain parenchyma constitute approximately 7% of cases with subarachnoid hemorrhage. Four varieties are recognized:

1. capillary telangiectasia
2. cavernous angioma
3. venous angioma
4. AVM

Capillary telangiectasias and both types of angiomas typically have a low bleeding risk (<0.5%/year).

Findings that suggest an AVM as the cause of subarachnoid hemorrhage include a history of previous focal seizures, slow stepwise progression of focal neurologic signs, and, occasionally, recurrent unilateral throbbing headache resembling migraine. In addition to meningeal irritation and focal neurologic signs reflecting bleeding, a bruit may be present over the orbit or skull in approximately 40% of patients.

Hypertensive intracerebral hemorrhages can be catastrophic events. Headache is the predominant feature at the onset in 40%–50% of hemorrhages. Generalized seizures are common with intracerebral hemorrhage and are less frequent with subarachnoid hemorrhage or cerebral infarction. The most important clues in the diagnosis of intracranial hemorrhage are explosive onset of headache, history of high BP, and early decline of the level of consciousness with evidence of a focal neurologic deficit.

Immediate CT examination shows blood in the subarachnoid space in approximately 95% of the cases of ruptured aneurysm within 24 hours of headache onset. CT scans identify the size and location of intracerebral hemorrhages, as well as the degree of surrounding edema and the amount and location of any distortion of the brain. If subarachnoid hemorrhage is suspected and CT results are negative, lumbar puncture is indicated. CT should always be carried out first to rule out a mass lesion. Cerebral arteriography remains the definitive procedure for identifying an aneurysm or AVM.

Control and maintenance of BP are mandatory in the treatment of ruptured aneurysms. Surgical intervention is best accomplished by placing a small clip or ligature across the neck of the sac. Coil embolization of the aneurysm is an alternative procedure that may be used. If the aneurysm cannot be directly obliterated, surgical ligation of a proximal vessel may be necessary. Symptomatic AVMs sometimes can be dissected and removed, depending on their location. Proton-beam irradiation remains controversial. Ligation of the feeding vessels, coupled with balloon catheter embolization, may be carried out. Results of surgical drainage or clot removal of parenchymal intracerebral hemorrhages are mostly unsatisfactory.

Furie KL, Kasner SE, Adams RJ, et al; American Heart Association Stroke Council, Council on Cardiovascular Nursing, Council on Clinical Cardiology, Interdisciplinary Council on Quality of Care and Outcomes Research. Guidelines for the prevention of stroke in patients with stroke or transient ischemic attack: a guideline for healthcare professionals from the American Heart Association/American Stroke Association. *Stroke.* 2011;42(1):227–276.

Goldstein LB, Bushnell CD, Adams RJ, et al; American Heart Association Stroke Council, Council on Cardiovascular Nursing, Council on Epidemiology and Prevention, Council for High Blood Pressure Research, Council on Peripheral Vascular Disease, Interdisciplinary Council on Quality of Care and Outcomes Research. Guidelines for the primary prevention of stroke: a guideline for healthcare professionals from the American Heart Association/American Stroke Association. *Stroke.* 2011;42(2):517–584.

The authors would like to thank Renee B. Van Stavern, MD, for her contributions to this chapter.

CHAPTER 7

Pulmonary Diseases

Recent Developments

- Sildenafil and tadalafil have been shown to be effective in patients with pulmonary arterial hypertension.
- Omalizumab can be used in adults and children 12 years of age and older for the treatment of severe asthma.
- Persons with chronic obstructive pulmonary disease who use inhaled corticosteroids are at increased risk for pneumonia.
- Obstructive sleep apnea syndrome can be associated with various ocular conditions. Treatment with continuous positive airway pressure can cause dry eye symptoms.

Introduction

The lungs can be affected by numerous pathologic processes, including inflammation (allergic, infectious, autoimmune, toxic), vascular insults, fibrosis, carcinoma, and changes secondary to cardiac or musculoskeletal problems. The functional consequences of the pathology can be divided into *obstructive* and *restrictive* ventilatory functions.

Symptoms of lung disease include dyspnea, cough, and wheezing. *Dyspnea* develops when the demand for gas exchange exceeds the capacity of the respiratory system, as in hypoxemia or hypercapnia. Dyspnea may also reflect the increased work of breathing, as occurs with airway obstruction or reduced compliance of the lungs or chest. *Cough* develops when mucus, inflammatory debris, or irritants stimulate the bronchi, causing reflex clearing expectoration, or when the lung parenchyma is infiltrated with fluid, cells, or fibrosis. *Wheezing* occurs when bronchospasm narrows the large airways and exhaled air is forced through narrowed passages.

Obstructive Lung Diseases

In obstructive lung disease, changes in the bronchi, bronchioles, and lung parenchyma can cause airway obstruction. Obstructive diseases can be categorized as reversible or irreversible, although many obstructive lung diseases may have some degree of both reversible and irreversible obstruction.

Reversible obstructive diseases are grouped under the term *asthma.* In asthma, the airways are hyperresponsive and develop an inflammatory response with bronchospasm to various stimuli, although the specific cause and duration of the bronchospasm vary. In some persons, allergic IgE-mediated reactions to defined antigens cause bronchospasm. In many patients, however, the cause of abnormal airway reactivity is unknown. Precipitating factors may include exercise, aspirin, sulfites, tartrazine dye, emotional stress, cold air, environmental pollutants, or viral infection. Bronchial smooth muscle constriction, mucosal edema, excess mucus accumulation, and epithelial cell shedding all contribute to airway obstruction. This obstruction may be reversible spontaneously or with treatment.

Irreversible obstructive disease (sometimes known as *chronic obstructive pulmonary disease [COPD]*) comprises a group of conditions in which forced expiratory flow is reduced in either a constant or a slowly progressive manner over months or years. COPD is the fourth leading cause of death in the United States. The Global Initiative for Chronic Obstructive Lung Disease (GOLD), an international consortium working to improve prevention and treatment of COPD, publishes a guide on the diagnosis, classification, and management of this condition. The guide is updated regularly and can be downloaded from the Internet (www.goldcopd.com). GOLD offers a framework for the management of COPD. Some conditions, such as *cystic fibrosis* or *bronchiectasis,* either secondary to recurrent necrotizing bacterial infections or occurring as part of Kartagener syndrome, have an identifiable cause. However, most irreversible obstructive diseases, such as *emphysema, chronic bronchitis,* and *peripheral airway disease,* cannot be ascribed to specific conditions; rather, they represent an individual response to cigarette smoking and various airborne pollutants. For example, such responses occur in the setting of either α_1-antitrypsin deficiency (in certain forms of emphysema) or airway hyperactivity and mucus hypersecretion (as in bronchitis). The pathologic consequences of the abnormal response result in specific damage to lung tissue. Emphysema is characterized by pathologic enlargement of the terminal bronchiole air spaces and by destruction of the alveolar connective tissue septa. Bronchitis is characterized by hypertrophied mucous glands in the bronchi; in peripheral airway disease, only the small airways demonstrate fibrosis, inflammation, and tortuosity.

Global Initiative for Chronic Obstructive Lung Disease. Global strategy for the diagnosis, management, and prevention of chronic obstructive pulmonary disease (updated 2014). www.goldcopd.org. Accessed August 20, 2014.

Restrictive Lung Diseases

The restrictive lung diseases encompass a diverse group of conditions that cause diffuse parenchymal damage. The physiologic consequences of this damage include a reduction in total lung volume, diffusing capacity, and vital capacity. Occasionally, patients without parenchymal involvement who have diseases of the chest wall, respiratory muscles, pleura, or spine may have similarly restricted lung volumes. A *fibrotic* parenchymal response can result from occupational exposure to various substances, including asbestos, silica dust, graphite, talc, coal, and tungsten. A *granulomatous* hypersensitivity reaction can develop in response to moldy hay, grains, birds, humidifiers, and cooling systems. Endogenous pulmonary disease can result from collagen vascular diseases, sarcoidosis, eosinophilic granuloma, granulomatosis with polyangiitis (formerly known as Wegener granulomatosis), Goodpasture syndrome, alveolar proteinosis, idiopathic pulmonary hemosiderosis, idiopathic pulmonary fibrosis, and other idiopathic parenchymal diseases. Therapeutic agents such as phenytoin, penicillin, gold, methotrexate, and radiation can also cause pulmonary disease.

Evaluation

Although all patients with respiratory problems should be under the care of a capable internist or pulmonologist, ophthalmologists and other physicians should be aware of the key components in the diagnosis and evaluation of patients with pulmonary diseases. The following should be considered:

- *Symptoms:* Dyspnea, orthopnea, chronic cough, and chronic sputum production.
- *History:* Occupational exposure to various substances, family history, cigarette use.
- *Signs:* Audible wheezing, cyanosis, finger clubbing, forced expiratory time greater than 4 seconds, increased anteroposterior diameter of the chest.
- *Laboratory studies:* Elevated hematocrit level and hypoxia or hypercapnia on arterial blood gas measurement.
- *Chest radiography:* Parenchymal disease, hyperinflation, diaphragmatic flattening, increased retrosternal lucency, and pleural abnormalities.
- *Computed tomography* of the chest can detect many abnormalities not seen on chest radiographs: small areas of adenopathy, pulmonary embolus, small nodules, infiltrative lung disease, and bronchiectasis.
- *Bronchoscopy, transbronchial biopsy,* and *bronchial lavage:* Used to obtain culture material, cytology material, and pathologic specimens for analysis.
- *Pulmonary function tests* measure the mechanical and gas exchange functions of the lungs. The *forced expiratory volume over 1 second* (FEV_1) represents the volume exhaled in the first second of exhalation; the *forced vital capacity (FVC)* represents the total volume that the patient can exhale. Both parameters and their serial rate of decline in a patient are objective measures of lung function as well as predictors of comorbidity and mortality from lung cancer and cardiovascular disease. An FEV_1/FVC ratio less than 70% of predicted suggests obstructive disease; total lung capacity less than 70% of predicted suggests restrictive disease.

Treatment

There are 2 major goals in the treatment of pulmonary disease. The first goal is to favorably alter the natural history of the disease. The second is to improve the patient's symptoms and functional status and minimize associated problems.

Nonpharmacologic Treatment

Smoking cessation is the single most efficacious and cost-effective intervention in reducing the risk of COPD and slowing its progression. Ophthalmologists should not underestimate the power of even a brief discussion about the impact of smoking and the beneficial effects of smoking cessation. Similarly, *avoiding precipitants* of airway obstruction is important in ameliorating asthmatic conditions. In patients with severe pulmonary hypertension and cor pulmonale, use of supplemental oxygen to maintain an arterial oxygen pressure above 60 mm Hg confers a modest reduction in pulmonary hypertension and improved survival. However, a patient receiving supplemental oxygen must be carefully monitored because such treatment may decrease the respiratory drive to eliminate carbon dioxide, aggravating the respiratory acidosis that may lead to carbon dioxide narcosis. *Breathing exercises* and *postoperative chest physiotherapy* have demonstrable short-term effects in improving respiratory function.

Noninvasive pressure support ventilation can be used to deliver increased airway pressure. Continuous positive airway pressure (CPAP) throughout the ventilation cycle improves alveolar oxygen exchange. In CPAP therapy, a tight, well-fitting mask is placed over the patient's mouth and nose or just over the nose. Noninvasive pressure support ventilation is best applied to patients with respiratory failure who are expected to quickly respond to medical therapy. Intubation and standard ventilation are preferred for patients who require total ventilatory support because the mask may slip and effective ventilation may cease. Nasal CPAP can be used in the management of obstructive sleep apnea syndrome (OSAS). See Chapter 3 for further discussion of this syndrome.

Ophthalmic considerations Floppy eyelid syndrome, keratoconus, and nonarteritic anterior ischemic optic neuropathy (NAION) can be associated with OSAS. Ophthalmologists should be aware that nasal CPAP, which is used in the nonpharmacologic treatment of OSAS and lung diseases, has been reported to modestly increase intraocular pressure in patients with glaucoma and that patients using this therapy can experience symptoms of dry eye.

Archer EL, Pepin S. Obstructive sleep apnea and nonarteritic anterior ischemic optic neuropathy: evidence for an association. *J Clin Sleep Med.* 2013;9(6):613–618.

Hayirci E, Yagci A, Palamar M, Basoglu OK, Veral A. The effect of continuous positive airway pressure treatment for obstructive sleep apnea syndrome on the ocular surface. *Cornea.* 2012;31(6):604–608.

Pharmacologic Treatment

Pharmacologic approaches include medications that are specific for the particular pulmonary condition and medications that improve the patient's symptoms and functional status. *Specific medications* directly alter the pathophysiologic mechanisms underlying pulmonary disease. Some examples include cyclophosphamide for granulomatosis with polyangiitis, corticosteroids for sarcoidosis, and plasmapheresis with immunosuppressive drugs in Goodpasture syndrome. There is some evidence suggesting that the use of statin medications is associated with a decreased risk of COPD exacerbation.

Symptomatic medications are designed to reduce the obstructive or restrictive components affecting the patient's lung function. Medications used to treat symptomatic bronchospastic airway obstruction include bronchodilators and inhibitors of inflammation (Table 7-1), as well as antibiotics during infection-precipitated airway closure.

Bronchodilators, which include theophylline, β-adrenergic agonists, and anticholinergics, act primarily by relaxing the tracheobronchial smooth muscle. *β-Adrenergic agonists* activate bronchial smooth muscle, resulting in bronchodilation. The selective β_2-adrenergics, which have greater bronchodilatory effect and less cardiostimulatory effect, are commonly used, often in metered-dose inhalers (they can also be administered orally or parenterally). These drugs have replaced the nonselective β-adrenergic agents such as isoproterenol. The short-acting β_2-agonists include fenoterol, salbutamol, and isoetharine. These drugs differ in onset and duration of action. For example, the onset of action of isoetharine is within 1–3 minutes, and its duration is 60–90 minutes. Common long-acting β_2-agonists include formoterol and salmeterol. Salmeterol, a particularly long-acting β_2-adrenergic, is helpful in maintenance treatment of asthma; it should not be

Table 7-1 Drugs for the Treatment of Asthma

Short-acting β_2-selective adrenergic agents
Albuterol
Levalbuterol
Pirbuterol acetate
Long-acting β_2-selective adrenergic agents
Formoterol
Terbutaline sulfate
Anticholinergics
Ipratropium bromide
Oxitropium bromide
Tiotropium
Xanthine derivative
Theophylline
Combination short-acting β_2-agonist plus anticholinergic in 1 inhaler
Albuterol/ipratropium
Fenoterol/ipratropium
Combination long-acting β_2-agonist plus corticosteroid in 1 inhaler
Salmeterol/fluticasone
Leukotriene inhibitors
Montelukast
Zafirlukast
Zileuton
Mast-cell stabilizer
Cromolyn sodium
Corticosteroids
Beclomethasone dipropionate
Budesonide
Flunisolide
Fluticasone
Triamcinolone acetonide
Immunosuppressive agent
Omalizumab

used for acute exacerbations. Although epinephrine causes predominantly β-adrenergic stimulation in the lungs, it also causes peripheral α-adrenergic stimulation, resulting in vasoconstrictive hypertension and tachycardia. Epinephrine is most often administered subcutaneously to help control an acute asthma attack.

Anticholinergic agents directly relax smooth muscle by competing for acetylcholine at muscarinic receptors. Atropine and similar agents have been replaced by poorly absorbing atropinic congeners such as ipratropium bromide, oxitropium bromide, and tiotropium. These inhalation agents have few systemic and minimal cardiac effects. They have an additive bronchodilator effect when combined with submaximal doses of β-adrenergic agonists.

Inhibitors of inflammation include corticosteroids, leukotriene inhibitors, mast-cell stabilizers (cromolyn sodium), and immunosuppressive agents. *Corticosteroids* not only suppress inflammation of the bronchioles but also potentiate the bronchodilator response to β-adrenergic receptors. Inhaled corticosteroids can be used for an extended period to reduce bronchial hyperreactivity; they are not used to manage acute attacks. Systemic corticosteroids are highly effective in managing acute episodes, but because of the potential adverse effects associated with their use, they should be used only when necessary for serious flare-ups. *Leukotriene inhibitors* suppress the effects of inflammatory mediators. They are especially useful for prophylaxis and long-term maintenance therapy in asthma. *Cromolyn sodium* prevents the release of chemical mediators from mast cells in the presence of IgE antibody and the specific antigen. *Immunotherapy* has been shown to be helpful for asthma triggered by a defined antigen.

Asthma treatment should be tailored to disease severity. Medication doses should be adequate to control symptoms rapidly and should later be reduced to the minimal level required to maintain control. The goals of therapy should include prevention of symptoms, reduction in frequency and severity of exacerbations, maintenance of normal (or near-normal) pulmonary function, maintenance of normal activity levels, and minimization of medication side effects. Maintenance medications include inhaled corticosteroids, chromones, leukotriene inhibitors, long-acting β_2-agonists, anticholinergic agents, and oral corticosteroids. Appropriately used supplemental oxygen increases survival among patients with chronic respiratory failure and has a beneficial effect on pulmonary arterial pressure, polycythemia, exercise capacity, lung mechanics, and mental state.

Baena-Cagnani CE, Gómez RM. Current status of therapy with omalizumab in children. *Curr Opin Allergy Clin Immunol.* 2014;14(2):149–154.

Wang MT, Lo YW, Tsai CL, et al. Statin use and risk of COPD exacerbation requiring hospitalization. *Am J Med.* 2013;126(7):598–606.

Perioperative Considerations

Before operating on a patient with lung disease, the surgeon should consult with an internist or pulmonologist to carefully define the patient's functional respiratory status, especially with respect to the supine position. The patient's respiratory function should be maximized with medications and nonpharmacologic means, as appropriate. He or she should be sedated only if necessary and, in that case, should be carefully monitored for arterial gas values. Also see the section Respiratory Diseases in Chapter 15.

CHAPTER 8

Hematologic Disorders

Recent Developments

- Iron deficiency anemia remains the most common cause of anemia worldwide. It can be distinguished from inflammatory anemia by differences in serum iron and ferritin levels, total iron-binding capacity, and transferring saturation (the ratio of iron to total iron-binding capacity).
- Allogeneic hematologic stem cell transplantation is the treatment of choice for β-thalassemia major and has increased survival rates for this disease. Patients who undergo transplantation also receive lifelong blood transfusion and iron chelation therapy.
- The best screening test for paroxysmal nocturnal hemoglobinuria remains flow cytometry.
- Parental diagnosis is available for couples at risk for producing a child with sickle cell anemia. Genetic counseling should be made available for such couples.
- Additional thrombotic risk factors (eg, factor V and prothrombin gene mutations, hyperhomocysteinemia) have been identified.
- Thrombophilia (the hypercoagulable state) is associated with recurrent fetal loss and preeclampsia.

Blood Composition

Formed elements—erythrocytes (red blood cells, or RBCs), white blood cells, and platelets—constitute approximately 45% of the total blood volume. The fluid portion, *plasma,* is about 90% water. The remaining 10% of the plasma consists of proteins (albumin, globulin, fibrinogen, and enzymes), lipids, carbohydrates, hormones, vitamins, and salts. If a blood specimen is allowed to clot, the fibrinogen is consumed and the resultant fluid portion is called *serum.*

Erythropoiesis

All blood cells originate from the uncommitted pluripotent stem cells. The latter give rise to lymphoid stem cells and myeloid stem cells. Myeloid stem cells are the precursors of RBCs, granulocytes, monocytes, and platelets. Hormones such as erythropoietin, thrombopoietin, and granulocyte colony-stimulating factor initiate the differentiation of the various cellular elements. The life span of a circulating RBC is 120 days.

Anemia

Anemia is the result of an insufficient quantity of erythrocytes to carry oxygen to the peripheral tissues. It can be divided into 3 pathophysiologic states: (1) blood loss, (2) underproduction of erythrocytes, and (3) destruction of erythrocytes (hemolysis). The normal hemoglobin level in men ranges from 14 to 17 g/dL, whereas the normal hemoglobin level in women is lower (12–16 g/dL). The higher level in men is due to the erythropoietic effects of androgens.

In the evaluation of a patient with anemia, it is important for the clinician to classify the anemia by reviewing the RBC indexes, including a complete blood count, the concentration of hemoglobin, the erythrocyte count, and the RBC indexes indicative of erythrocyte size: specifically, the mean corpuscular volume (MCV) of erythrocytes and size distribution (red cell distribution width). Reviewing these indexes and observing the morphology on a peripheral blood smear help the clinician determine whether the anemia is microcytic (MCV <80 fL), normocytic (MCV 80–100 fL), or macrocytic (MCV >100 fL). The differential diagnoses of microcytic and macrocytic anemias are limited; thus, a focused diagnostic approach is possible for patients determined to have either of these anemias. In addition to the peripheral blood smear, the reticulocyte count gives an indication of erythrocyte production. Patients with normal bone marrow who have lost blood or undergone hemolysis have increased reticulocyte counts, whereas patients with underproduction anemia have low reticulocyte counts for their degree of anemia.

Iron Deficiency Anemia

By far the most common type of anemia worldwide, *iron deficiency anemia* is diagnosed when the serum ferritin concentration is less than 15 μg/L. Iron deficiency anemia is also characterized by low hepcidin levels. Hepcidin is a peptide hormone produced by the liver. It inhibits iron transport across the intestinal mucosa, thereby preventing excess iron absorption and maintaining normal iron levels within the body. Hepcidin also inhibits the transport of iron out of macrophages, that is, the site of iron storage and transport. Every adult with iron deficiency anemia is suspected to be bleeding until proven otherwise. Menstrual blood loss in women plays a major role, as does gastrointestinal bleeding in both men and women. Aspirin can cause gastrointestinal bleeding.

Patients with mild iron deficiency anemia may experience fatigue, lack of a sense of well-being, irritability, decreased exercise tolerance, and headaches before symptoms of overt anemia occur. Patients with iron deficiency anemia typically have normal findings on physical examination. However, abnormal findings, such as facial pallor, glossitis, stomatitis, and conjunctival pallor, can be observed in severe iron deficiency anemia. Occasionally, patients with severe iron deficiency anemia exhibit pica, a tendency to eat ice, clay, starch, paper, or crunchy materials. Once the etiology of iron deficiency anemia has been identified, it may be treated with oral ferrous sulfate 325 mg 3 times daily. This is the least expensive preparation for treating iron deficiency anemia. For patients unable to absorb oral iron, parenteral iron preparations are available.

Inflammatory Anemia

Inflammatory anemia can occur in chronic conditions such as chronic infections (eg, tuberculosis, osteomyelitis), malignancies, collagen-vascular diseases, and liver disease. Chronic renal failure can also cause a more severe type of anemia, primarily due to the decrease in erythropoietin production. For patients on dialysis, current guidelines recommend the use of erythropoiesis-stimulating agents (ESAs) to achieve a target hemoglobin value of 11–12 g/dL. Adverse effects of ESAs include hypertension, thrombosis, and cardiovascular events. Therefore, it is very important to gradually increase hemoglobin levels when these agents are used.

The Thalassemias

The thalassemias are a group of hereditary anemias characterized by a reduced rate of synthesis of hemoglobin polypeptide chains alpha or beta. This decreased synthesis in turn leads to reduced hemoglobin and a hypochromic microcytic anemia. *α-Thalassemia* is due to a gene deletion that reduces synthesis of alpha hemoglobin chains. *β-Thalassemia* is caused by a point mutation rather than a deletion. In the absence of beta chains, the excess of alpha chains leads to instability in the RBC and hemolysis. The bone marrow becomes hyperplastic, and in severe cases this may lead to bone deformities and fractures. Transfusion and iron chelation are performed to minimize iron overload. Allogeneic hematologic stem cell transplantation has become the treatment of choice for β-thalassemia major, improving the survival rate of these patients to more than 80%.

Sideroblastic Anemia

If the incorporation of iron into the heme molecule is defective, hemoglobin synthesis is reduced; this condition is called *sideroblastic anemia (SA)*. Diagnosis of SA is made primarily based on results of the bone marrow examination with Prussian blue stain. (A normal sideroblast is an erythroblast that has few granules of hemosiderin in the cytoplasm.) In SA, iron accumulates, particularly in the mitochondria, creating the "ring sideroblast." Sideroblastic anemia may be caused by a genetic disorder, or it may develop indirectly as part of a myelodysplastic syndrome, which can progress to acute myelogenous leukemia or other hematologic malignancies. Other causes of SA are usually acquired and include chronic alcoholism and lead poisoning.

Vitamin B_{12} Deficiency

Vitamin B_{12} comes from the diet and is available in all foods of animal origin. To be absorbed, it requires an intrinsic factor produced by the gastroparietal cells. This complex is absorbed in the terminal ileum and stored in the liver. It takes 3 years to deplete the reserves of vitamin B_{12} in the liver. Strict vegetarians (vegans), patients with a history of abdominal surgery or gastrectomy, and individuals with parasitic or pancreatic disease are at increased risk for vitamin B_{12} deficiency. *Pernicious anemia* is an autoimmune disease that leads to lack of vitamin B_{12} absorption due to atrophic gastritis and, consequently, intrinsic-factor deficiency. Megaloblastic anemia, a type of macrocytic anemia due to inhibition of DNA synthesis in RBCs, is the result. When B_{12} levels are in the low normal range, the physician should examine levels of serum cobalamin B_{12} (<170 pg/mL is abnormal), folate, homocysteine, and methylmalonic acid. An elevated serum methylmalonic acid level is more sensitive and specific for diagnosing vitamin B_{12} deficiency than is a low vitamin B_{12} level. Often, leukopenia and thrombocytopenia accompany the anemia. Even in the absence of hematologic changes, vitamin B_{12} deficiency can cause a neurologic syndrome; peripheral nerves are affected first, while balance problems and alteration of cerebral function (eg, dementia, neuropsychiatric changes) occur in more severe cases. Parenteral B_{12} is used for treatment of pernicious anemia; otherwise, daily oral B_{12} is effective and is less expensive and cumbersome than parenteral B_{12}.

Folic Acid Deficiency

Folic acid deficiency is another etiology of megaloblastic, or macrocytic, anemia. Macro-ovalocytes and hypersegmented neutrophils are seen on peripheral smear. The serum vitamin B_{12} concentration is normal. The most common etiology of folate deficiency is inadequate dietary intake of folate due to generalized malnutrition or poor nutrition associated with alcohol dependence. Other causes of folate deficiency include malabsorption, pregnancy and lactation, certain anemias, kidney dialysis, and liver disease. It is important to exclude vitamin B_{12} deficiency in these patients because although treatment with folate can correct anemia in patients with vitamin B_{12} deficiency, it does not reverse the neuropsychiatric symptoms that can occur in severe cases (see the subsection Vitamin B_{12} Deficiency). Once vitamin B_{12} deficiency is excluded, a therapeutic trial of folate in patients with presumed folate deficiency may be the most cost-effective way of establishing the diagnosis.

Hemolytic Anemias

In *hemolytic anemia,* the life span of the RBC is reduced, and the bone marrow responds to this reduced survival by increasing production of RBCs. An increased reticulocyte count, increased indirect bilirubin levels, increased L-lactate dehydrogenase levels, decreased haptoglobin levels, and morphologic changes in the RBCs may aid diagnosis.

Treatment depends on the etiology, but regardless of the cause of hemolytic anemia, folic acid supplementation is required. In hereditary spherocytosis, the RBC has an autosomal dominant membrane abnormality that causes it to become spherical. This abnormal shape leads to lack of RBC strength and to RBC deformability, trapping of the RBC in the spleen, and hemolysis. The treatment of choice is splenectomy, which eliminates the site of hemolysis. Uninterrupted supplementation of folic acid is also needed.

In paroxysmal nocturnal hemoglobinuria (PNH), the RBC membrane is sensitive to lysis by complement. The best screening test is flow cytometry, which has largely replaced the classic sucrose hemolysis test. The use of eculizumab, a humanized monoclonal antibody against the terminal complement component 5 (C5), has decreased transfusion requirements, improved quality of life, and potentially decreased thrombosis in transfusion-dependent patients with PNH. Glucose-6-phosphate dehydrogenase (G6PD) deficiency, an X-linked hereditary enzyme defect occurring primarily in males, causes hemolytic anemia due to decreased ability of the RBC to deal with oxidative stresses. Oxidized hemoglobin precipitates and forms precipitants called *Heinz bodies.* The RBC is then removed by the spleen. The triggering factor is usually an infection or exposure to a specific drug. Specific G6PD assays are available. Treatment during an acute crisis is usually supportive and includes the withdrawal and avoidance of the responsible drug and/or treatment of underlying infection. Severe reactions may be treated with RBC transfusions.

Sickle cell disease

In *sickle cell anemia,* abnormal hemoglobin leads to chronic hemolytic anemia, an autosomal recessive disorder causing an amino acid substitution on the beta chain. The new hemoglobin is called *hemoglobin S,* and it appears after several months of life. This in turn damages the RBC membrane and leads to sickling. Parental diagnosis is available for couples at risk for producing a child with sickle cell anemia; genetic counseling should be made available for such couples. One out of 400 black persons born in the United States, 1 out of 250 black persons born in the West Indies, and 1 out of 4000 born in France has sickle cell anemia. Chronic hemolytic anemia can produce jaundice, gallstones, poorly healing ulcers over the lower tibia, and splenomegaly (which rapidly disappears after a few years because of repeated splenic infarction).

Sickle cell disease is manifested by acute painful episodes caused by the sickling of the RBCs; these episodes can be precipitated by infection, dehydration, and/or hypoxia. Vascular occlusion can lead to necrosis of bone and to infection. Hematuria can be caused by infarction of the renal papillae. Sickle cell retinopathy can lead to vision loss in severe cases. With improved supportive care, an affected person now has an average life expectancy of 40 to 50 years. Most clinical laboratories offer a screening test for sickle cell hemoglobin. For patients who have a positive screening test, the diagnosis is confirmed by hemoglobin electrophoresis, which can detect the presence and measure the amount of hemoglobin S. Sickle cell disease is a systemic multiorgan disease that requires lifelong routine medical care, which includes regular updating of vaccinations, annual ophthalmologic examinations, and screening for hypertension, proteinuria, and pulmonary hypertension. Management of an uncomplicated sickle cell episode includes hydration, nonopioid analgesia, and incentive spirometry to avoid acute chest syndrome. Notably, hydroxyurea therapy has decreased mortality in patients with sickle cell disease and is indicated for recurrent painful episodes, acute chest syndrome, and symptomatic anemia. Patients should be given folic acid supplements, pneumococcal vaccination, and, if infections arise, specific treatment for infections. Patients should be kept well hydrated, and they should be given oxygen if they are hypoxic. Allogeneic hematologic stem cell transplantation is a possible curative option for severely affected young patients. See also BCSC Section 12, *Retina and Vitreous.*

Autoimmune hemolytic anemia

In autoimmune hemolytic anemia, either an immunoglobulin G (80% of cases) or immunoglobulin M (20% of cases) autoantibody is formed and binds to the RBC membrane, leading to formation of a spherocyte and sequestration and destruction by macrophages in the spleen. Half of all cases of autoimmune hemolytic anemia are idiopathic; others are associated with autoimmune diseases or lymphoproliferative, malignant, infectious, or drug-related processes. The Coombs test is positive in cases of autoimmune hemolytic anemia. Treatment consists of administration of prednisone and, if the disease is recurrent, splenectomy.

Disorders of Hemostasis

Disorders of hemostasis may be due to defects in platelet number or function or to problems in formation of a fibrin clot (coagulation). A basic understanding of the hemostatic process and the manifestations associated with specific abnormalities helps the ophthalmologist with both medical and surgical management. (See Fig 8-1 for a diagram of blood-clotting pathways.) For the purpose of laboratory test interpretation, the coagulation cascade can be divided into intrinsic and extrinsic pathways. However, it is now understood that this is an oversimplification. For example, factor IX (an intrinsic factor) can be activated by factor VII (an extrinsic factor).

Hemostasis is initiated by damage to a blood vessel wall. This event triggers constriction of the vessel, followed by accumulation and adherence of platelets at the site of injury. Coagulation factors in the blood are activated, leading to formation of a fibrin clot. Slow

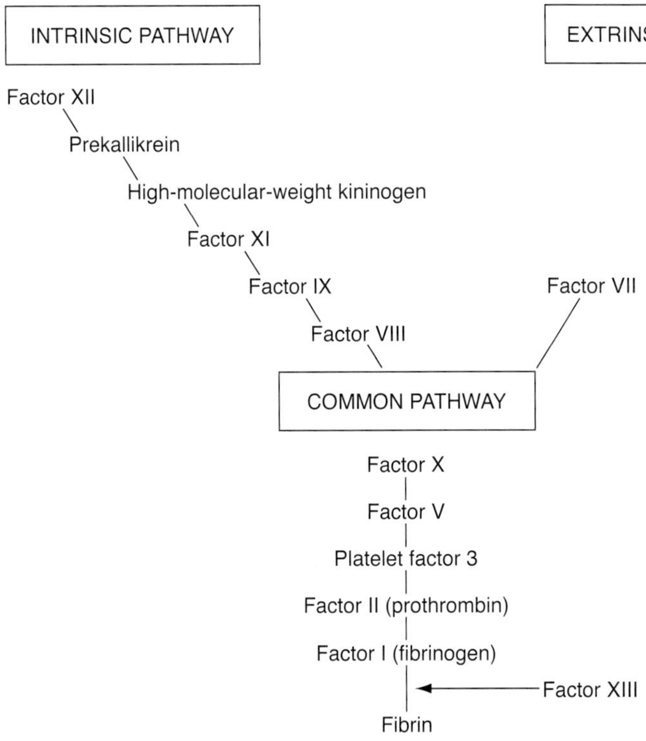

Figure 8-1 Blood-clotting pathways.

fibrinolysis ensues, dissolving the clot while the damage is repaired. Circulating inhibitors are also present, modulating the process by inactivating coagulation factors to prevent widespread clotting. Normal endothelium plays a critical role in naturally anticoagulating blood by preventing fibrin accumulation. The following physiologic antithrombotic components can produce this effect:

- antithrombin III
- protein C and/or protein S
- tissue factor pathway inhibitor
- the fibrinolytic system

Antithrombin III (AT III) inactivates thrombin. Activated protein C (APC), with its cofactor protein S, functions as a natural anticoagulant by destroying factors Va and VIIa. Thrombin itself activates protein C. Although inherited deficiencies of AT III, protein C, or protein S are associated with a lifelong thrombotic tendency, tissue factor pathway inhibitor deficiency has not yet been related to the hypercoagulable state (see the discussion of thrombotic disorders later in the chapter).

Laboratory Evaluation of Hemostasis and Blood Coagulation

Various techniques are used to assess the status of a patient's hemostatic mechanisms. Following are some of the most common tests:

- *Platelet count.* Minor bleeding may occur at platelet counts below 50,000/μL. Abnormal bleeding at higher platelet counts suggests abnormal platelet function. Below 20,000/μL, spontaneous bleeding may be serious.
- *Bleeding time.* A small dermal wound is created, excess blood is blotted away to identify when bleeding stops, and the duration of bleeding is recorded. This evaluates primary hemostasis rather than fibrin formation. In many hospital laboratories, bleeding time is no longer an available test, having been replaced by the automated platelet function analyzer. Because bleeding-time test results can be affected by operator-dependent factors, use of the platelet function analyzer with a small amount of blood has been found to be more accurate in screening for primary hemostasis. Because disorders of blood vessels are rare, the results essentially reflect platelet number and function. Bleeding time is rarely prolonged when platelet counts are above 50,000/μL.
- *Activated partial thromboplastin time (aPTT).* The aPTT test incorporates factors I, II, V, VIII, IX, X, XI, and XII; prekallikrein; and high-molecular-weight kininogen. The aPTT test is most commonly used to measure the effect of heparin therapy. Platelet abnormalities do not affect the result of this test.
- *Prothrombin time (PT).* The PT test measures the integrity of factors I, II, V, VII, and X. It requires a 30% concentration of the vitamin K–dependent factors II, VII, and X (but not factor IX, a part of the intrinsic pathway) and therefore is prolonged in conditions affecting these factors (see Disorders of Blood Coagulation later in this chapter). The PT test is most commonly used to monitor anticoagulant therapy. The action of heparin may slightly prolong PT.

Efforts have been made to tailor anticoagulation therapy to the problem being treated. For example, treatment or prevention of deep venous thrombosis is thought to require less oral anticoagulation therapy than treatment of endocardial mural thrombi or cardiac replacement valves. However, because of variation in test results among and within laboratories, it has been difficult to standardize therapeutic dosages. To solve this problem, the international normalized ratio (INR) was developed. The INR modifies the standard PT ratio (patient PT to control PT) to reflect the particular thromboplastin reagent used by a laboratory. The resulting reported INR value is an expression of the ratio of the patient's PT to the laboratory's mean normal PT. Thus, for prevention or treatment of deep venous thrombosis, the recommended INR value (comparable to subsequent values measured over time or across laboratories) is 2.0–3.0; for tissue replacement valves, 2.0–3.0; and for mechanical replacement valves, 2.5–3.5.

Genetic testing in the form of a DNA assay is also available to determine the correct warfarin dose for an individual patient, especially in cases in which resistance to the drug is suspected. This knowledge has substantially reduced the risk of bleeding and clotting events.

Clinical Manifestations of Hemostatic Abnormalities

Hemorrhage resulting from hemostatic derangement must be differentiated from hemorrhage caused by localized processes. The presence of generalized or recurrent bleeding suggests abnormal hemostasis. *Petechiae* (small capillary hemorrhages of the skin and mucous membranes) and *purpura* (ecchymoses) are typical of platelet disorders and vasculitis. Subcutaneous hematomas and hemarthroses characterize coagulation abnormalities. Bleeding due to trauma may be massive and life-threatening in coagulation disorders, whereas bleeding is more likely to be slow and prolonged when platelet function is impaired.

Vascular Disorders

A number of inherited and acquired disorders of blood vessels and their supporting connective tissues result in pathologic bleeding. *Hereditary hemorrhagic telangiectasia* (Rendu-Osler-Weber disease) is an autosomal dominant condition characterized by localized dilation of capillaries and venulae of the skin and mucous membranes. The lesions increase in size and number over a period of decades, often leading to profuse bleeding.

Several inherited connective tissue disorders are associated with hemorrhage. *Ehlers-Danlos syndrome* is characterized by hyperplastic fragile skin and hyperextensible joints; it is dominantly inherited. In *osteogenesis imperfecta,* also a dominant trait, bone fractures and otosclerosis (leading to deafness) are common. In both of these conditions, easy bruising and hematomas are common. *Pseudoxanthoma elasticum,* a recessive disorder, is much rarer but is often complicated by gastrointestinal hemorrhage. *Marfan syndrome* is sometimes associated with mild bleeding as well as with aortic dissection.

Scurvy, the result of severe ascorbic acid deficiency, is associated with marked vascular fragility and hemorrhagic manifestations resulting from abnormal synthesis of collagen.

In addition to the classic findings of perifollicular petechiae and gingival bleeding, intradermal, intramuscular, and subperiosteal hemorrhages are common. *Amyloidosis* is another acquired disorder in which petechiae and purpura are common.

Ophthalmic considerations All of the inherited vascular disorders have associated ocular findings. Conjunctival lesions occur in hereditary hemorrhagic telangiectasia. Blue sclerae are typical of osteogenesis imperfecta. Ocular manifestations of Ehlers-Danlos syndrome include microcornea, myopia, and angioid streaks; retinal detachment and ectopia lentis have also been reported. Angioid streaks also occur in patients with pseudoxanthoma elasticum. Fifty percent of patients with Marfan syndrome have ectopia lentis; severe myopia and retinal detachment are common.

Platelet Disorders

By far the most common cause of abnormal bleeding, platelet disorders may result from an insufficient number of platelets, inadequate function, or both. Mild derangement of platelet function may be asymptomatic or may cause minor bruising, menorrhagia, or bleeding after surgery. More severe dysfunction leads to petechiae, purpura, and gastrointestinal bleeding and other types of serious bleeding.

Thrombocytopenia

The number of platelets may be reduced by decreased production, increased destruction, or abnormal distribution. Production may be suppressed by many factors, including radiation, chemotherapy, alcohol use, malignant invasion of the bone marrow, aplastic anemia, and vitamin B_{12} or folic acid deficiency.

Accelerated destruction may occur because of immunologic or nonimmunologic causes. *Idiopathic thrombocytopenic purpura (ITP)* is the result of platelet injury by antiplatelet antibodies. The acute form of ITP usually occurs in children and young adults, often following a viral illness, and commonly undergoes spontaneous remission. Chronic ITP is more common in adults and is characterized by mild manifestations; spontaneous remission is uncommon. Initial treatment consists of corticosteroid therapy. Patients with ITP who do not respond to corticosteroid therapy should receive intravenous immunoglobulin, anti-D immunoglobulin, rituximab, or mycophenolate mofetil. In 2008, the US Food and Drug Administration approved 2 thrombopoietin agonists for the treatment of ITP, romiplostim and eltrombopag. Splenectomy can be considered in patients with refractory disease. A neonatal form occurs in babies born to women with ITP; this form results from transplacental passage of antiplatelet antibodies. Recovery follows physiologic clearance of the antibodies from the child's circulation.

Many drugs and other substances, including quinine, quinidine, digitalis, procainamide, thiazide-type diuretics, sulfonamides, phenytoin, aspirin, penicillin, heparin, and gold compounds, have been implicated as causes of immunologic platelet destruction.

Drug-induced thrombocytopenia is common, and discontinuation of the offending drug should result in platelet recovery.

Nonimmunologic causes of thrombocytopenia include *thrombotic thrombocytopenic purpura (TTP)* and the syndromes of intravascular coagulation and fibrinolysis (see "Disseminated intravascular coagulation" later in the chapter). In addition to causing symptoms of thrombocytopenia, TTP is characterized by thrombotic occlusions of the microcirculation and hemolytic anemia. Fever, neurologic symptoms, anemia, and renal dysfunction occur with abrupt onset, with death occurring in days to weeks in the majority of untreated cases. Early treatment with exchange plasmapheresis has improved the survival rate to over 80%. Refractory cases may be treated with antiplatelet drugs, corticosteroids, immunosuppressive agents, and most recently, eculizumab.

Abnormal distribution of platelets is most commonly caused by splenic sequestration. The usual clinical setting is hepatic cirrhosis, and the level of thrombocytopenia is mild. Patients with severely depressed platelet counts probably also have accelerated platelet destruction in the spleen.

Platelet dysfunction

Patients with platelet dysfunction usually come to the physician's attention because of easy bruising, epistaxis, menorrhagia, or excessive bleeding after surgery or dental work. Unlike patients with marked thrombocytopenia, patients with platelet dysfunction rarely have petechiae.

Hereditary disorders of platelet function are rare. Much more important clinically are the acquired forms, of which drug ingestion is the most common cause. As with drugs causing antiplatelet antibodies, the list of causative agents is very long. A single aspirin tablet taken orally irreversibly inhibits platelet aggregation for the life span of the circulating platelets present, causing a modest prolongation of bleeding time for at least 48–72 hours following ingestion. This reaction has remarkably little effect in otherwise healthy individuals, although intraoperative blood loss may be slightly increased. However, in patients with hemophilia, severe thrombocytopenia, or uremia and in those on warfarin or heparin therapy, bleeding may be significant.

Nonsteroidal anti-inflammatory drugs cause reversible inhibition of platelet function in the presence of the drug; the effect disappears as the drug is cleared from the blood. Other commonly used drugs that may affect platelet function include ethanol, tricyclic antidepressants, and antihistamines.

In addition to uremia, clinical conditions associated with abnormal platelet function include liver disease, multiple myeloma, systemic lupus erythematosus, chronic lymphocytic leukemia, and Hermansky-Pudlak syndrome (an autosomal recessive form of oculocutaneous albinism).

Disorders of Blood Coagulation

Hereditary coagulation disorders

Inherited coagulation abnormalities involve all of the coagulation factors except factors III and IV. The most common and most severe is factor VIII deficiency, called *hemophilia A*, or *classical hemophilia*. Typical manifestations of this X-linked disease include severe and protracted bleeding, after even minor trauma, and spontaneous bleeding into joints (hemarthroses), the central nervous system, and the abdominal cavity.

Treatment involves infusion of coagulation factor VIII. In the past, transfusion of pooled human factor VIII always carried a significant risk of hepatitis B virus transmission; in the 1980s, transmission of the human immunodeficiency virus became a major problem as well. With the availability of recombinant factor VIII, however, those risks have now been mostly eliminated. Up to 10% of patients with hemophilia A develop antibodies, presumably due to sensitization following administration of factor VIII. These anticoagulants can also develop in healthy older patients, in nonhemophilic patients after drug reactions, and in those with collagen vascular diseases. Clinical manifestations range from mild bleeding to full-blown hemophilia. The aPTT is prolonged, and the PT is normal. Treatment involves various regimens of coagulation factor replacement and immunosuppression to try to eliminate the inhibitor. Gene therapy is currently in the developmental phase but could further transform the outlook for these patients.

Von Willebrand disease (vWD) is the most common inherited bleeding disorder: low levels of von Willebrand factor (vWF) are found in 1% of the population. It is an autosomal dominant disorder; mild disease is codominant, and more severe disease is recessive. The 2 main functions of vWF are (1) stabilization of factor VIII to prevent degradation and (2) platelet adhesion. Many women with vWD have significant menorrhagia, endometriosis, and postpartum hemorrhage. In patients with acquired vWD, autoantibodies bind to vWF and the resulting complex is rapidly cleared from the circulation. A form of vWD also occurs in patients with aortic valve stenosis, leading to gastrointestinal bleeding. Thrombocythemia is another cause of acquired vWD simply because of the vast number of platelets sequestering vWF.

Acquired coagulation disorders

Vitamin K deficiency Vitamin K is required for the production of factors II (prothrombin), VII, IX, and X in the liver. Normal diets contain large amounts of vitamin K, which is also synthesized by intestinal flora. Causes of vitamin K deficiency include biliary obstruction and various malabsorption syndromes (including sprue, cystic fibrosis, and celiac disease), in which intestinal absorption of vitamin K is reduced. Suppression of endogenous gastrointestinal flora, seen commonly in hospitalized patients on prolonged broad-spectrum antibiotic therapy, decreases intestinal production of vitamin K. However, clinical deficiency occurs only if dietary intake is also diminished. Nutritional deficiency is unusual but may occur with prolonged parenteral nutrition. Laboratory evaluation reveals prolongation of both PT and, later in the course of the disease, aPTT. Most forms of vitamin K deficiency respond to subcutaneous or intramuscular administration of 20 mg of vitamin K_1; coagulation defects normalize within 24 hours. Vitamin K_1 should not be given intravenously because of the risk of sudden death from an anaphylactoid reaction. One special form of vitamin K deficiency is *hemorrhagic disease of the newborn,* which is the result of a normal mild deficiency of vitamin K–dependent factors during the first 5 days of life and the absence of the vitamin in maternal milk. This condition is now rare in developed countries because of the routine administration of vitamin K to newborns. (See also Antiphospholipid Antibody Syndrome in Chapter 9.)

Liver disease Hemostatic abnormalities of all types may be associated with disease of the liver, the site of production of all the coagulation factors. As liver dysfunction develops, levels of the vitamin K–dependent factors decrease first, followed by those of factors V, XI, and XII; both PT and aPTT are prolonged. Thrombocytopenia, primarily the result of hypersplenism, and a prolonged bleeding time due to platelet dysfunction are common. In addition, intravascular coagulation and fibrinolysis are common, further complicating the clinical picture.

Mild hemorrhagic symptoms are common in patients with significant liver disease. Severe bleeding is usually gastrointestinal in origin, arising from peptic ulcers, gastritis, or esophageal varices. Treatment is difficult at best and consists of blood and coagulation factor replacement. Local measures, such as vasopressin infusion or balloon tamponade of bleeding varices, can sometimes control potentially catastrophic bleeding.

Disseminated intravascular coagulation *Disseminated intravascular coagulation (DIC)* is a complex syndrome involving widespread activation of the coagulation and fibrinolytic systems within the general circulation. Utilization and consumption of coagulation factors and platelets produce bleeding; formation of fibrin and fibrin degradation products (fibrin split products) leads to occlusion of the microcirculation, various forms of organ failure, and occasionally thrombosis of larger vessels. Laboratory findings may vary but usually include thrombocytopenia, hypofibrinogenemia, and elevated levels of fibrin split products. PT and aPTT are usually, but not invariably, prolonged.

Clinically, 2 forms of DIC are recognized. *Acute DIC* is characterized by the abrupt onset of severe, generalized bleeding. The most common causes are obstetric complications (most notably abruptio placentae and amniotic fluid embolism), septicemia, shock, massive trauma, and major surgical procedures. Treatment, other than specific measures aimed at the underlying disease, is controversial. Among the modalities used are heparinization and replacement of blood, platelets, and fibrinogen.

Chronic DIC is associated with disseminated neoplasms, some acute leukemias, and autoimmune diseases. Laboratory values range from normal to moderately abnormal; levels of coagulation factors may even be elevated. Bleeding and thrombosis (especially leg vein thrombosis and pulmonary embolism) may occur, but in most patients the syndrome remains undiagnosed unless renal failure results from intravascular coagulation in the kidney. Many patients with chronic DIC do not require specific therapy for the coagulopathy because it is not severe enough to present a major risk of bleeding or thrombosis. On occasion, chronic DIC may convert to the acute form.

Thrombotic disorders

The hypercoagulable states encompass a group of inherited and acquired thrombotic disorders that increase the risk of thrombosis *(thrombophilia).* The primary hypercoagulable states are caused by abnormalities of specific coagulation proteins involving inherited mutations in one of the antithrombotic factors. The trigger for a thrombotic event is often the development of one of the acquired secondary hypercoagulable states superimposed on an inherited state of hypercoagulability. The secondary hypercoagulable states cause a thrombotic tendency by complex and often multifactorial mechanisms.

Primary Hypercoagulable States

Antithrombin III deficiency

Antithrombin III deficiency leads to increased fibrin accumulation and a lifelong propensity for thrombosis.

Protein C deficiency

Protein C deficiency leads to unregulated fibrin generation because of impaired inactivation of factors VIIIa and Va, 2 essential cofactors in the coagulation cascade.

Protein S deficiency

Protein S is the principal cofactor of APC, and therefore its deficiency mimics that of protein C.

Activated protein C resistance

Inherited APC resistance causing thrombophilia was originally detected by the finding that the aPTT in affected individuals could not be appropriately prolonged by the addition of exogenous APC in vitro. It is now recognized that the great majority of these subjects harbor a single specific point mutation in the factor V gene, termed *factor V Leiden.* This mutation is remarkably frequent (3%–7%) in healthy white populations but appears to be far less prevalent or even absent in certain black and Asian populations.

Prothrombin gene mutation

The prothrombin gene mutation has been associated with elevated plasma levels of prothrombin; it is second only to factor V Leiden as a genetic risk factor for venous thrombosis.

Hyperhomocysteinemia

Hyperhomocysteinemia, which is due to elevated blood levels of homocysteine, leads to severe neurologic developmental abnormalities in the homozygous state. Adults with the heterozygous state may have only thrombotic tendencies. Acquired causes of hyperhomocysteinemia in adults commonly involve nutritional deficiencies of pyridoxine, vitamin B_{12}, and folate, all cofactors in homocysteine metabolism. High blood concentrations of homocysteine constitute an independent risk factor for both venous and arterial thrombosis; in contrast, all of the other primary hypercoagulable states are associated only with venous thromboembolic complications, usually involving the lower extremities. The initial treatment of acute venous thrombosis in these patients is not different from treatment in those without genetic defects.

Ophthalmic considerations Primary hypercoagulable states, particularly factor V Leiden mutation and subsequent APC resistance, are risk factors for central and branch retinal vein occlusion, especially in young patients. However, routine screening for clotting factors is not presently recommended.

Secondary Hypercoagulable States

Malignancy may stimulate thrombosis directly by elaborating procoagulant substances that initiate chronic DIC. This appears to be most prominent in patients with pancreatic cancer, adenocarcinoma of the gastrointestinal tract or lung, or ovarian cancer. *Myeloproliferative disorders* (polycythemia vera, essential thrombocythemia, chronic myelogenous leukemia, and myelofibrosis) are major causes of thrombosis and paradoxical bleeding, as is *paroxysmal nocturnal hemoglobinuria,* a related stem cell disorder.

Antiphospholipid antibody syndrome is characterized by both venous and arterial thrombosis, including recurrent spontaneous abortions, deep venous thrombosis, and thrombotic events involving the cerebrovascular arteries. Ophthalmic complications include retinal vein and artery occlusion, retinal vasculitis, choroidal infarction, and anterior ischemic optic neuropathy. Tests for patients with this syndrome include tests for anticardiolipin antibodies and lupus anticoagulants. See the section Antiphospholipid Antibody Syndrome in Chapter 9 for additional discussion.

The hypercoagulability associated with *pregnancy* involves a progressive state of DIC throughout the course of pregnancy, activated in the uteroplacental circulation. *Oral contraceptives* induce similar changes. The *postoperative state* and *trauma* are significant causes of venous thrombosis. Detailed discussion of treatment of these various and complex disorders is beyond the scope of this text.

Therapeutic anticoagulation

Many clinical situations require intentional disruption of the hemostatic process. The effect of aspirin on platelet function has already been discussed.

Unfractionated heparin (UFH) is a mucopolysaccharide that binds antithrombin III, inhibiting the formation of thrombin. It is given intravenously or subcutaneously, and therapy is assessed by measuring the aPTT. Aspirin should not be given to patients receiving heparin because the resultant platelet dysfunction may provoke bleeding. Additional parenteral anticoagulants are low-molecular-weight (LMW) heparins. LMW heparins have a number of advantages over UFH, including greater bioavailability when given by subcutaneous injection and greater duration of anticoagulant effect, permitting once or twice daily administration. The dose is highly correlated with body weight, allowing administration of a fixed dose, and laboratory monitoring is not necessary. In addition, the risk of heparin-induced thrombocytopenia is lower. Direct thrombin inhibitors, such as lepirudin, argatroban, and bivalirudin, are reserved for the treatment of heparin-induced thrombocytopenia.

There are 2 novel groups of oral anticoagulants, factor Xa inhibitors (eg, rivaroxaban, apixaban) and direct thrombin inhibitors (eg, dabigatran). These are fixed-dose oral agents that, unlike vitamin K antagonists, do not require routine laboratory monitoring and dose adjustments. Another advantage is that they reach their peak efficacy within 1–4 hours after ingestion; therefore, a period of bridging therapy is not required when switching from the initial treatment (eg, heparin) to these agents. Their major disadvantage is that unlike vitamin K antagonists, none of these newer agents have a readily available antidote for bleeding events. Fondaparinux, which binds to antithrombin, is a synthetic anticoagulant that is very similar to UFH and LMW heparin. It exclusively catalyzes antithrombin inhibition of factor Xa. Because it is eliminated in the kidney, it should be used cautiously in patients with renal disease.

The orally administered warfarin derivatives, of which warfarin sodium is the most widely used, inhibit the production of normal vitamin K–dependent coagulation factors (II, VII, IX, and X). Therapeutic effect is assessed by measuring the patient's INR. One critical issue is the long list of commonly used drugs that interact with warfarin. These interactions may cause an unintended increase or decrease in the INR, depending on the drug.

Heparin and the warfarin derivatives are used to prevent the formation of new thrombi and the propagation of existing thrombi, but neither affects the original clot. Thrombolytic agents such as streptokinase, urokinase, and tissue plasminogen activator (tPA) are used to dissolve existing thrombi, most notably in the very early stages of myocardial infarction resulting from coronary artery thrombosis. These agents are also currently being used for early treatment of thrombotic stroke; this form of treatment increases the risk of converting a thrombotic stroke into a hemorrhagic stroke.

Hall C, Richards S, Hillmen P. Primary prophylaxis with warfarin prevents thrombosis in paroxysmal nocturnal hemoglobinuria (PNH). *Blood.* 2003;102(10):3587–3591.

Hematology and oncology. In: *Medical Knowledge Self-Assessment Program (MKSAP) 16.* Philadelphia: American College of Physicians; 2012. Available at https://mksap16.acponline.org.

Schafer AI. Approach to the patient with bleeding and thrombosis. In: Goldman L, Schafer AI, eds. *Cecil Medicine.* 24th ed. Philadelphia: Elsevier/Saunders; 2012:chap 174.

Schafer AI. Thrombotic disorders: hypercoagulable states. In: Goldman L, Schafer AI, eds. *Cecil Medicine.* 24th ed. Philadelphia: Elsevier/Saunders; 2012:chap 179.

The authors would like to thank Liborio Tranchida, MD, for his review of this chapter.

CHAPTER 9

Rheumatic Disorders

Recent Developments

- Several new biologic agents are either in use or being developed for the treatment of rheumatologic diseases. These agents include drugs that interfere with tumor necrosis factor α (TNF-α), interleukin-1, interleukin-6, and T-cell receptor CD28. Also in use are biologic agents that were initially employed in chemotherapy.
- Anti–TNF-α agents may cause uncommon but significant adverse effects, such as lymphoma, opportunistic infections, and demyelinating disease that can include optic neuritis. One such agent, etanercept, has also been implicated as a possible cause of uveitis.
- Many rheumatologic diseases continue to undergo reclassification to allow a more uniform approach to defining treatment and prognosis.

Introduction

The rheumatic disorders are a heterogeneous collection of autoimmune and inflammatory diseases that include rheumatoid arthritis, the spondyloarthropathies, connective tissue diseases, and the vasculitides. Ocular involvement is common with autoimmune diseases but varies among the different disorders. Ophthalmologists should be aware of such underlying conditions, their potential for ocular involvement, and the pharmacotherapy used to treat not only the rheumatologic but also the ophthalmic manifestations. Treatment of rheumatic conditions commonly involves systemic anti-inflammatory and immunosuppressive therapy, discussed at the end of this chapter. See Medical Therapy for Rheumatic Disorders for descriptions of many of the drugs mentioned in the following sections.

Rheumatoid Arthritis

Rheumatoid arthritis (RA) is the most common rheumatic disorder, affecting approximately 1% of adults worldwide. RA is classically an additive, symmetric, deforming, peripheral polyarthritis characterized by synovial hypertrophy and chronic joint inflammation. This disorder may involve all joints, but it affects primarily the small joints of the hands and feet. Typically, affected joints are swollen, tender, and show decreased range of motion. Hand deformities include ulnar deviation, Boutonnière deformity (abnormally flexed proximal interphalangeal [PIP] joint and extended distal interphalangeal [DIP] joint), and swan-neck deformity (abnormally hyperextended PIP and flexed DIP).

Elevated levels of rheumatoid factor (RF), an antibody directed against immunoglobulin G (IgG), occur in 60%–80% of patients with RA. Seropositive RA aggregates in families, particularly those with the human leukocyte antigen (HLA) DRB1 alleles. Recent studies have shown that anti–cyclic citrullinated peptide (anti-CCP) antibodies and anti–mutated citrullinated vimentin (anti-MCV) are highly specific and sensitive for RA. The anti-CCP antibodies are directed toward certain peptides in the skin that contain the amino acid citrulline. The presence of these antibodies can help predict the transformation of undifferentiated arthritis into RA. In addition, patients who are positive for anti-CCP antibodies tend to have more erosive disease.

Extra-articular disease in RA may affect a wide variety of nonarticular tissues. Rheumatoid nodules, located subcutaneously on extensor surfaces, occur in approximately 25% of patients with RA. RA may also cause pleural effusions, pulmonary nodules, and interstitial fibrosis. Cardiac disease includes pericarditis and rheumatoid nodules involving the conducting system, heart valves, or both. Mild anemia of chronic disease is the rule. *Felty syndrome* is a triad of RA, splenomegaly, and neutropenia. Patients with Felty syndrome can also have hyperpigmentation, chronic leg ulcers, and recurrent infections. Rheumatoid vasculitis affects less than 1% of patients with RA. It generally presents as peripheral polyneuropathy or as refractory skin ulcers. Patients may develop digital gangrene or, occasionally, visceral ischemia. The most common neuropathy is median nerve compression caused by synovitis of the wrist. RA may cause ocular disease such as dry eye syndrome, scleritis, episcleritis, and marginal corneal ulcers. The ocular manifestations of RA are discussed in BCSC Section 8, *External Disease and Cornea,* and Section 9, *Intraocular Inflammation and Uveitis.*

RA causes significant joint damage early in the course of the disease. Thus, clinicians try to identify and aggressively treat even subtle evidence of disease. Treatment of RA reflects an integrated approach including nonpharmacologic interventions such as diet, exercise, physical therapy, and massage, as well as pharmacologic therapy and occasionally surgery.

The goal of pharmacologic therapy is disease remission. Clinicians treat the symptoms of pain and joint stiffness with analgesics and *nonsteroidal anti-inflammatory drugs (NSAIDs),* but these medications do not alter the long-term prognosis. Rheumatology standards of care include treatment of early disease using *disease-modifying antirheumatic drugs (DMARDs).* These agents slow disease progression, reduce potential joint destruction, and maintain joint function. Methotrexate, discussed later in this chapter, is the gold standard. Patients who are intolerant of methotrexate may be initiated on an alternative agent, such as leflunamide, sulfasalazine, or injectable gold. In patients whose disease progresses on monotherapy, clinicians may employ combination therapy with 2 separate DMARDs; glucocorticoids; or adjunctive agents, such as a TNF-α antagonist. More aggressive disease may require biologic agents such as abatacept, tocilizumab, or rituximab.

Smolen JS, Landewé R, Breedveld FC, et al. EULAR recommendations for the management of rheumatoid arthritis with synthetic and biological disease-modifying antirheumatic drugs. *Ann Rheum Dis.* 2010;69(6):964–975.

Spondyloarthropathies

Textbooks previously described the spondyloarthropathies as the *seronegative spondyloarthropathies;* the term *seronegative* referred to a negative rheumatoid factor test. As newer and more specific clinical definitions are created, however, that term has become redundant. The defining clinical term is *spondyloarthropathy* (or *spondyloarthritis*), which refers to a spectrum of diseases that share a predilection for axial (spinal and sacroiliac joint) inflammation and HLA-B27 positivity. As with RA, clinicians try to identify and treat early disease. Enthesitis, or inflammation of the entheses, the sites where tendons or ligaments insert into bone; and dactylitis, painful inflammation of a finger or toe, are commonly seen with spondyloarthropathy. Diagnostic classification criteria are variable; however, the presence of any of the following findings suggests a possible spondyloarthropathy: peripheral arthritis, enthesitis, dactylitis, inflammatory bowel disease, HLA-B27 positivity, uveitis, psoriasis, or inflammatory back pain. The often-late development of radiographic sacroiliitis is not required for diagnosis. The presence of these additional features helps distinguish among the various types of spondyloarthropathies, although there may be a great deal of overlap.

The spondyloarthropathy family comprises (1) undifferentiated spondyloarthropathy, (2) ankylosing spondylitis, (3) psoriatic arthritis, (4) reactive arthritis (formerly Reiter syndrome), and (5) inflammatory bowel disease (ulcerative colitis and Crohn disease). Clinicians use the term *undifferentiated spondyloarthropathy* to describe the disease in patients who do not have clear findings of the last 4 categories. Undifferentiated spondyloarthropathy may represent an early or incomplete phase of another spondyloarthropathy, and 20%–25% of these cases are HLA-B27 positive. Undifferentiated spondyloarthropathy also encompasses cases deemed preradiographic, which carry a similar burden of disease despite the normal findings.

Ophthalmologists need to be aware of these diseases because they commonly manifest with acute HLA-B27–positive anterior uveitis. In some cases, the characteristic uveitis may be the presenting feature of a spondyloarthropathy; therefore, ophthalmologists may be crucial in referring such patients for early diagnosis and treatment, preventing future morbidity. See BCSC Section 9, *Intraocular Inflammation and Uveitis,* for further discussion of the ophthalmic manifestations.

Ankylosing Spondylitis

Ankylosing spondylitis (AS) causes bony fusion (ankylosis) of the axial skeleton. The cause of AS is unknown, but its strong association with HLA-B27 (90% of white patients with AS are positive for HLA-B27) suggests a genetic predisposition. AS affects men 3 times more often than women, and men have a higher rate of radiologic manifestations.

The classic features of AS are inflammatory low back pain, ankylosis, and sacroiliitis on x-ray examination. The last stage of this process is a completely fused and immobilized spine, also known as a *bamboo* or *poker spine.* In addition to the spinal arthritis that is the hallmark of the disease, patients may develop arthritis of peripheral joints, limited chest expansion, and restrictive lung disease. Other extra-articular features include apical pulmonary fibrosis, ascending aortitis, aortic valvular incompetence, and heart block. AS is surprisingly resistant to the usual rheumatologic therapeutics. The most effective agents seem to be sulfasalazine and TNF-α inhibitors such as infliximab.

The primary ocular manifestation of AS is recurrent, acute, nongranulomatous iridocyclitis, which affects 25% of patients. Ocular manifestations do not correlate with the activity of the joint disease.

Reactive Arthritis

In the broadest sense, the term *reactive arthritis* implies an autoimmune response to an antecedent infection that usually involves the genitourinary or gastrointestinal system. The classic triad of symptoms includes arthritis, urethritis, and conjunctivitis; however, only one-third of patients present with the full triad at the time of diagnosis. Similar to AS, reactive arthritis has a clear genetic predisposition in that 63%–95% of patients are positive for HLA-B27. Reactive arthritis is at least 5 times as common in men as in women. Precipitating agents include *Chlamydia trachomatis* in the genitourinary tract and *Salmonella, Shigella, Yersinia,* or *Campylobacter* organisms in the gastrointestinal tract. Microbial components have been identified in the synovial tissues of patients with reactive arthritis, but intact organisms have not been cultured, hence the designation *reactive* and not *infective.*

The arthritis of reactive arthritis typically appears within 1 month of the inciting urethritis or diarrhea. It is an asymmetric, episodic oligoarthritis that affects primarily the lower extremities, in particular the large joints such as the knees or ankles. Other features include inflammatory spinal pain; enthesitis; interphalangeal arthritis of the toes and fingers, which produces "sausage digits"; and sacroiliitis. Mucocutaneous lesions include urethritis in men and cervicitis in women, shallow ulcers on the glans penis (circinate balanitis), painless oral ulcers, nail lesions, and skin lesions on the soles and palms (keratoderma blennorrhagicum). Patients may also have systemic symptoms, including fever and malaise. The disease tends to follow an episodic course, and most patients go into remission within 2 years. Those who develop long-term disease may be treated with NSAIDs, sulfasalazine, or alternative immunomodulatory agents in addition to appropriate antibiotic therapy if an active infection is still present after initial treatment.

Ophthalmic considerations Conjunctivitis is one of the most common manifestations of reactive arthritis. It tends to be mild and bilateral with a mucopurulent discharge. Follicular or papillary changes may occur. Cultures are negative, and the conjunctivitis typically resolves within 10 days without treatment. A more serious ocular manifestation is uveitis, which occurs in 15%–25% of patients with reactive arthritis. It is often the acute, nongranulomatous, recurrent iridocyclitis that is characteristic of HLA-B27 disease. The uveitis may also be chronic; some patients require long-term immunosuppressive therapy.

The conjunctivitis and urethritis of reactive arthritis are, by definition, sterile autoimmune phenomena that can occur after either gastrointestinal tract or genitourinary infections. Confusion may arise because *C trachomatis* can cause both conjunctivitis and urethritis, and a *Chlamydia* infection can stimulate a genetically predisposed individual to develop reactive arthritis. It is important to rule out an infectious cause via urine analysis or urethral discharge culture in a patient with presumed reactive arthritis, especially because chlamydial urethritis may be asymptomatic. Usually, however, the precipitating infection will have resolved by the time the reactive autoimmune response supervenes. See BCSC Section 9, *Intraocular Inflammation and Uveitis,* for additional information on reactive arthritis.

Other Spondyloarthropathies

Spondyloarthropathies may also occur in association with ulcerative colitis or with Crohn disease. *Ulcerative colitis* is an inflammatory disorder of the gastrointestinal mucosa with diffuse involvement of the colon. *Crohn disease* is a focal granulomatous disease that involves all areas of the bowel and affects both the large and the small intestine. Crohn disease is also known as *regional enteritis, granulomatous ileocolitis,* and *granulomatous colitis.* Symptoms of inflammatory bowel disease include diarrhea, bloody diarrhea, and cramping abdominal pain.

Extraintestinal manifestations of inflammatory bowel disease include dermatitis, mucous membrane disease, ocular inflammation, and arthritis. Arthritis associated with inflammatory bowel disease is referred to as *enteropathic arthritis* and may include peripheral arthritis, a spondyloarthropathy, or both. Multiple studies have shown that 50%–75% of patients with inflammatory bowel disease–associated spondyloarthropathy are positive for HLA-B27, which also predisposes them to iridocyclitis. The activity of the spondyloarthropathy is unrelated to the activity of the bowel disease. Enteropathic arthritis that involves the peripheral joints is not associated with HLA-B27, and disease activity tends to parallel the activity of the bowel disease.

Psoriasis is another systemic disease that may be associated with spondyloarthropathy. Psoriatic arthritis may have multiple presentations, including oligoarthritis, distal polyarthritis, and a destructive type of arthritis known as *arthritis mutilans.* Spondyloarthropathy is often seen in psoriatic arthritis, and the frequency of HLA-B27 in these patients is higher, although the frequency of HLA-B27 in psoriatic arthritis is not as high as it is in AS or reactive arthritis. Uveitis in patients with psoriatic arthritis tends to be more insidious in onset, smoldering, posterior, and bilateral compared with the more typical HLA-B27–positive anterior uveitis.

Spondyloarthropathies may occur in childhood, although their occurrence is rare before the second decade. Clinicians may misdiagnose the findings as the result of trauma because the radiographic findings are similar. Patients may develop all the features of AS (juvenile ankylosing spondylitis), or they may have systemic diseases similar to those found in adults (eg, inflammatory bowel disease, reactive arthritis, or psoriasis). As in adults, most young patients are HLA-B27 positive, and more men than women seem to be affected. These patients may develop acute uveitis characteristic of HLA-B27–positive uveitis. The juvenile-onset spondyloarthropathies are considered to be a separate category of juvenile idiopathic arthritis referred to as *enthesitis-related arthritis.*

Sieper J, Rudwaleit M, Baraliakos X, et al. The Assessment of SpondyloArthritis International Society (ASAS) handbook: a guide to assess spondyloarthritis. *Ann Rheum Dis.* 2009;68 (Suppl 2):ii1–ii44.

Juvenile Idiopathic Arthritis

The term *juvenile idiopathic arthritis (JIA)* has replaced the older term *juvenile rheumatoid arthritis (JRA)*. The word *rheumatoid* is not considered accurate because, for most children, the arthritides that constitute JIA have no relationship to adult-onset RA. The juvenile arthritides have classically been divided into 3 subsets based on associated symptoms and the number of joints involved.

In patients with *pauciarticular-onset* (or *oligoarticular-onset*) *JIA*, fewer than 5 joints are involved during the first 6 months of illness. This subset accounts for approximately 50% of JIA cases. The antinuclear antibody (ANA) test is positive in many of these patients, and there is a strong predilection for females. The arthritis tends to remit, but 10%–50% of patients may develop chronic iridocyclitis. Thus, ophthalmologists should perform periodic eye examinations on these patients to detect occult ocular inflammation. (See BCSC Section 6, *Pediatric Ophthalmology and Strabismus,* and Section 9, *Intraocular Inflammation and Uveitis.*)

Responsible for 30%–40% of JIA cases, *polyarticular-onset JIA* is defined by the involvement of more than 4 joints during the first 6 months of illness. As with pauciarticular-onset JIA, females are more commonly affected. The arthritis tends to be severe, but uveitis is rare.

Systemic-onset JIA (formerly Still disease) is responsible for approximately 10%–15% of JIA cases. Patients with systemic-onset JIA have fever, rash, and arthritis of any number of joints. They may also have hepatosplenomegaly and lymphadenopathy. In contrast to the other variants, males and females are equally affected. Ocular disease is generally not associated with this variant.

A new classification system of the idiopathic arthritides of childhood has been proposed that will allow differentiation of etiologic mechanisms, prognostication, and response to therapy. This classification system includes systemic arthritis, polyarthritis, pauciarthritis, psoriatic arthritis, and enthesitis-related arthritis. Each category is further subdivided according to, for instance, ANA positivity and the presence of uveitis. Because there is currently no universal agreement regarding this approach, several different classification systems remain. Therefore, the older terminology will likely persist at the interface of pediatric rheumatology and ophthalmology, at least for now, because the screening and treatment guidelines for uveitis are based on the classic categories.

Systemic Lupus Erythematosus

Systemic lupus erythematosus (SLE) is generally regarded as the prototypical autoimmune disease; the many clinical manifestations reflect the multiple areas in which the immune system can malfunction. The cause of SLE is unknown, but familial aggregation of autoimmune diseases and association with HLA types DR2 and DR3 suggest a genetic predisposition. Pathogenically, SLE is characterized by B-cell hyperreactivity, polyclonal B-cell activation, hypergammaglobulinemia, and a plethora of autoantibodies. These autoantibodies include ANAs, antibodies to DNA, and antibodies to cytoplasmic components. SLE has classically been considered an immune complex disease, in which immune complexes incite an inflammatory response and lead to tissue damage.

Women, especially in their 20s and 30s, are affected far more frequently than men. The presentation and course of disease are highly variable, ranging from mild to fulminant. Patients may present with single-organ involvement, such as nephritis or cytopenia, or multiorgan disease. The characteristic cutaneous manifestation of SLE is development of a butterfly rash across the nose and cheeks, also known as a *malar rash,* which appears in 70%–80% of patients. Other cutaneous manifestations include discoid lesions, vasculitic skin lesions such as cutaneous ulcers or splinter hemorrhages, purpuric skin lesions, and alopecia. Mucosal lesions, characteristically painless oral ulcers, occur in 30%–40% of patients. Photosensitivity, acute or chronic, occurs in many patients.

Approximately 80%–85% of patients with SLE will experience articular disease, either a polyarthralgia or a nondeforming, migratory polyarthritis. Systemic features—including fatigue, fever, and weight loss—occur in more than 80% of patients with lupus. Renal disease is present in approximately 50%–75% of patients, presenting clinically as either proteinuria with nephrotic characteristics or glomerulonephritis with active urinary sediment. Lupus nephritis is a major cause of the morbidity and mortality of SLE.

Raynaud phenomenon occurs in 30%–50% of patients with SLE (Fig 9-1), and hepatosplenomegaly and adenopathy occur in more than 50%. Cardiac disease includes pericarditis, occasionally myocarditis, and Libman-Sacks endocarditis. Higher rates of valvular vegetation are found in patients with SLE and antiphospholipid antibodies. Pulmonary involvement includes pleuropulmonary lesions, which cause pleuritic chest pain and, less commonly, pneumonitis. Gastrointestinal symptoms, particularly nausea and dyspepsia, are also common.

Central nervous system (CNS) involvement occurs in more than 35% of patients with SLE, and manifestations are typically transient. The most common manifestations of CNS lupus are headache, seizures, and psychosis. Transverse myelitis with spastic paresis and

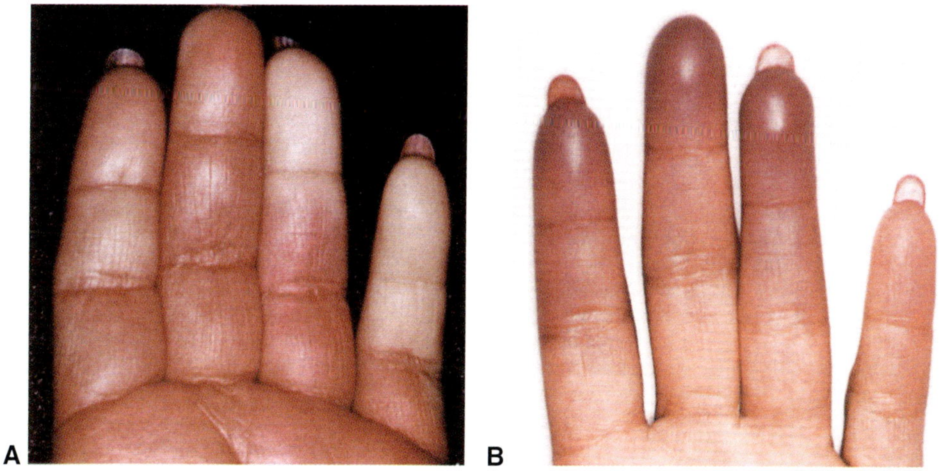

Figure 9-1 Raynaud phenomenon. **A,** Sharply demarcated pallor resulting from the closure of digital arteries. **B,** Digital cyanosis of the fingertips in a patient with primary Raynaud phenomenon. *(Reproduced with permission from Wigley FM. Clinical Practice. Raynaud's phenomenon.* N Engl J Med. *2002;347(13):1001. Copyright ©2002 Massachusetts Medical Society.)*

sensory loss is an uncommon manifestation in patients with SLE, but it can occur in association with optic neuritis in active disease. Idiopathic intracranial hypertension may also be associated with SLE.

SLE frequently affects the hematologic system. Patients often have anemia of chronic disease but may also develop autoimmune hemolytic anemia. Leukopenia, in particular lymphopenia, is characteristic. Thrombocytopenia occurs in approximately one-third of patients.

Diagnosis

Table 9-1 lists the diagnostic criteria for SLE. New diagnostic criteria emphasize the importance of viewing SLE as an autoantibody-driven clinical disease. Patients must satisfy at least 4 criteria with the requirement of at least 1 clinical and 1 immunologic criterion. Alternatively, SLE can be diagnosed in the setting of biopsy-proven nephritis with positive ANAs or anti–double-stranded DNA (anti-dsDNA) antibodies. The updated criteria attempt to retain simplicity while reflecting the current understanding of SLE pathogenesis.

The ANA criterion remains unchanged; however, additional antibodies are separated as individual immunologic criteria. Clinicians should perform a laboratory test for ANA positivity whenever they suspect SLE. Virtually all patients with SLE have a significant titer of ANA (usually 1:160 or higher). Three additional antibodies that are highly specific for SLE are anti-dsDNA, anti-Smith (anti-Sm), and antiphospholipid antibodies. The presence of any one of these is considered an acceptable immunologic criterion. There

Table 9-1 SLICC Criteria for Diagnosis of Systemic Lupus Erythematosus

Clinical criteria
Acute cutaneous lupus
Chronic cutaneous lupus
Oral ulcers*
Nonscarring alopecia*
Synovitis
Serositis*
Renal findings
Neurologic findings*
Hematologic findings, hemolytic anemia
Hematologic findings, leukopenia*
Hematologic findings, thrombocytopenia*
Immunologic criteria
ANA
Anti-dsDNA antibody
Anti-Sm antibody
Antiphospholipid antibody
Low levels of complement
Direct Coombs test

ANA = antinuclear antibody; dsDNA = double-stranded DNA; SLICC = Systemic Lupus International Collaborating Clinics; Sm = Smith.
*In the absence of an alternative cause.

Modified with permission from Petri M, Orbai AM, Alarcón GS, et al. Derivation and validation of the Systemic Lupus International Collaborating Clinics Classification criteria for systemic lupus erythematosus. *Arthritis Rheum.* 2012;64(8):2682. Copyright ©2012 by the American College of Rheumatology.

are other autoantibodies (anti-Ro/SS-A, anti-La/SS-B, anti-RNP, and anti-RA33) that may indicate a predisposition to SLE or another autoimmune disease, but they are not included within the classification system.

Unfortunately, clinicians order ANA testing for patients who are unlikely to have SLE (such as patients with uveitis but no systemic symptoms). The test is very nonspecific under these circumstances. Furthermore, analysis of the pattern of ANA staining is subjective and is therefore of limited diagnostic strength. False-positive ANAs are commonly found in the normal population; 1 study found that 32% of individuals without SLE had an ANA titer above 1:40. The combination of very low titers of antibody (<1:80) and no signs or symptoms of disease suggests that the patient should simply be monitored.

SLE can have a varied clinical course, ranging from a relatively benign illness to fulminant organ failure and death. Most patients have a relapsing and remitting course that requires frequent titration of medications. Treatment depends on disease severity.

The most commonly employed agent is hydroxychloroquine. Alternatively, treatment may include NSAIDs, glucocorticoids, and immunosuppressive drugs. Refractory cases and severe disease with CNS involvement may require high-dose pulse therapy with glucocorticoids and cyclophosphamide or rituximab.

Petri M, Orbai AM, Alarcón GS, et al. Derivation and validation of the Systemic Lupus International Collaborating Clinics classification criteria for systemic lupus erythematosus. *Arthritis Rheum.* 2012;64(8):2677–2686.

Ophthalmic considerations The major ocular manifestations of SLE include discoid lesions of the skin of the eyelids, keratitis sicca from secondary Sjögren syndrome, and retinal and choroidal microvascular lesions. Retinal lesions include cotton-wool spots, hemorrhages, vascular occlusions, and neovascularization. The prevalence of ocular manifestations varies from 3% of outpatients to 29% of hospitalized patients. The inflammatory vasculopathy of SLE should be distinguished from vascular damage due to secondary problems such as hypertension from renal disease or occlusions due to embolic disease or antiphospholipid antibodies. Typical anterior or intermediate uveitis is not a common feature of SLE. Neuro-ophthalmic involvement in SLE includes cranial nerve palsies, lupus optic neuropathy, and central retrochiasmal disorders of vision. The cerebral disorders of vision include hallucinations, visual field defects, and cortical blindness. (See also BCSC Section 9, *Intraocular Inflammation and Uveitis,* and Section 12, *Retina and Vitreous.*)

Antiphospholipid Antibody Syndrome

The *antiphospholipid antibody syndrome (APS)* is a potential cause of vascular thrombosis. The diagnosis of APS requires the presence of 1 clinical and 1 laboratory criterion. The clinical features include 1 or more episodes of arterial and/or venous thrombosis or complications of pregnancy such as fetal death, spontaneous abortion, and premature birth. Laboratory criteria include anticardiolipin antibodies present at moderate to high levels and/or lupus anticoagulant activity. Abnormalities in laboratory tests must be detected on at least 2 different occasions at least 12 weeks apart.

APS can occur in association with SLE and other rheumatic diseases and can be caused by certain infections and drugs. When it occurs alone, it is referred to as *primary APS*. The main clinical manifestation is venous or arterial thrombosis. Deep venous thrombosis is the most common type of thrombosis, occurring in approximately one-third of patients. Patients may also have pulmonary embolism and superficial thrombophlebitis. This syndrome can complicate pregnancy. Patients may have multiple first-trimester abortions and premature births due to preeclampsia or placental insufficiency and late-term fetal death. CNS disease can include strokes, transient ischemic attacks, dementia, and even psychosis. APS should be considered when cerebrovascular disease occurs in a young patient without other risk factors for stroke.

Episodes of thrombosis can recur; this recurrence may be more likely in patients with high antiphospholipid antibody titers. Additional manifestations of APS include thrombocytopenia, hemolytic anemia, nephropathy, and livedo reticularis. Cardiac manifestations include valvular thickening and vegetations, both of which are caused by thrombotic endocardial deposits. In rare instances, a severe form of APS can occur with multiple vessel occlusion and multiorgan failure. This form of the disease is referred to as *catastrophic antiphospholipid syndrome* and carries a mortality rate of 48%.

Diagnosis

Testing for antiphospholipid antibodies can be divided into 2 broad categories: (1) tests for anticardiolipin antibodies and (2) tests for lupus anticoagulants. Medium to high levels of anticardiolipin antibodies are more clinically significant. Among blood donors without APS, 5%–10% may have some level of positive anticardiolipin antibodies, and this percentage can be higher among older donors. However, repeatedly positive results are required for a diagnosis of APS. In 1 study, less than 2% of the population without APS remained positive for a period of 9 months. Antiphospholipid antibodies also occur in association with other conditions, such as infections or cancer, and with the use of some drugs. In these cases, the antibodies are present at low levels and are not typically associated with thrombotic events.

Testing for lupus anticoagulant activity involves looking for evidence of a functional inhibition of clotting. Whereas testing for antiphospholipid antibodies simply indicates whether such antibodies are present, testing for lupus anticoagulant activity determines whether the antibodies have an identifiable effect on phospholipid-dependent clotting pathways. With lupus anticoagulant positivity, there seems to be a somewhat greater risk for thrombosis than with isolated antiphospholipid positivity. Lupus anticoagulants prolong in vitro clotting assays such as the activated partial thromboplastin time (aPTT); the dilute Russell viper venom time (dRVVT); the kaolin plasma clotting time (KCT); and in rare cases, the prothrombin time. More than 1 test for lupus anticoagulant is often needed because patients with negative results for 1 test may have positive results for another.

The antibodies detected by assays for antiphospholipid antibodies may or may not be the same antibodies responsible for lupus anticoagulant activity, hence the need to perform both types of testing when APS is suspected. The remarkable complexity of the coagulation system is demonstrated by the apparent paradox of lupus anticoagulants. The in vitro effect of these substances is to inhibit clotting, yet in vivo the effect is to enhance thrombosis.

Ophthalmic considerations Ophthalmic manifestations of APS include amaurosis fugax, ischemic optic neuropathy, and retinal and choroidal vascular occlusion. Visual field loss, diplopia, and even proliferative retinopathy have also been reported. Some studies have suggested that the prevalence of antiphospholipid antibodies is increased in patients with retinal vaso-occlusive disease, but it is difficult to assign a definite causative etiology, given the prevalence of antiphospholipid antibodies in the population without APS. Furthermore, in a study looking for ophthalmic findings in a population of patients with known APS, none had definite vaso-occlusive disease and only 13% had identifiable changes, which consisted largely of mild retinopathy. Patients in this series were more likely to have vision symptoms from neurologic disease.

Clinicians should consider APS with atypical ocular vaso-occlusive disease (occurring in patients who are younger than 50 years or who have bilateral presentation) or neurologic disease. However, testing may show false-positive results, and establishing a cause-and-effect relationship is difficult. This caveat is important because treatment of APS may include long-term anticoagulation, which carries a significant risk, and it may be very difficult for a consulting specialist to determine whether an isolated ophthalmic vascular occlusion represents the type of thrombotic episode that warrants such treatment. In such cases, it has been proposed that repeatedly positive levels of antiphospholipid antibodies suggest the presence of APS. More studies are needed to determine the prevalence of ophthalmic disease in APS, as well as the significance of positive laboratory test results in patients with ocular vaso-occlusive disease without systemic features of APS.

Treatment

Therapy for thrombosis usually consists of heparin, followed by warfarin. The optimal duration of treatment is not known. Some experts believe that anticoagulation can be discontinued if the antiphospholipid antibody titers decrease, but lifelong treatment is recommended for patients with recurrent disease. Treatment of pregnant patients remains controversial and may include some combination of heparin or low-molecular-weight heparin and aspirin (warfarin is teratogenic). Patients with antiphospholipid antibodies but no prior history of thrombosis may benefit from prophylactic aspirin. Trials of rituximab in the treatment of APS are currently in progress.

Systemic Sclerosis

Systemic sclerosis (SSc), formerly known as scleroderma, is a connective tissue disease characterized by fibrous and degenerative changes in the viscera, skin, or both. It is subcategorized into diffuse SSc, limited SSc, transitory SSc, systemic sclerosis sine scleroderma, and malignant scleroderma. The disease seems to be mediated by the activation of fibroblasts that produce excessive collagen deposition and fibrosis. Except for malignant scleroderma, which typically affects elderly males, SSc is much more common in women. Sclerosis sine scleroderma affects only internal organs. The limited form of SSc, known as *CREST* (*c*alcinosis, *R*aynaud phenomenon, *e*sophageal involvement, *s*clerodactyly, and *t*elangiectasias), infrequently affects internal organs and carries a better prognosis, often with normal life span.

The hallmark of systemic sclerosis is changes to the skin, namely thickening, tightening, and induration, with subsequent loss of mobility and contracture. The disease usually begins peripherally and involves the fingers and hands, subsequently spreading centripetally up the arms to involve the face and body. Telangiectasia and calcinosis are common. Vascular effects also occur; more than 95% of SSc patients experience Raynaud phenomenon (see Fig 9-1). Although Raynaud phenomenon usually represents a short-duration, reversible vasospasm, SSc may also create permanent damage to blood vessels with subsequent digital ulcers or infarcts.

Organ involvement is common and includes esophageal dysmotility with gastroesophageal reflux secondary to stricture formation and submucosal fibrosis in more than 90% of patients. The small and large intestine may be involved, with decreased motility, malabsorption, and diverticulosis. Cardiopulmonary disease is manifested primarily by pulmonary vascular fibrosis, which results in restrictive lung disease with a decreased diffusing capacity, pulmonary hypertension, and right-sided heart failure. Conduction abnormalities and arrhythmias arise from cardiac fibrosis. Musculoskeletal features include polyarthralgias, tendon friction rubs, and occasionally myositis.

Most patients with SSc have positive ANA test results. Rheumatologists recommend testing for specific ANAs, such as anticentromere, anti–topoisomerase I (anti–Scl-70), and anti–RNA polymerase. These specific ANAs help define the disease and various syndromes that overlap with SSc. The best-known overlap syndrome is *mixed connective tissue disease,* which has features of SLE and myositis. This syndrome is characterized by a specific autoantibody directed at the U1-ribonucleoprotein complex.

There is no known cure for SSc. Treatment is aimed at controlling problems related to organ-system involvement. Pulmonary arterial hypertension and renal disease are major causes of morbidity. Despite the lack of controlled trials, angiotensin-converting enzyme (ACE) inhibitors are recommended for the treatment of renal crisis. Bosentan, a dual endothelin receptor antagonist, increases exercise capacity in patients with severe pulmonary hypertension. Patients with digital vasculopathy associated with SSc benefit from calcium-channel blockers; intravenous prostanoids are also effective in resistant cases and in the treatment of digital ulcers. Immunosuppressive agents, including methotrexate and cyclophosphamide, have proven beneficial in the treatment of diffuse SSc cutaneous manifestations and may slow the progression of disease.

Kowal-Bielecka O, Landewé R, Avouac J, et al. EULAR recommendations for the treatment of systemic sclerosis: a report from the EULAR Scleroderma Trials and Research group (EUSTAR). *Ann Rheum Dis.* 2009;68(5):620–628.

van den Hoogen F, Khanna D, Fransen J, et al. 2013 classification criteria for systemic sclerosis: an American College of Rheumatology/European League Against Rheumatism collaborative initiative. *Arthritis Rheum.* 2013;72(11):1747–1755.

Ophthalmic considerations Ocular manifestations of systemic sclerosis include eyelid involvement that causes tightness and blepharophimosis (but only rarely corneal exposure); conjunctival vascular abnormalities, including telangiectasia and vascular sludging; and keratoconjunctivitis sicca. Patchy choroidal nonperfusion can be seen on fluorescein angiography as part of the diffuse microvascular damage caused by systemic sclerosis. Occasionally, as a result of scleroderma renal crisis, a patient develops retinopathy of malignant hypertension, with cotton-wool spots, intraretinal hemorrhages, and optic disc edema.

Sjögren Syndrome

Sjögren syndrome is a systemic chronic inflammatory disorder characterized by lymphocytic infiltration of exocrine glands. It may present as a triad of dry eyes, dry mouth, and parotid gland enlargement. Sjögren syndrome can coexist with a variety of other connective tissue diseases, including SLE and SSc (in which case it is known as secondary Sjögren syndrome), or without a definable connective tissue disease (primary Sjögren syndrome). The ophthalmologist is often the first physician to see these patients once they become symptomatic.

Sjögren syndrome classification criteria incorporate laboratory blood testing, ocular examination findings, and tissue biopsy evaluation. Suggestive findings include positive anti-SS-A and/or anti-SS-B antibody results, dry eye syndrome, and minor salivary gland biopsy demonstrating inflammation.

Patients with primary Sjögren syndrome may have a number of systemic manifestations, including upper-airway dryness, mucous plug development, purpuric vasculitis, and hyperglobulinemia. CNS inflammation may be present and mimic multiple sclerosis or psychiatric symptoms. Treatment is aimed at relief of symptoms and substitution of the missing secretions, although immunosuppression may be necessary for patients with systemic manifestations. (See also BCSC Section 8, *External Disease and Cornea.*)

Shiboski SC, Shiboski CH, Criswell LA, et al; Sjögren's International Collaborative Clinical Alliance (SICCA) Research Groups. American College of Rheumatology Classification Criteria for Sjögren's Syndrome: a data-driven, expert consensus approach in the SICCA cohort. *Arthritis Care Res (Hoboken).* 2012;64(4):475–487.

Polymyositis and Dermatomyositis

Polymyositis and *dermatomyositis* are inflammatory diseases of skeletal muscle characterized by progressive weakness affecting proximal muscular groups, particularly those of the shoulders and hips. Dermatomyositis is distinguished from polymyositis by the presence of cutaneous lesions. These skin lesions are an erythematous to violaceous rash variably affecting the eyelids (heliotrope rash), cheeks, nose, chest (V-neck sign), and extensor surfaces (Gottron sign). Pathogenically, dermatomyositis is associated with immune complex deposition in the vessels, whereas polymyositis appears to reflect direct

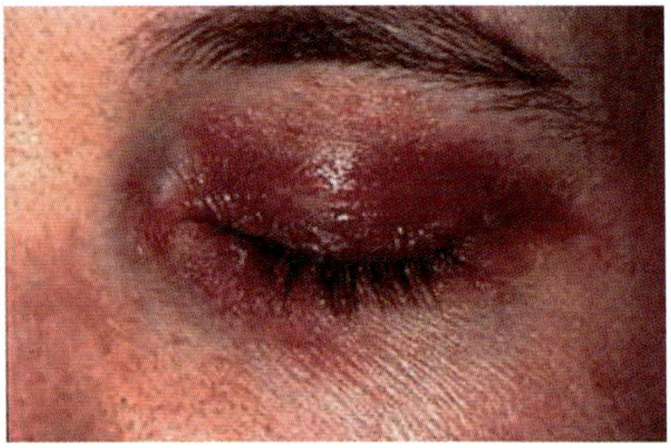

Figure 9-2 Heliotrope rash in dermatomyositis. A reddish-purple eruption on the upper eyelid (the heliotrope rash) is accompanied by swelling of the eyelid in a patient with dermatomyositis (DM). This is the most specific rash in DM, although it is present only in a minority of patients. *(Reproduced with permission from Miller ML, MD. Clinical manifestations and diagnosis of adult dermatomyositis and polymyositis. In:* UpToDate, *Rose BD (ed), Waltham, MA. Available at www.uptodate.com.)*

T-cell–mediated muscle injury. Laboratory findings include elevated serum levels of skeletal muscle enzymes and abnormal electromyography results. Muscle biopsy may confirm the muscle damage from inflammation. These entities may overlap with other connective tissue diseases or be associated with a malignancy.

Ocular involvement is relatively uncommon in inflammatory myositis, other than the heliotrope rash of dermatomyositis, which is very specific but not often present (Fig 9-2). Occasionally, ophthalmoplegia may occur because of involvement of the extraocular muscles, which myositis can provoke. Such cases often respond to systemic corticosteroids or immunomodulatory agents.

Relapsing Polychondritis

Relapsing polychondritis is an episodic autoimmune disorder characterized by widespread, potentially destructive inflammation of cartilage, the cardiovascular system, and the organs of special sense. The most common clinical features are auricular inflammation, arthropathy, and nasal cartilage inflammation. Nasal chondritis, leading to saddle-nose deformity, and auricular chondritis are the features that most often suggest the diagnosis. Laryngotracheobronchial disease may lead to a fatal complication from laryngeal collapse. Involvement of the internal ear, cardiovascular system, and skin is less common. Cardiovascular lesions include aortic insufficiency (due to progressive dilation of the aortic root) and vasculitis. Skin lesions are most often due to cutaneous vasculitis.

Relapsing polychondritis can be associated with other autoimmune diseases such as SLE or RA; spondyloarthropathies; or any of the systemic vasculitides, such as granulomatosis with polyangiitis, polyarteritis nodosa, and Behçet disease. Ocular manifestations occur in approximately 50% of patients with relapsing polychondritis. The most common ocular conditions are conjunctivitis, scleritis, uveitis, and retinal vasculitis.

Treatment focuses on reducing symptoms and preserving the integrity of cartilaginous structures. Pharmacotherapy includes systemic corticosteroids, dapsone, methotrexate, and cyclophosphamide. Patients may require surgical interventions such as tracheostomy, aortic aneurysm repair, and cardiac valve replacement.

Vasculitis

The primary systemic vasculitides are a group of diseases whose principal pathology involves autoimmune damage to blood vessels. In 2012, an updated classification of these entities reflected the size of the vessel involved, organ distribution, and etiology. Table 9-2 outlines the definitions created by the Chapel Hill Consensus Conference on these diseases.

Several other diseases can cause vasculitis as part of their clinical spectrum; these are considered to be *secondary vasculitides.* Secondary vasculitis can occur as part of an autoimmune disorder or arise from an exogenous factor such as infection, neoplasia, or medication. The following subsections emphasize the primary vasculitides that are more likely to have ophthalmic involvement.

Jennette JC, Falk RJ, Bacon PA, et al. 2012 Revised International Chapel Hill Consensus Conference Nomenclature of Vasculitides. *Arthritis Rheum.* 2013;65(1):1–11.

Table 9-2 Names of Vasculitides Adopted by the Chapel Hill Consensus Conference on the Nomenclature of Systemic Vasculitides*

Large-vessel vasculitis
Giant cell (temporal) arteritis
Takayasu arteritis
Medium-sized–vessel vasculitis
Polyarteritis nodosa†
Kawasaki disease
Small-vessel vasculitis
ANCA-associated small-vessel vasculitis
Granulomatosis with polyangiitis (Wegener granulomatosis)
Eosinophilic granulomatosis with polyangiitis (Churg-Strauss syndrome)
Microscopic polyangiitis
Immune complex vasculitis
IgA vasculitis (Henoch-Schönlein purpura)
Cryoglobulinemic vasculitis
Anti-GBM disease
Variable-vessel vasculitis
Behçet disease
Cogan syndrome

ANCA = antineutrophil cytoplasmic antibody; GBM = glomerular basement membrane; IgA = immunoglobulin A.

* *Large vessel* refers to the aorta and the largest branches directed toward major body regions (eg, to the extremities and the head and neck); *medium-sized vessel* refers to the main visceral arteries (eg, renal, hepatic, coronary, and mesenteric arteries); and *small vessel* refers to venules, capillaries, arterioles, and the intraparenchymal distal arterial radicals that connect the arterioles.

†Strongly associated with antineutrophil cytoplasmic autoantibodies.

Modified with permission from Jeanette JC, Falk RJ, Bacon PA, et al. 2012 Revised International Chapel Hill Consensus Conference Nomenclature of Vasculitides. *Arthritis Rheum.* 2013;65(1):1–11. Copyright ©2013 by the American College of Rheumatology.

Large-vessel Vasculitis

Giant cell arteritis

Giant cell (temporal) arteritis affects older adults with potentially blinding, granulomatous inflammatory disease affecting the aorta and its branches. It is of particular concern to ophthalmologists and is discussed thoroughly in BCSC Section 5, *Neuro-Ophthalmology.*

Takayasu arteritis

Takayasu arteritis, like giant cell arteritis, affects large arteries, particularly branches of the aorta, but occurs primarily in children and young women. The disease is rare in the West but common in Asia, particularly Japan. Other names for Takayasu arteritis include *aortic arch arteritis, aortitis syndrome,* and *pulseless disease.*

This disease may involve the entire aorta or be localized to any segment of the aorta or its primary branches. The inflammatory process is characterized by panarteritis with granulomatous inflammation. The involved vessels may ultimately become narrowed or obliterated, resulting in ischemia to the supplied tissues. Areas of weakened vascular walls may develop dissections or aneurysms.

Systemic features such as fatigue, headache, weight loss, and low-grade fever are common. Evidence of vascular insufficiency due to large-artery narrowing leads to the characteristic pulseless phase. Angiography is the gold standard for diagnosis. Treatment is generally with systemic corticosteroids, which may successfully suppress the disease. Cyclophosphamide or methotrexate is added in resistant cases. Surgical reconstruction of stenotic vessels may be necessary.

Ophthalmic considerations Patients with Takayasu arteritis may report transient visual disturbances and blindness due to decreased perfusion. The most characteristic ocular findings are retinal arteriovenous anastomoses, best demonstrated by fluorescein angiography. Milder changes found earlier in the course of the disease include small-vessel dilation and microaneurysm formation; more severe ischemia may result in peripheral retinal nonperfusion, iris and retinal neovascularization, and vitreous hemorrhage.

Medium-sized–vessel Vasculitis

Polyarteritis nodosa

Classic *polyarteritis nodosa (PAN)* is characterized by necrotizing vasculitis of the medium-sized and small muscular arteries. The lesions are segmental, and aneurysms may develop, which can be detected by angiography. One of the most common presenting symptoms is mononeuritis multiplex, which is simultaneous or sequential ischemic damage to anatomically unrelated peripheral nerves. CNS lesions can also occur. Renal involvement is common, and hypertension develops as a consequence of renal disease. Gastrointestinal disease with infarction of the viscera is also common. PAN may be limited to a single organ, such as the appendix, uterus, or testes. Hepatitis B virus (HBV) infection is strongly linked to PAN, seemingly via immune complex–induced disease.

The mean age of onset of PAN is 40–50 years; men are affected more often than women. Survival in patients with untreated PAN is poor. However, most patients are now treated with a combination of corticosteroids and an immunosuppressive drug such as cyclophosphamide. Therapy appears to improve disease control and long-term outcomes. Studies are currently investigating the treatment of HBV-related PAN with systemic antivirals.

Ophthalmic considerations Ocular manifestations occur in approximately 10%–20% of patients with PAN and may include hypertensive retinopathy, retinal vasculitis, and visual field loss from CNS lesions. Cranial nerve palsies can occur, as well as scleritis and marginal corneal ulceration. Choroidal vasculitis is often overlooked in PAN and may cause transient visual symptoms, exudative retinal detachments, and pigment changes. Fluorescein angiography may be necessary to identify choroidal involvement. There is no specific test to diagnose PAN. Rather, the diagnosis depends on characteristic clinical features, angiographic findings, and biopsy results. Results of HBV studies may be positive in a subset of patients.

Kawasaki disease

Kawasaki disease, also known as mucocutaneous lymph node syndrome, is a condition associated with inflammation in the walls of medium-sized vessels throughout the body, including the coronary arteries. The disease typically affects infants and young children. Patients often develop a high, persistent fever; swollen lymph nodes; bilateral conjunctivitis; and truncal rash. A characteristic feature of Kawasaki disease is a strawberry tongue—an extremely red, swollen tongue.

Kawasaki disease is a leading cause of acquired heart disease in children. Cardiac complications include coronary artery aneurysms, myocarditis, and dysrhythmias. Prompt treatment reduces the potential for lasting damage. Treatment includes intravenous immunoglobulin and aspirin. Given the potential for serious complications, initial treatment is typically performed in a hospital.

Small-vessel Vasculitis

Inflammation in small-vessel vasculitis predominantly affects the arterioles, venules, and capillaries. This group of vasculitides is further categorized based on the presence or relative absence of vessel wall deposition of immunoglobulin and/or complement components. The subcategories are immune complex small-vessel vasculitis and antineutrophil cytoplasmic antibody (ANCA)–associated small-vessel vasculitis. This text focuses on the ANCA-associated small-vessel vasculitides.

ANCA-associated vasculitis

Granulomatosis with polyangiitis Formerly known as Wegener granulomatosis, granulomatosis with polyangiitis (GPA) was originally described as a triad of necrotizing granulomatous vasculitis of both the upper and lower respiratory tract and focal segmental glomerulonephritis. The clinical features of GPA include granulomatous inflammation of the paranasal sinuses in 90% of cases, nasopharyngeal disease in 63%, cutaneous vasculitis in 45%, and vasculitis affecting the nervous system in 25%. Ocular disease occurs in up to 60% of patients and may be the presenting feature. Ocular findings include scleritis with or without peripheral keratitis, idiopathic orbital inflammatory disease, and vasculitis-mediated retinal vascular or neuro-ophthalmic lesions. Limited forms of the disease may occur without significant systemic involvement, making diagnosis difficult. Approximately 80% of patients with GPA are seropositive for a cytoplasmic pattern of antineutrophil cytoplasmic antibody (c-ANCA). Because this cytoplasmic pattern is usually caused by the presence of autoantibodies to proteinase 3, the specificity of positive findings for c-ANCA may be enhanced by testing for these antibodies. (See also BCSC Section 7, *Orbit, Eyelids, and Lacrimal System,* and BCSC Section 9, *Intraocular Inflammation and Uveitis.*)

Before immunosuppressive drugs were used to treat GPA, this disease was uniformly fatal, with a mean untreated survival rate of 5 months. Corticosteroid treatment increased the mean survival time to 12.5 months, but long-term survival occurred only in patients with limited disease. Recently, the use of weekly rituximab for 1 month in conjunction with high-dose corticosteroids has been effective in inducing and maintaining remission of disease. Previously, cytotoxic drugs, specifically cyclophosphamide, were initiated, with eventual transition to long-term therapy with a less toxic immunosuppressive agent such as methotrexate. Trimethoprim-sulfamethoxazole may also help maintain remission and prevent relapses.

Microscopic polyangiitis Microscopic polyangiitis (MPA) is a systemic necrotizing vasculitis that affects small vessels and is associated with necrotizing glomerulonephritis. Characteristic features include constitutional symptoms, renal disease, pulmonary involvement, arthralgias, rash, and neuropathy. Patients with MPA often have positive findings for ANCA, with peripheral staining around the nucleus (p-ANCA). This particular staining pattern is nonspecific and must be confirmed by testing for autoantibodies to myeloperoxidase (MPO-ANCA). Peripheral ulcerative keratitis may be a presenting feature of this entity. As with GPA, cyclophosphamide and rituximab have successfully induced remission in some patients.

Eosinophilic granulomatosis with polyangiitis An allergic diathesis, particularly asthma, is present in eosinophilic granulomatosis with polyangiitis (EGPA), formerly known as Churg-Strauss syndrome. Pathologic examination often shows granulomas with eosinophilic tissue infiltration of smaller vessels. Asthma and eosinophilia are the principal features of the disease, and systemic vasculitis may also involve the heart, skin, kidneys, and gastrointestinal tract. CNS disease may also occur, and mononeuritis multiplex is common. Ophthalmic manifestations include conjunctival granulomas, retinal vasculitis and occlusion, uveitis, and cranial nerve palsies. The diagnosis depends on the presence of several criteria, including asthma, eosinophilia, eosinophilic vasculitis, transient pulmonary infiltrates, and neuropathy. Also, in patients with EGPA, p-ANCA titers may be positive. Patients without severe vasculitis can be treated with systemic corticosteroids alone; severe disease may require combination therapy with corticosteroids and immunosuppressants.

Variable-vessel Vasculitis

Variable-vessel vasculitides represent vasculitis in which no predominant type of vessel is involved. Two examples are Behçet disease and Cogan syndrome vasculitis.

Behçet disease

Behçet disease was initially described as a triad of oral ulcers, genital ulcers, and uveitis with hypopyon. It is now recognized as a multisystem vasculitis of unknown etiology that can affect vessels of any size. The disease is most common in the Middle East and Asia, particularly Japan. Oral ulcers are the most common clinical feature, affecting 98%–99% of patients. Genital ulcers occur in 80%–87%. Skin disease occurs in 69%–90% of affected patients and includes erythema nodosum, superficial thrombophlebitis, and pyoderma. Pathergy (pustular response to skin injury) may be seen. Up to 60% of patients have asymmetric, nondeforming arthritis, most commonly affecting the knees.

Vascular disease can present as migratory superficial thrombophlebitis, major-vessel thrombosis, arterial aneurysms, or even peripheral gangrene. CNS disease, found in 10%–30% of patients, includes 3 types: (1) brainstem syndrome, (2) meningoencephalitis, and (3) confusional states. Most often, patients have combinations of these 3 types. The major causes of mortality in Behçet disease are CNS involvement and large-vessel disease including arterial aneurysm.

Behçet disease may include a number of nonspecific abnormalities in laboratory findings, including an elevated erythrocyte sedimentation rate (ESR), C-reactive protein, and circulating immune complexes. Patients may also have serologic evidence of a hypercoagulable state and greater prevalence of HLA-B51. However, no specific laboratory tests define Behçet disease. The diagnosis is based on clinical criteria including oral ulcers and any 2 of the following: uveitis, genital ulcers, skin involvement, and pathergy. Other criteria may be used, depending on regional differences in disease presentation.

Treatment varies according to disease severity. Patients with mild disease may benefit from colchicine for treatment of arthritis and ulcers. Oral and genital lesions may respond to topical steroid solutions or require systemic therapy if severe. The use of corticosteroids alone may control acute exacerbations but does not seem to alter outcome. As a result, 1 or more immunosuppressive agents are usually added as therapy. Treatment of ocular disease typically begins with azathioprine. If severe or resistant disease exists, combination therapy with corticosteroids or alternative treatment with cyclosporine and infliximab is indicated. Alkylating agents such as cyclophosphamide and chlorambucil may be used in refractory cases, although these drugs may have significant toxicity. Newer agents that may hold promise include interferon alfa-2a, especially for treatment of ophthalmic disease.

Hatemi G, Silman A, Bang D, et al. EULAR recommendations for the management of Behçet disease. *Ann Rheum Dis.* 2008;67(12):1656–1662.

Ophthalmic considerations Ophthalmic disease is a significant cause of morbidity in Behçet disease. The most common ocular manifestations are iridocyclitis, with or without hypopyon, and retinal vasculitis. The natural history of retinal vasculitis in Behçet disease is poor. Most untreated patients lose all or part of their vision within 5 years of onset. Also see BCSC Section 9, *Intraocular Inflammation and Uveitis.*

Cogan syndrome

Cogan syndrome is characterized by inflammatory lesions of the eye and inner ear. Patients may present with nonspecific symptoms such as fatigue, fever, and weight loss. Ophthalmic findings may include uveitis, interstitial keratitis, and scleritis. Dizziness and hearing problems may reflect inner ear disease such as vestibular dysfunction and sensorineuronal hearing loss, respectively. Recurrent, untreated inflammation may lead to blindness and deafness. Patients are commonly treated with oral corticosteroids and other immunosuppressive medications, including methotrexate, cyclophosphamide, and cyclosporine. See BCSC Section 8, *External Disease and Cornea,* for further discussion.

Medical Therapy for Rheumatic Disorders

Medications are used in rheumatology for a number of purposes, including analgesia, an anti-inflammatory effect, and immunosuppression. These drugs and their use in treating ocular inflammatory diseases are also discussed in BCSC Section 9, *Intraocular Inflammation and Uveitis.*

Corticosteroids

Glucocorticoids decrease inflammation by inhibiting phospholipid breakdown to arachidonic acid, blocking downstream production of inflammatory mediators including prostaglandins and leukotrienes. In addition to their anti-inflammatory activity, glucocorticoids have a variety of other systemic effects. Gluconeogenesis is promoted, with a concomitant negative nitrogen balance and reduction in protein production. Fat oxidation, synthesis, storage, and mobilization are also affected. The number of circulating neutrophils increases because mature neutrophils are released from bone marrow and their movement from blood to other tissues decreases, whereas the number of other circulating leukocytes decreases after glucocorticoid administration. Associated mineralocorticoid activity increases sodium retention and potassium excretion.

Table 9-3 lists the relative potency of commonly used glucocorticoid preparations. The molecular structure of the corticosteroid nucleus can be modified to dissociate glucocorticoid from mineralocorticoid activity. Unfortunately, the goal of dissociating beneficial anti-inflammatory effects from the harmful manifestations of glucocorticoid activity has not been achieved. The ophthalmologist must be aware of the ocular and systemic toxicities associated with systemic corticosteroids. Ocular adverse effects of systemic corticosteroids include posterior subcapsular cataracts, glaucoma, mydriasis, ptosis, papilledema associated with idiopathic intracranial hypertension, reactivation or aggravation of ocular infection, and delay of wound healing. Systemic complications may include peptic ulceration, osteoporosis, aseptic necrosis of the femoral head, and muscle and skin atrophy. Steroids may also cause hyperglycemia, hypertension, edema, weight gain, and changes

Table 9-3 **Potency of Commonly Used Glucocorticoids**

Glucocorticoid	Approximate Equivalent Dose, mg	Relative Anti-inflammatory Potency
Hydrocortisone	20	1.0
Cortisone	25	0.8
Prednisone	5	4.0
Prednisolone	5	4.0
Methylprednisolone	4	5.0
Triamcinolone	4	5.0
Dexamethasone	0.75	25.0

in body fat distribution with cushingoid habitus. Other adverse effects include hyperosmolar nonketotic coma, hypokalemia, and growth delay in children. Mental changes are a common problem and may range from mild mood alterations to severe psychological reactions, including psychological dependence.

Osteoporosis is a particularly insidious problem that may increase the risk of fractures as early as a few months after beginning treatment with corticosteroids. Bone mineral density testing is used to assess the degree of osteoporosis. Patients can be treated with calcium and vitamin D supplementation. More sophisticated interventions include hormone replacement therapy and the use of bisphosphonates. Patients should consult with a specialist to optimize the identification and management of this disease.

Another frequently overlooked complication of systemic corticosteroid therapy is rapid withdrawal. The rate of corticosteroid withdrawal should be determined by 2 criteria: (1) the degree of hypothalamic-pituitary-adrenal (HPA) suppression, which in turn is related to dose and duration of therapy, and (2) the response of the underlying disease to the corticosteroid withdrawal. Various schedules have been suggested. High-dose glucocorticoids given for 1–3 weeks probably suppress HPA function only temporarily, so they can be withdrawn suddenly or gradually over 1 week. After 1 or more months of treatment, a dosage-reduction protocol is usually followed. Otherwise, sudden withdrawal of corticosteroid therapy may result in adrenal insufficiency, with symptoms such as fatigue, weakness, arthralgias, nausea, orthostatic hypotension, and hypoglycemia. In severe cases, adrenal suppression may be fatal. After corticosteroid therapy has been discontinued, adrenal function may not return to normal for 1 year or more; thus, supplementary corticosteroids may be needed if the patient has a serious illness or undergoes surgery during this recovery period. Because of the likelihood of withdrawal symptoms, even physiologic doses of long-term corticosteroids (eg, 5 mg of prednisone a day) should be gradually reduced.

Ophthalmologists may occasionally initiate corticosteroid therapy for ophthalmic diseases and should consider the assistance of the primary care provider to monitor for systemic adverse effects. Physicians may become complacent with the use of corticosteroids because of their effectiveness and relative ease of use to control symptoms. However, studies have shown that even a dosage as low as 5 mg a day is associated with increased adverse events over time. For patients who require high-dose or extended corticosteroid treatment, clinicians should strongly consider early use of other immunosuppressive medications, which can decrease patient dependency on corticosteroids. The ophthalmologist may need to be responsible for initiating this discussion if the corticosteroids are being used solely to treat localized ocular disease. The other physicians involved in the patient's care may be unaware of or uninterested in making relatively onerous changes in the management of a disease viewed as being a part of the ophthalmologist's area of focus.

Nonsteroidal Anti-inflammatory Drugs

Clinicians use a wide variety of NSAIDs to treat RA and other rheumatic diseases. All of these agents decrease synthesis of inflammatory mediators such as the prostaglandins by inhibiting the enzyme cyclooxygenase (COX), and all of them are analgesic, antipyretic, and anti-inflammatory. Their relative efficacy remains largely untested, and the response of individual patients to these drugs varies.

Complications from the use of NSAIDs cause approximately 100,000 hospitalizations and 10,000–20,000 deaths per year in the United States. The most significant adverse effects from use of oral NSAIDs are gastrointestinal bleeding, renal failure, worsening hypertension, and heart failure, as well as onset of asthma in aspirin-sensitive individuals. Oral NSAIDs can interfere with platelet function and can cause bone marrow suppression; hepatic toxicity; and CNS symptoms, including headache, dizziness, and confusion. In rare cases, NSAIDs have been associated with ocular adverse effects such as nonspecific blurred vision and diplopia. There have also been reports of possible optic neuropathy and macular edema, especially with use of ibuprofen.

There are 2 isoforms of the COX enzyme. COX-1 is present in most cells and appears to be involved in various aspects of cellular metabolism, such as gastric cytoprotection, platelet aggregation, and renal function. COX-2 is present in some tissues, such as brain and bone, but is also expressed in other sites in response to inflammation. The traditional NSAIDs, including meloxicam, inhibit both enzyme forms. Selective COX-2 inhibitors reduce the risk of gastrointestinal damage and have less effect on platelet function. Unfortunately, 2 of these drugs (rofecoxib and valdecoxib) have been removed from the market worldwide because of adverse cardiovascular events; however, parecoxib, a prodrug of valdecoxib, remains available in many European countries. Similar concerns have been raised about celecoxib, and although it is still available, this drug carries significant warnings. It has been proposed that the selective blocking of COX-2 decreases the production of prostacyclins, which cause vasodilation and inhibit platelet aggregation, leading to increased prothrombotic activity. Another COX-2–selective class member, etoricoxib, is available outside the United States. Ophthalmologists should be aware that conjunctivitis, temporary blindness, and vague vision blurring have been reported with use of COX-2 inhibitors.

The exact role of oral NSAIDs in treating ocular inflammation remains uncertain. For instance, systemic NSAIDs may be useful in partially controlling uveitis or scleritis in some patients. In general, however, these drugs are not as effective as corticosteroids. Several topical NSAIDs have been approved for ocular use, and these are discussed in BCSC Section 8, *External Disease and Cornea,* and Section 9, *Intraocular Inflammation and Uveitis.*

Methotrexate

Methotrexate, a structural analogue of folic acid, interferes both with folate-dependent metabolic pathways such as purine and with pyrimidine metabolism. Its disease-modifying effect may be mediated partly via increased extracellular adenosine, which has intrinsic anti-inflammatory activity. Methotrexate is given weekly, usually beginning at a dose of 7.5–10 mg and gradually increasing to a maximum dose of 25 mg, depending on disease response. All patients are supplemented with folic acid; folic acid therapy decreases the adverse effects associated with methotrexate therapy. Minor adverse effects can include gastric upset, stomatitis, and rash. Major adverse effects include hepatic fibrosis, interstitial lung disease, marrow toxicity, teratogenicity, and sterility. Patients are closely followed with laboratory investigations to rule out potential bone marrow toxicity.

Leflunomide

Traditional immunosuppressive drugs work by interfering with lymphocyte proliferation. *Leflunomide* inhibits pyrimidine synthesis, targeting rapidly dividing cell populations such as activated lymphocytes. Potential adverse effects include liver toxicity, neuropathy, and birth defects. This drug is about as effective as methotrexate, and the two are often combined when methotrexate is ineffective alone.

Hydroxychloroquine

Hydroxychloroquine is an antimalarial compound commonly used to treat rheumatologic diseases (chloroquine is a related drug that has an increased risk of retinal toxicity and is now rarely used). The drug seems to work by slightly raising the pH of various cellular compartments. The increase in pH has multiple subtle effects, including decreased cytokine production and decreased lymphocyte proliferation. The response to treatment may take weeks to months, in part because of the drug's half-life (1–2 months) and the time required to achieve steady-state levels.

Hydroxychloroquine is one of the safest immunomodulating drugs. Gastrointestinal symptoms and, in rare cases, myopathy may occur. When the drug is first started, patients may report a self-limited decrease in accommodation, which is probably mediated by a transient effect on ciliary muscle function. Retinopathy (bull's-eye maculopathy) due to use of hydroxychloroquine is relatively unusual. Researchers have developed a screening protocol that assigns a patient's level of risk for retinopathy on the basis of factors such as duration of drug use, age, the presence of preexisting retinal disease, and the presence of renal or liver disease. Dosing greater than 6.5 mg/kg/day also increases the risk. Hydroxychloroquine is not retained in fatty tissues, so the dosage limit refers to lean body weight—not the patient's actual weight. That is, a short, obese patient with reduced lean body mass may actually be at greater risk for toxicity than a taller, leaner patient of similar weight. Recent practice guidelines recommend annual examinations that include central visual field testing and 1 of the following: spectral domain optical coherence tomography, multifocal electroretinography, or fundus autofluorescence. Retinopathy is discussed more fully in BCSC Section 12, *Retina and Vitreous.*

Marmor MF, Kellner U, Lai TY, Lyons JS, Mieler WF; American Academy of Ophthalmology. Revised recommendations on screening for chloroquine and hydroxychloroquine retinopathy. *Ophthalmology.* 2011;118(2):415–422.

Sulfasalazine

Sulfasalazine is effective in treating RA, although the exact mechanism of action is unclear. Similar to those of other sulfa drugs, the adverse effects of sulfasalazine may be due to idiosyncratic hypersensitivity (skin reactions, aplastic anemia) or may be dose related (gastrointestinal tract symptoms, headache). Sulfasalazine is often used in combination with other drugs, such as hydroxychloroquine and methotrexate.

Gold Salts

Gold salts are rarely used because of their limited efficacy and considerable adverse effects, including hematologic, renal, and dermatologic reactions.

Anticytokine Therapy and Other Immunosuppressive Agents

An improved understanding of the immune response has enabled the development of drugs targeting specific mediators. Cytokines, which are compounds generated by activated immune cells, can enhance or inhibit the immune response. TNF-α is a major proinflammatory cytokine involved in the pathogenesis of inflammatory diseases. Five TNF-α antagonists have been approved by the US Food and Drug Administration (FDA). They include *etanercept, adalimumab, infliximab, certolizumab pegol,* and *golimumab. Infliximab* is given as an intravenous infusion every 4–8 weeks, whereas the other agents are administered subcutaneously. Certolizumab pegol is classified as a category B drug by the US FDA (Table 9-4) and is therefore a treatment option for patients who are pregnant or nursing.

The drugs are usually well tolerated, but there is potential for severe adverse effects. These include the development of opportunistic infections such as tuberculosis or atypical

Table 9-4 US FDA Drug Formulary Pregnancy Categories

A	Adequate and well-controlled studies have failed to demonstrate a risk to the fetus in the first trimester of pregnancy; no evidence in later trimesters.
B	Animal reproduction studies have failed to demonstrate a risk to the fetus, and there are no adequate and well-controlled studies in pregnant women.
C	Animal reproduction studies have shown an adverse effect on the fetus, and there are no adequate and well-controlled studies in humans, but potential benefits may warrant use of the drug in pregnant women despite potential risks.
D	There is positive evidence of human fetal risk based on adverse reaction data from investigational or marketing experience or studies in humans, but potential benefits may warrant use of the drug in pregnant women despite potential risks.
X	Studies in animals or humans have demonstrated fetal abnormalities and/or there is positive evidence of human fetal risk based on adverse reaction data from investigational or marketing experience, and the risks involved in use of the drug in pregnant women clearly outweigh the potential benefit.
N	Not classified

FDA = Food and Drug Administration.

Modified from FDA Pregnancy Categories. University of Washington. http://depts.washington.edu/druginfo/Formulary/Pregnancy.pdf.

mycobacteria; a possible association with demyelinating disease; and a possible association with lymphoma, especially in the pediatric population. Other associations include cytopenias, heart failure, shingles, and a lupuslike syndrome. Ophthalmologists should be aware that these drugs have been reported to cause optic neuritis due to demyelination. Also, etanercept has been implicated in actually exacerbating uveitis in some patients. The drugs are also very expensive; the cost of infliximab, for example, is approximately $12,000 per year based on an average of 8 treatments. Despite these problems, these drugs can be very effective in the treatment of autoimmune diseases, and they herald the onset of immunomodulatory therapies that target specific aspects of the immune response. All patients on immunosuppressive therapy require regular hematologic chemomonitoring to detect life-threatening adverse effects.

Biologic agents used to treat autoimmune disease can affect pathways other than TNF-α. *Anakinra* and *canakinumab* are anticytokine drugs that inhibit interleukin-1 (IL-1) by binding to IL-1 receptors on the cell surface. *Tocilizumab* is an anti–IL-6 receptor antibody recently approved by the FDA for the treatment of RA and JIA. It works best when combined with other disease-modifying agents such as methotrexate. *Abatacept* has recently been approved in the United States for the treatment of RA that is poorly responsive to other therapies. This drug blocks the T-cell receptor CD28, which is involved in T-cell activation and can be very effective in treating refractory disease.

Rituximab is a B-cell–depleting monoclonal antibody used primarily for chemotherapy but also in cases of RA that are unresponsive to other agents. *Belimumab* is a human monoclonal antibody that inhibits B-cell activation. The FDA has approved it for the treatment of SLE, but clinicians use it infrequently because of its marginal effectiveness, the risk of infection, and increased mortality. *Alemtuzumab* is a monoclonal antibody that binds to CD52, a protein on mature lymphocytes; it is used to treat chronic lymphocytic leukemia and has shown promise in the treatment of autoimmune diseases.

Cyclophosphamide and *chlorambucil* are alkylating agents that are very potent immunosuppressive drugs. Their primary mechanism of action involves the cross-linking of DNA molecules, which blocks DNA replication. They also have potentially severe adverse effects, including infertility, bone marrow suppression, increased risk of infection, and late malignancy. Consequently, these drugs are reserved for very resistant or life-threatening diseases such as GPA, for which the benefits outweigh the risks. Cyclophosphamide is available as an oral or intravenous agent; the oral form is associated with increased rates of bladder cancer.

Azathioprine is an antimetabolite that ultimately interferes with purine metabolism. The most common adverse effects are gastrointestinal tract symptoms, risk of infection, and bone marrow suppression. Up to 10% of the population may have decreased levels of the enzyme thiopurine methyltransferase (TPMT), which is important in the metabolism of this drug. Because decreased levels of TPMT may lead to more pronounced bone marrow suppression and toxicity, measuring the levels of this enzyme may help identify patients at risk.

Cyclosporine and *tacrolimus* inhibit the transcription of IL-2 and other cytokines, primarily in helper T cells. They are used primarily to prevent rejection in patients who have undergone transplants, but clinicians are increasingly recognizing their utility in treating autoimmune diseases. The chief adverse effects of both drugs are nephrotoxicity and hypertension. Other potential problems include infections and nonmelanoma skin cancers. Because of such risks, these agents are reserved for recalcitrant cases that do not respond to standard therapies.

Mycophenolate mofetil inhibits the production of guanosine in lymphocytes and thereby decreases cellular proliferation and antibody production. It was initially used in transplant patients in the United States and is increasingly used in patients with immunologic diseases. The primary adverse effects include gastrointestinal symptoms, bone marrow suppression, and increased risk of infection. An alternative formulation, mycophenolate, typically reduces the incidence of gastrointestinal adverse effects. Overall, the drug seems to be well tolerated by patients and may serve as an adjunct to other medications.

Firestein GS, Budd RC, Harris ED Jr, McInnes IB, Ruddy S, Sergent JS. *Kelley's Textbook of Rheumatology.* 8th ed. 2 vols. Philadelphia: Elsevier/Saunders; 2008.

Fraunfelder FT, Fraunfelder FW, Chambers WA. *Clinical Ocular Toxicology: Drug-Induced Ocular Side Effects.* Philadelphia: Elsevier/Saunders; 2008.

CHAPTER 10

Geriatrics

The median age of the world's population is increasing almost exponentially. In the United States, the proportion of the population aged 65 years and older is projected to increase from 12.4% in 2000 to 19.6% in 2030, and the number of persons aged 80 years and older is expected to increase from 9.3 million in 2000 to 19.5 million in 2030. Worldwide, over the same period, the population aged 65 years and older is projected to increase by approximately 550 million, to 973 million, from 6.9% to 12.0%. In some regions, projected increases are still greater: from 15.5% to 24.3% in Europe, 12.6% to 20.3% in North America, 6.0% to 12.0% in Asia, and 5.5% to 11.6% in Latin America and the Caribbean. An expanding older population presents a growing challenge to primary care physicians and medical subspecialists in the United States and Western Europe.

Ophthalmology is one specialty that is already significantly affected by this demographic shift. Cataracts, age-related macular degeneration (AMD), ischemic optic neuropathy, giant cell arteritis, diabetic retinopathy, and glaucoma are all diseases that disproportionately affect older persons.

Ophthalmologists may be expert in dealing with ophthalmic problems in the geriatric population, but they do not identify and manage geriatric problems in general. In the past, most medical specialties (including ophthalmology) followed the traditional medical paradigm of diagnosis of illness, treatment of disease, and measurement of objective outcomes. The subspecialty of geriatrics emphasizes a different medical paradigm of functional assessment and a more holistic approach to patient care. Geriatricians focus on the unique needs of older individuals, distinguishing between disease and the effects of normal aging. Ophthalmologists are specifically qualified to work with the geriatrician or primary care physician in evaluating and managing older patients with impaired vision.

The ophthalmologist's role in this multidisciplinary evaluation is to communicate the visual limitations and visual needs of the older patient to the geriatrician and to contribute to the integrated goals of the care plan. The ophthalmologist should also be able to recognize the effect of vision loss on function. Referral for vision rehabilitation is appropriate for patients with acuity less than 20/40, central scotomata, visual field loss, or contrast sensitivity loss. The SmartSight patient handout, available on the American Academy of Ophthalmology website, can be given to patients to assist in seeking Medicare-funded multidisciplinary vision rehabilitation or other vision rehabilitation services in their community. The Academy's Preferred Practice Pattern *Vision Rehabilitation* outlines how comprehensive vision rehabilitation addresses reading, activities of daily living, patient safety, continued community participation, and patient well-being.

American Academy of Ophthalmology. *SmartSight.* San Francisco: American Academy of Ophthalmology; 2012. Available at: one.aao.org/smart-sight-low-vision.

American Academy of Ophthalmology Vision Rehabilitation Committee. Preferred Practice Pattern Guidelines. *Vision Rehabilitation.* San Francisco: American Academy of Ophthalmology; 2013. Available at: one.aao.org/preferred-practice-pattern/vision-rehabilitation-ppp--2013.

US Census Bureau. International Data Base [database online]. Midyear population, by age and sex. Revised December 19, 2013. http://www.census.gov/population/international/data/worldpop/table_population.php. Accessed September 2, 2014.

Physiologic Aging and Pathologic Findings of the Aging Eye

Changes in the eye due to aging affect everyone, but there are marked differences among individuals. The periorbital and eyelid skin and soft tissues atrophy with age. Dermatochalasis and levator dehiscence may produce secondary ptosis. Eyelid laxity may cause entropion, ectropion, and trichiasis. Lacrimal gland dysfunction, decreased tear production, meibomian gland disease, and goblet cell dysfunction may cause dry eye symptoms. As a person ages, the conjunctiva undergoes atrophic changes and corneal sensitivity is reduced. The pupils become progressively miotic and less reactive to light. There is an increasing incidence of presbyopia, cataract, glaucoma, AMD, and diabetic retinopathy. Contrast sensitivity and visual field sensitivity are reduced. In addition, refractive error (of some type) is present in more than 90% of older patients and remains a significant cause of visual disability in the nursing home patient.

The 4 leading causes of vision loss in the older population are AMD, glaucoma, cataract, and diabetic retinopathy. It is estimated that by 2020, 2.95 million persons in the United States will have AMD. Glaucoma becomes more common with increasing age; thus, screening is recommended for patients older than 50 years. It is also estimated that by 2020, 30.1 million Americans will have cataracts and 9.5 million will be pseudophakic/aphakic, an increase of 50% and 60%, respectively, from the year 2000. Diabetic retinopathy is a leading cause of new cases of legal blindness among working-aged Americans. The prevalence of retinopathy in persons aged 40 years and older in the United States is 3.4% (4.1 million persons), and the prevalence of vision-threatening retinopathy is 0.75% (899,000 persons). Assuming a similar prevalence for diabetes mellitus, the projected numbers in 2020 would be 6 million persons with diabetic retinopathy and 1.34 million persons with vision-threatening diabetic retinopathy.

American Academy of Ophthalmology Retina/Vitreous Panel. Preferred Practice Pattern Guidelines. *Diabetic Retinopathy.* San Francisco: American Academy of Ophthalmology; 2008 (4th printing 2012). Available at: one.aao.org/preferred-practice-pattern/diabetic-retinopathy-ppp--september-2008-4th-print.

Congdon N, O'Colmain B, Klaver CC, et al; Eye Diseases Prevalence Research Group. Causes and prevalence of visual impairment among adults in the United States. *Arch Ophthalmol.* 2004;122(4):477–485.

Congdon N, Vingerling JR, Klein BE, et al; Eye Diseases Prevalence Research Group. Prevalence of cataract and pseudophakia/aphakia among adults in the United States. *Arch Ophthalmol.* 2004;122(4):487–494.

Outpatient Visits

Ophthalmology is largely an outpatient specialty. For older patients, access to the ophthalmologist's office can be a major physical barrier to eye care. The ideal outpatient office should be designed to accommodate older patients with various disabilities. The geriatric-friendly office environment should include the following:

- a safe, well-lit office that is close to drop-off areas and parking
- automatic or assisted doors (doorways with pull levers or handles, not doorknobs)
- large-print, legible, well-placed signs
- wheelchair-accessible entryways and waiting rooms
- obstacle-free and well-lit, high-contrast walkways, hallways, and waiting areas (free of rugs, electrical cords, and tripping hazards, such as toys)
- accessible bathrooms with elevated toilet seats, grab bars, and a wheelchair-accessible sink
- staff trained to assist patients with disabilities to and from the examination room
- a private area where patients with decreased hearing and vision can receive assistance from staff in completing forms

Elder Abuse

Elder abuse is a violation of human rights and a significant cause of illness, injury, loss of productivity, isolation, and despair, according to the World Health Organization. The ophthalmologist may be the first physician to see an older patient who is being abused or neglected. The signs may be subtle, and early recognition is key. In the United States, the prevalence of elder maltreatment has been reported as 7.6%–10% of study participants and is estimated to affect 11.4% of adults aged 60 years and older. The National Elder Abuse Incidence Study, the first major investigation of mistreatment of the elderly in the United States, found that 449,924 persons aged 60 years or older had been physically abused, neglected, or in some way mistreated in 1996. However, the study did not solicit data directly from older adults; rather, it assessed Adult Protective Service records and sentinel (eg, community professionals') reports. Thus, it is very likely that the results greatly underestimated the true scope of the problem of abuse of older Americans, because a large majority of cases are unreported and are undetected by monitoring agents.

Major risk factors for elder abuse include external stresses due to marital, financial, and legal difficulties; dependent relationships (eg, the abuser may be dependent on the older patient for finances or housing, or vice versa); mental illness and substance abuse; social isolation; and misinformation about normal aging or about the patient's medical or nutritional needs. Maltreatment can occur at home, in assisted living, or in nursing homes. It can take the form of physical or psychological abuse, material misappropriation, neglect, or sexual attack.

Physical neglect includes withholding of food or water, medical care, medication, or hygiene. Neglect may be intentional or unintentional and may be related to financial constraints or lack of other resources (eg, transportation, supervision). Elder abuse also includes financial abuse or exploitation, deprivation of basic rights (eg, decision making for care, privacy), and abandonment. Actual physical abuse in the form of slapping, restraining, and hitting may cause physical pain or injury.

The ophthalmologist should suspect elder abuse in the following circumstances:

- bruises, black eyes, and fractures
- broken eyeglasses and report by the patient of being slapped or abused
- repeated visits to the emergency department or office
- conflicting or noncredible history from caregiver or patient
- unexplained delay in seeking treatment
- unexplained, inconsistent, vague, or poorly explained injuries
- history of being "accident prone"
- expressions of ambivalence, anger, hostility, or fear by the patient toward the caregiver
- poor adherence to follow-up or care instructions
- evidence of physical abuse (eg, lacerations, wounds in various stages of healing, burns, welts, patches of hair loss, or unexplained subconjunctival, retinal, or vitreous hemorrhage)

Sometimes it is necessary to obtain the history with the caregiver out of the room. Directed questions for the patient include "Has anyone at home tried to harm you?" "Has anyone tried to make you do things that you don't wish to do?" and "Has anyone taken anything from you without your consent?"

Any suspected case of elder neglect or abuse should prompt a complete written report. Documentation of any suspicious injuries is mandatory, including type, size, location, and characteristics of injury and stage of healing. Requirements for reporting elder abuse vary from state to state, and many localities have abuse hotlines for reporting maltreatment. The physician should be aware of local services for adult protection, community social services, and law enforcement agencies.

Acierno R, Hernandez MA, Amstadter AB, et al. Prevalence and correlates of emotional, physical, sexual, and financial abuse and potential neglect in the United States: the National Elder Mistreatment Study. *Am J Public Health.* 2010;100(2):292–297.

Perioperative Considerations in the Management of Elderly Patients

There are a number of considerations that the ophthalmologist should take into account in the preoperative evaluation and perioperative management of elderly patients. First, loss of vision alone may not be an appropriate sole indication for surgical intervention (eg, cataract surgery). Functional assessment includes determining how vision loss affects instrumental activities of daily living (IADLs) such as reading, driving, taking medications properly, and using the telephone independently. Documentation of impaired IADLs is important for the preoperative assessment. It is also important to document any prescription medications that the patient is taking to ensure that they do not interact with perioperative medications. An elderly patient may have multiple medical conditions that require use of numerous prescription medications. Further, the clinician should be aware that management of informed consent may be different in patients with mild dementia and in those who have legal guardians or caregivers, as they will need to participate in the process.

Elderly patients undergoing surgery may be prone to confusion or delirium perioperatively. Delirium is estimated to occur in approximately 4%–5% of patients after cataract surgery. There are numerous causes for confusion in this setting, but many are preventable. Minimization of preoperative sedation or psychotropic medications, appropriate patient and family orientation by nursing or ancillary staff, and careful supervision and reassurance in the postoperative period can diminish confusion. Often, a confused older patient simply needs a familiar face or reassurance to regain calm. The use of restraints should be minimized.

Confusion may be exacerbated in patients with vision loss or in those who require vision rehabilitation. In a monocular older patient, patching of the eye after surgery may aggravate confusion and disorientation. Having a family member in the recovery room can be very helpful. The patch should be removed as soon as possible and the patient provided with appropriate eye protection. Topical anesthetic may not be indicated because of comorbidities such as cognitive impairment and inability to cooperate during surgery. In addition, patients with decreased vision following intraocular surgery may experience limited mobility or be at increased risk for falls. Bed rest and immobilization can lead to disuse of extremities, development of pressure ulcers, and other problems. For these patients, active rehabilitation should be encouraged as soon as possible.

Though rare in outpatient ophthalmic surgery, surgical or anesthesia complications may result in life-threatening conditions. The surgeon must pay careful attention to any preexisting directives (eg, do-not-resuscitate order or living will) prior to any surgical intervention (including laser treatments and periocular injections or anesthetics). By discussing possible treatment decisions with the patient and family members early on—preferably before any serious illness arises or, if a serious illness is present, early in its course—the surgeon can avoid emergency decisions.

Some potential issues for discussion include limits of treatment, antibiotics, and changes in the patient's living situation. Candidly and openly discussing these important issues with the patient and the family (especially in cases of dementia) in the preoperative period allows them to consider these matters in the context of their belief systems and without the disorientation and confusion created by an emergency. The content, context, time, and date of such discussions should be well documented in the medical record and communicated to the patient, the family, and the primary care physician or geriatrician.

Psychology of Aging

The psychology of aging is influenced by a wide range of factors, including physical changes, adaptive mechanisms, and psychopathology. Each older patient has a unique psychological profile and social life history. Deleterious changes are not universal; in fact, in the absence of disease, growth of character and the ability to learn continue throughout life.

As we age, the issue of loss becomes more prevalent. Losses—of status, physical abilities, loved ones, and income—become more frequent. A fear of loss of social and individual power, and the attendant loss of independence, is common. In addition, the reality of death has increasing influence on a person's psychological status. All of these losses increase the incidence of depression.

Normal Aging Changes

Age-related changes in sensation and perception can have great influence, isolating an individual from the surrounding environment and triggering complex psychological reactions. There may be diminution of hearing and vision, slowing of intellectual and physical response time, and increasing difficulty with memory.

Many physical and intellectual abilities, however, are retained throughout life, and their loss should not be assumed to be part of the normal aging process. These include the senses of taste and smell, intelligence, the ability to learn, and sexuality. Any change in physical, intellectual, or emotional capabilities may reflect underlying organic or psychological disease.

Depression

Depression is the most frequent psychiatric problem in the older population. Approximately one-quarter of older patients seen in primary care settings are clinically depressed. The prevalence of depression in patients with macular degeneration is even higher, at 30%–40%. The suicide rate in white American men older than 65 years is 5 times greater than that of the general population; loneliness is the main reason cited, along with financial problems and poor health. Successful suicide is much less common in older American women, but older women attempt suicide more often than do men.

The criteria set forth in the *Diagnostic and Statistical Manual of Mental Disorders, Fifth Edition* (DSM-5), require that depressive symptoms as a result of a general medical condition or the medication used to treat it be separated out from late-life depression. An alternative diagnosis of mood disorder is preferred for the former.

Major depressive disorder is characterized by episodes of at least 2 weeks of depressed mood or loss of interest or pleasure in activities with 4 or more of the following symptoms:

- changes in appetite with associated weight loss or gain
- significant weight loss or gain
- sleep disturbance
- agitation
- diminished libido
- retardation (slowing down)
- loss of energy
- feelings of worthlessness or guilt
- difficulties in concentration and decision making
- recurrent thoughts of suicide or death

The signs and symptoms of depression in older individuals are similar to those seen in younger age groups, although older depressed patients are *more likely* than younger patients to have somatic or hypochondriacal complaints, minimize depression symptoms (masked depression), and have psychotic delusional disease. However, they are *less likely* to report symptoms of guilt. The most frequent presentations of subclinical depression include new medical complaints, fatigue, poor concentration, exacerbation of existing symptoms and medical problems, preoccupation with health, and diminished interest in pleasurable activities.

The ophthalmologist's role is to recognize and refer the patient with depression or to be aware of precipitating factors. For instance, loss of function, such as moderate or severe vision loss, can precipitate depression, as can recent death of a spouse. Red flags may include frequent visits to the ophthalmology office and unexplained vision loss. Though not prevalent in the ophthalmology setting, testing for depression would be enormously helpful in attaining care for those patients who have this disorder.

Many case-finding instruments ask about depressed mood and *anhedonia,* the latter defined as a psychological condition characterized by inability to experience pleasure in acts that normally produce it. Most of these instruments require more time than is available in the typical office practice. A brief case-finding instrument, the Patient Health Questionnaire-2 (PHQ-2), is a suggested screening device. It is sensitive, but not specific. It does not suggest or establish a final diagnosis or monitor depression severity, but screens for depression in a "first step" approach. The self-report questionnaire consists of 2 questions:

1. During the past month, have you been bothered by feeling down, depressed, or hopeless?
2. During the past month, have you often been bothered by little interest or pleasure in doing things?

If the first question is answered in the affirmative, it is highly likely that the patient has depression. The added sensitivity and greater specificity provided by the second question, if answered in the affirmative, makes it worthwhile to ask the questions. A positive response to this 2-question test is a score of 2 or 3 on either question, which is in line with DSM criteria for depression. Further information on the PHQ-2 is available on the website of the Center for Quality Assessment and Improvement in Mental Health (http://www.cqaimh.org; see STABLE Resource Toolkit). The ophthalmologist may conclude that further evaluation by the primary care physician is necessary.

Durso SC, Sullivan GM, eds. *Geriatrics Review Syllabus: A Core Curriculum in Geriatric Medicine.* 8th ed. New York: American Geriatrics Society; 2013.

Fraunfelder FW, Fraunfelder FT. Adverse ocular drug reactions recently identified by the National Registry of Drug-Induced Ocular Side Effects. *Ophthalmology.* 2004;111(7): 1275–1279.

Kroenke K, Spitzer RL, Williams JB. The Patient Health Questionnaire-2: validity of a two-item depression screener. *Med Care.* 2003;41(11):1284–1292.

Whooley MA, Avins AL, Miranda J, Browner WS. Case-finding instruments for depression. Two questions are as good as many. *J Gen Intern Med.* 1997;12(7):439–445.

Alzheimer Disease and Dementia

Alzheimer disease and dementia are discussed in Chapter 11.

Osteoporosis

Osteoporosis is defined by the World Health Organization as a disease "characterized by low bone mass and micro-architectural deterioration of bone tissue, leading to bone fragility and a consequent increase in risk of fracture." Osteoporosis is a significant, worldwide public health problem that is becoming increasingly common. It is estimated that 1 of every 2 women and 1 of every 4 men older than 50 years will have an osteoporosis-related fracture. In the United States, 1.5 million fractures related to osteoporosis occur annually, with the estimated cost of caring for these patients approaching $18 billion. This number is expected to triple by the year 2040. In older patients, a broken hip can increase mortality fourfold. Those with hip fractures have a 20% risk of entering a nursing home within a year of their fracture, and it is estimated that almost 50% of women with hip fractures do not fully regain previous function. Many patients with hip fractures experience a decline in function, along with increased feelings of isolation, depression, and fear of falling. In the context of osteoporosis, the potential for falling becomes even more important.

For the ophthalmologist, it is important to note what medications are being taken by a patient with osteoporosis. One of the drugs that can affect eye health is the class of drugs known as bisphosphonates, which are often prescribed for postmenopausal women to inhibit bone resorption. These drugs are associated with inflammatory disease of the eye, including conjunctivitis, uveitis, and episcleritis. Scleritis has also been reported, which can be vision threatening. On the other hand, a study of veterans revealed that the rates of uveitis/scleritis following dispensing of a bisphosphonate drug were low and did not differ significantly from those of the control group.

French DD, Margo CE. Postmarketing surveillance rates of uveitis and scleritis with bisphosphonates among a national veteran cohort. *Retina.* 2008;28(6):889–893.

Falls

The incidence and severity of falls rises with increasing age. Approximately one-third of US adults older than 65 years fall each year, yet less than half talk to their physicians about it. Falls are the leading cause of nonfatal and fatal injuries. In 2010, about 21,700 older adults in the United States died as a result of unintentional fall injuries. In 2010, direct medical costs of falls, adjusted for inflation, was $30 billion. Traumatic brain injury (TBI) in the older adult is most commonly caused by falls. In 2000, 46% of fatal falls among older adults in the United States were due to TBI. Men are more likely to die from a fall. Older whites are 2.4 times more likely to die from falls than are older blacks. Also, there are differences in fatal fall rates among ethnic groups; older non-Hispanic persons have higher fatal fall rates than do older Hispanic persons. Fear of falling causes elderly persons to limit activities, leading to reduced physical fitness, which, in turn, increases the actual risk of falling.

Prevention of falls is key. Older adults may reduce their chances of falling by

- exercising regularly
- increasing leg strength and balance

- asking their physician or pharmacist to review their medications that might cause dizziness or drowsiness
- having their eyes checked annually to update glasses or evaluate for eye diseases that limit vision
- getting assistance to make their living areas safer by
  - removing tripping hazards
  - installing grab bars in the bathroom and railings on the side of stairways (such as the entry to the home)
  - improving lighting

Visual disorders are the cause of up to 4% of falls. The ophthalmologist's role in fall prevention is twofold:

- ask the patient appropriate questions about the activities listed above that might reduce fall risk
- recognize and treat visual disorders, including refractive errors to identify and minimize ocular reasons for falls

It is the responsibility of the ophthalmologist to inquire, during the intake history, if the patient has fallen during the past year. Those patients with reduced vision from eye disease, most often macular degeneration, are at the highest risk of falling. Once a history of falls is obtained, it is incumbent upon the ophthalmologist to notify the patient's primary care physician about this finding or refer the patient to a multidisciplinary medical facility with resources for managing falls in the elderly.

Centers for Disease Control and Prevention. Injury Prevention & Control: Data & Statistics. Web-based Injury Statistics Query and Reporting System (WISQARS). www.cdc.gov/injury/wisqars/. Accessed July 10, 2014.

Stevens JA. Fatalities and injuries from falls among older adults—United States, 1993–2003 and 2001–2005. *Morb Mortal Wkly Rep.* 2006;55(45):1221–1224.

Stevens JA, Ballesteros MF, Mack KA, Rudd RA, DeCaro E, Adler G. Gender differences in seeking care for falls in the aged Medicare population. *Am J Prev Med.* 2012;43(1):59–62.

Stevens JA, Dellinger AM. Motor vehicle and fall related deaths among older Americans 1990–98: sex, race, and ethnic disparities. *Inj Prev.* 2002;8(4):272–275.

CHAPTER 11

Behavioral and Neurologic Disorders

Recent Developments

- Newer therapeutic agents for psychiatric diseases allow more effective treatment with generally fewer adverse effects compared with older agents.
- Ophthalmologists should be aware that newer antipsychotic agents have also been associated with an increased risk for diabetes mellitus.
- A meta-analysis of the literature on the pharmacologic treatment of dementia indicates that none of the currently available agents can significantly improve cognition, although there may be a mild effect in some patients.
- The Medicare Improvements for Patients and Providers Act and the Mental Health Parity and Addiction Equity Act of 2008 represent attempts to ensure that psychiatric conditions are given parity with other medical conditions when it comes to insurance coverage.
- The antiepileptic medications topiramate and vigabatrin are associated with adverse ophthalmic effects. Topiramate can cause angle-closure glaucoma, and vigabatrin can cause visual field loss.

Introduction

Since the 1980s, the World Health Organization (WHO) has focused its efforts on behavioral and neurologic disorders that occur frequently; cause substantial disability; and create a burden on individuals, families, communities, and societies. The WHO approach has been based on epidemiologic evidence: the assessment of disease burden using disability-adjusted life-years. This approach has emphasized the public health importance of behavioral and neurologic disorders, which in 2000 accounted for 12.3% of the worldwide disease burden. It is estimated that such disorders will account for 15% of disability-adjusted life-years in 2030. In addition to behavioral disorders, neurologic disorders that significantly affect this disease burden include epilepsy, dementias (in particular, Alzheimer disease), multiple sclerosis, Parkinson disease and other motor system disorders, stroke, pain syndromes, and brain injury.

Behavioral Disorders

Behavioral disorders encompass a wide variety of conditions in which the common factor is disordered functioning of thinking, behavior, and/or interpersonal relationships. Such disorders may profoundly affect the diagnosis and treatment of ophthalmic diseases. In addition, some of the medications used to treat psychiatric disorders may have significant adverse ophthalmic effects.

It is estimated that, in the United States, only 20%–25% of patients with depression and other mental health conditions receive effective care. Coverage for mental health services has been substantially improved following the passage of 2 pieces of legislation: the Medicare Improvements for Patients and Providers Act, in which Medicare began reimbursing outpatient mental health treatment services at parity with other Part B services, and the Mental Health Parity and Addiction Equity Act of 2008, which bans employers and insurers from imposing stricter limits on coverage for mental health and substance-use conditions compared with those set for other health problems.

Mental Disorders Due to a General Medical Condition

Formerly called organic mental syndromes, mental disorders due to a general medical condition are psychological or behavioral abnormalities associated with transient or permanent dysfunction of the brain. Causes include any disease, drug, or trauma that directly affects the central nervous system and systemic illnesses that indirectly interfere with brain function; Alzheimer disease is included in the latter category. Orientation, memory, and other intellectual functions are impaired, often with subsequent behavioral manifestations. Psychiatric symptoms such as hallucinations, delusions, depression, obsessions, and personality changes may occur.

Patients with a mental disorder due to a general medical condition, either with or without cognitive impairment, are often unable to remember instructions and therefore unable to adhere to treatment regimens. This general inability to understand instructions, integrate information, and perform tasks is referred to as *executive function deficit.* Depression, which frequently accompanies the syndrome, can complicate the situation. Medications with adverse effects on the central nervous system, such as β-blockers, steroids, and carbonic anhydrase inhibitors, must be used with care because patients are often sensitive to these agents. Alzheimer disease is discussed later in this chapter.

Schizophrenia

Schizophrenia is a mental disorder that alters thought processes and impairs emotional responses. It is one of the most devastating mental illnesses in terms of personal and societal costs, causing significant dysfunction. Schizophrenia usually begins when patients are young and continues to a greater or lesser extent throughout their lives. The prevalence is estimated at 1.1% of the population.

The hallmarks of schizophrenia include hallucinations, delusions, disorganized thinking, and "negative" symptoms such as emotional and cognitive blunting and social and occupational dysfunction. Motor disturbances range from uncontrolled, aimless activity to catatonic stupor, in which the patient may be immobile, mute, and unresponsive yet fully conscious. Repetitive, purposeless mannerisms and an inability to complete goal-directed tasks are also common. Patients may have other mental health conditions, such as major depression and anxiety disorders. Alternatively, manifestations of schizophrenia can be confused with symptoms of depression or anxiety. The lifetime occurrence of substance abuse is almost 50%. Associated illnesses include *schizophreniform disorder,* in which schizophrenic manifestations occur for less than 6 months, and *brief psychotic disorder,* which lasts less than 1 month. Patients with *schizoaffective disorder* have a significant mood disorder, such as depression, in addition to the psychotic disorder.

Mood Disorders

Mood disorders, also referred to as affective disorders, range from appropriate reactions to negative life experiences to severe, recurrent, debilitating illnesses. Common to all of these disorders is depressed mood, elevated mood (mania), or alternations between the two.

Major depression refers to the condition of patients who have major depressive episodes without any manic symptoms and is far more common than mania. The lifetime risk for major depressive disorder is 10% for men and 20%–25% for women. Major depression may occur at any age, but people are most likely to suffer their first episode from 30 to 40 years of age, and it is most common in middle-aged and older persons. Affective changes include pervasive and persistent low mood, slowed thought processes, low self-esteem, and loss of interest or pleasure in normal activities. Social withdrawal and psychomotor retardation are observed, although agitation also occurs. Major depression is a disabling condition that causes impairment of basic physical functions, as manifested by sleep disturbances, changes in appetite with associated weight loss or gain, diminished libido, and an inability to experience pleasure *(anhedonia)*. Patients commonly report somatic symptoms such as fatigue and headache, as well as other, nonspecific symptoms. Around 3%–4% of patients with major depression die by suicide, and 60% of all persons who die by suicide had depression or another mood disorder. Patients with *dysthymic disorder* have chronic, less severe depressive symptoms that do not meet the criteria for major depression.

Mania is a period of abnormally and persistently elevated or irritable mood that is sufficiently severe to impair social or occupational functioning. Typical symptoms include euphoria or irritability, grandiosity, decreased need for sleep, increased talkativeness, flight of ideas, and increased goal-directed activity. Formally called manic depression, *bipolar disorder* is found in approximately 4% of people. It manifests in 2 forms. Bipolar I disorder describes any illness in which mania is present, whether or not depression occurs. Bipolar II disorder refers to patients with major depressive episodes and at least 1 mild manic episode (hypomania). *Cyclothymic disorder* describes cyclical episodes of mania and mild depression.

For the nonpsychiatric clinician, depression creates a number of problems. In some patients, mood change may not be apparent, and the illness may manifest in somatic symptoms, leading to time-consuming, expensive workups. Conversely, in patients known to be depressed, an organic disease may be overlooked as psychosomatic. Appropriate recommendations for psychotherapeutic intervention may be met with resistance, anger, or denial, disrupting the patient–physician relationship. Patients may have difficulty adhering to diagnostic and treatment regimens for medical disorders and surgical procedures. A screening study of older patients attending an ophthalmology clinic showed that 1 in 5 patients suffered from depression. Visual impairment almost doubles the risk of depression. It is estimated that as many as 30%–40% of patients with macular degeneration meet the criteria for depressive disorder. The American Academy of Ophthalmology's Preferred Practice Pattern Guidelines recommend screening and providing referrals for depression in all macular degeneration patients.

Casten RJ, Rovner BW. Update on depression and age-related macular degeneration. *Curr Opin Ophthalmol.* 2013;24(3):239–243.

Somatoform Disorders

Somatoform disorders are mental conditions characterized by symptoms suggesting physical illness or injury in the absence of physical findings or a known physiological mechanism. The symptoms are considered to be outside the patient's voluntary control. The practicing ophthalmologist should be aware of these syndromes because encounters with these patients are common.

Several somatoform disorders are recognized. *Conversion disorders* are characterized by temporary and involuntary loss or alteration of physical functioning due to psychosocial stress. Symptoms are typically neurologic and include functional vision loss. The *Diagnostic and Statistical Manual of Mental Disorders, Fifth Edition,* has renamed 2 variants of somatoform disorders. *Somatic symptom disorder (SSD),* formerly called somatization disorder, includes predominantly somatic complaints; SSD with pain features, formerly called somatoform pain disorder, includes prolonged, severe pain as the only symptom. Psychotherapy is the primary treatment. Diagnosis may be difficult because of the subjective nature of the symptoms.

Formerly called hypochondriasis, *illness anxiety disorder* is a preoccupation with the fear of having or developing a serious disease. Physical examination fails to support the patient's belief, and reassurance by the examining physician fails to allay the fear. In *body dysmorphic disorder,* the patient believes that his or her body is deformed, even though there is no physical defect, or the patient has an exaggerated concern about a mild physical anomaly. Ophthalmologists performing reconstructive and cosmetic surgery should be aware of this disorder because surgical repair of the "defect" is rarely successful in the patient's mind.

Two other conditions that are not actually somatoform disorders bear mentioning here. *Factitious disorders* are characterized by willful production, feigning, or exaggeration of physical or psychological signs or symptoms in the absence of external incentives. Treatment requires discovery of the true nature of the physical illness, a carefully planned confrontation, and psychotherapy. Prognosis for recovery is guarded. Chronic conjunctivitis, keratitis, and even scleritis are the usual ophthalmic presentations of factitious disease. *Malingering* is the intentional fabrication or exaggeration of physical or psychological symptoms for the purpose of identifiable secondary gain. Malingering is not considered a primary psychiatric illness. Ophthalmologists should be familiar with techniques for detecting malingerers who feign loss of vision because such persons are occasionally encountered in practice. (See BCSC Section 5, *Neuro-Ophthalmology,* for a description of some of these techniques.)

Anxiety disorders represent another group of diseases that can significantly interfere with normal functioning. *Generalized anxiety disorder (GAD)* is the most common anxiety disorder; it is characterized by unrealistic or excessive anxiety and worry not focused on one particular life event. GAD is also correlated with depression. Pharmacologic therapy and psychotherapy may be successful in treating this disease.

Patients with *panic disorder* report discrete periods of intense terror and impending doom with associated physical symptoms (trembling, difficulty breathing) that are almost intolerable. These episodes can occur abruptly, either in certain predictable situations or without any situational trigger. Mild cases may be treated with psychotherapy, but more significant disease is often treated with antidepressant medication, especially selective serotonin reuptake inhibitors (SSRIs).

Post-traumatic stress disorder (PTSD) occurs after an individual has been exposed to a traumatic event that is associated with intense fear. When exposed to reminders of the event, the patient then persistently re-experiences the event through intrusive recollections, nightmares, flashbacks, or distress. The prevalence of PTSD is 8% in the general population and increases to 60% in combat soldiers and victims of assault. Treatment usually includes cognitive behavioral therapy, psychotherapy, and use of antidepressants. Other anxiety-related conditions that may require pharmacologic intervention include obsessive–compulsive disorder and social phobia.

Personality disorders merit discussion here because they may be associated with poor adherence to treatment and substance abuse. Personality disorders are diagnosed when personality traits become inflexible and maladaptive to the point where they create significant occupational and/or interpersonal dysfunction. Patients usually have little or no insight into their disorder. There are 3 types of personality disorders:

- *cluster A personality disorders,* which are related to a tendency to develop schizophrenia and include paranoid, schizotypal, and schizoid disorders
- *cluster B personality disorders,* which include antisocial, borderline, histrionic, and narcissistic personality disorders; patients with these disorders may display dramatic or irrational behavior and may be very disruptive in clinical settings
- *cluster C personality disorders,* which often stem from maladaptive attempts to control anxiety and include avoidant, dependent, and obsessive–compulsive personality disorders

Psychotherapy is generally the treatment of choice for all of these entities. In prior versions of the *Diagnostic and Statistical Manual of Mental Disorders,* the personality disorders were placed on Axis II and have often been referred to as Axis II disorders. In the fifth edition of this manual, Axis II has been eliminated, and all mental disorders are diagnosed on the same axis. (As part of this process, the multiaxial system of diagnosis in psychiatry has been eliminated.)

Miller NR. Functional neuro-ophthalmology. *Handb Clin Neurol.* 2011;102:493–513.

Substance Abuse Disorders

Drug dependence is the abuse of a drug to the point that one's physical health, psychological functioning, or ability to exist within the demands of society is threatened. Drug abuse and addiction are often considered strictly social problems. However, scientific research provides overwhelming evidence that in addition to short-term effects, drug abuse has long-term effects on brain metabolism and activity. At some point, changes occur in the brain, turning drug abuse into the illness of addiction. Patients who are addicted to drugs have a compulsive drug craving and frequently are unable to quit by themselves. Treatment is necessary to end the compulsive behavior.

Ophthalmic considerations Pupil changes can occur with drug abuse. For instance, pupil constriction is common with the use of opiates, and pupil dilation occurs with the use of cocaine, amphetamines, or lysergic acid diethylamide (LSD). Pupil dilation may also be observed with opiate withdrawal.

Sustained horizontal gaze-evoked nystagmus can be a sign of sedative or ethanol use. Toxic optic neuropathy is observed in patients with alcohol dependence as a direct effect of the disease or in association with the malnutrition that often accompanies alcoholism. Wernicke disease occurs most often in patients with alcoholism. It is caused by thiamine deficiency, and findings include ocular palsies, nystagmus, memory disturbance, and peripheral neuropathy. Alcohol also crosses the placental barrier, and children born to mothers with alcoholism may be affected by fetal alcohol syndrome. Some ocular manifestations of this syndrome are blepharophimosis, telecanthus, ptosis, optic nerve hypoplasia or atrophy, and tortuosity of the retinal arteries and veins. (See also BCSC Section 6, *Pediatric Ophthalmology and Strabismus.*)

Vascular occlusion and endophthalmitis can occur in association with intravenous drug abuse, and patients who use intravenous drugs are more likely to have HIV infection and associated eye findings. (See BCSC Section 9, *Intraocular Inflammation and Uveitis.*) Optic neuropathy can occur in association with cocaine-induced nasal pathology; intracranial microinfarcts causing internuclear ophthalmoplegia and visual field defects have been reported with cocaine abuse. Cocaine addiction during pregnancy can cause intrauterine growth retardation, microcephaly, developmental delay, and learning disabilities. Affected infants also have an increased risk of strabismus, and neonatal retinal hemorrhages have been reported. Crack cocaine use in particular should be considered in young patients who present with corneal ulcers or epithelial defects without an obvious cause.

Marijuana has a transient lowering effect on intraocular pressure; thus, many patients assume that marijuana is good for treating or relieving the symptoms of glaucoma and other eye problems. However, marijuana has only a temporary (3–4 hour) effect on ocular pressure, and the response diminishes with time. Furthermore, the ocular hypotensive effect cannot be isolated from the psychological effect, making this drug clinically useless in ophthalmology.

Pharmacologic Treatment of Psychiatric Disorders

Antipsychotic Drugs

The antipsychotics may be broadly divided into 2 groups—namely, first-generation ("typical") drugs and second-generation ("atypical") drugs (Table 11-1). The distinction between first-generation and second-generation antipsychotics is based on differences in receptor activity, side effects, and overall efficacy. The first-generation drugs are primarily dopamine receptor blockers; the second-generation antipsychotics, in contrast, have an inhibitory effect on serotonin receptors as well as dopamine-blocking activity. With regard to adverse effects, most second-generation drugs are better tolerated than are first-generation drugs. The second-generation antipsychotics are also increasingly administered for off-label uses such as treatment of major depression, anxiety disorders, and Alzheimer disease, though often with little substantial supporting data. The US Food and Drug Administration (FDA) has issued a warning that such off-label use has been associated with increased mortality, usually due to heart-related events or infections.

Antipsychotic medications effectively reduce many symptoms of acute and chronic psychoses and have allowed many more patients to function outside psychiatric institutions. A wide range of adverse effects may occur with these agents, including extrapyramidal reactions, drowsiness, orthostatic hypotension, anticholinergic effects, tardive dyskinesia, and weight gain. Less common problems include cholestatic jaundice, blood dyscrasias, photosensitivity, and a rare idiosyncratic reaction known as *neuroleptic malignant syndrome (NMS).* NMS is characterized by "lead-pipe" muscle rigidity and

Table 11-1 Antipsychotic Medications

First-generation agents (or typical antipsychotics or classic neuroleptics)	
Chlorpromazine	Molindone
Fluphenazine	Perphenazine
Haloperidol	Pimozide
Loxapine	Thioridazine
Mesoridazine	Thiothixene
Second-generation (atypical) agents	
Aripiprazole	Olanzapine
Asenapine	Paliperidone
Clozapine	Quetiapine
Iloperidone	Risperidone
Lurasidone	Ziprasidone
Anticholinergic agents used to minimize extrapyramidal adverse effects	
Benztropine	Diphenhydramine
Biperiden	Trihexyphenidyl

hyperthermia, and it can lead to death if not recognized and treated and the offending agent discontinued. The second-generation antipsychotics are far less likely to cause these adverse effects, although higher doses may still cause problems.

Ophthalmic considerations The second-generation antipsychotics—especially olanzapine, quetiapine, and clozapine—may be associated with initiating or worsening diabetes mellitus; thus, the possibility of secondary refractive and retinal vascular changes should be considered in patients taking these drugs. Results from animal studies suggested that the atypical agent quetiapine increases the risk of cataracts. However, because a true causal relationship is unlikely, annual ophthalmic screening examinations are sufficient. The second-generation agents can cause anticholinergic problems such as dry eye symptoms, accommodative symptoms, and precipitation of angle-closure glaucoma. Such effects may be exacerbated if patients are given additional anticholinergic medications to minimize extrapyramidal adverse effects of the antipsychotics (see Table 11-1). Potential ocular adverse effects of the first-generation drugs include corneal deposition, lens pigmentation, and vision loss from retinal pigmentary degeneration. These adverse effects are most common with use of thioridazine, especially long-term use at high doses (usually higher than 800 mg/day). Blepharospasm and other ocular motility problems can occur in association with extrapyramidal side effects.

Fraunfelder FW. Twice-yearly exams unnecessary for patients taking quetiapine. *Am J Ophthalmol.* 2004;138(5):870–871.

Antianxiety and Hypnotic Drugs

Benzodiazepines

The benzodiazepines are usually the drugs of choice when a short-term antianxiety, sedative, or hypnotic action is needed. Other indications for selected benzodiazepines include preanesthetic medication, alcohol withdrawal, seizures, spasticity, localized skeletal muscle spasm, insomnia, and nocturnal myoclonus. The benzodiazepines have distinct advantages over other agents with respect to adverse reactions, drug interactions, and lethality. The pharmacokinetics of these medications greatly affects their efficacy and adverse reactions and thus influences drug selection (Table 11-2). Because of their enhanced safety profile, benzodiazepines have largely supplanted barbiturates when antianxiety or hypnotic drugs are required. Barbiturates have been relegated to treatment of seizure disorders and use in anesthesia. For chronic anxiety, SSRIs or serotonin–norepinephrine reuptake inhibitors are used, as they may be safer than benzodiazepines.

Benzodiazepines alleviate the uncomplicated anxiety of GAD and improve symptoms of situational anxiety. Cognitive behavioral therapy can be effective for these conditions as well. The treatment of insomnia is another common indication for these drugs. Short-acting nonbenzodiazepines, such as zaleplon, zolpidem, and eszopiclone, are preferred for this purpose because there is less residual somnolence. All of these drugs, however, have the potential to cause retrograde amnesia and rebound insomnia.

Table 11-2 Antianxiety and Hypnotic Drugs

Benzodiazepines	
Compounds with active metabolites	Compounds with weakly active, short-lived, or inactive metabolites
Chlordiazepoxide	Alprazolam
Clorazepate	Clonazepam
Diazepam	Estazolam
Flurazepam	Lorazepam
Halazepam	Midazolam
	Oxazepam
	Quazepam
	Temazepam
	Triazolam
Barbiturates	
Amobarbital	Phenobarbital
Pentobarbital	Secobarbital
Nonbenzodiazepine Nonbarbiturates	
Antianxiety agents	Hypnotic agents
Buspirone	Chloral hydrate
Hydroxyzine	Eszopiclone
Meprobamate	Ethchlorvynol
	Paraldehyde
	Zaleplon
	Zolpidem

Sedation is the most common initial adverse effect of the benzodiazepines. Other common dose-related adverse effects with oral use include dizziness and ataxia. All of these drugs have the potential to cause retrograde amnesia. Respiratory depression can occur, especially if these agents are combined with alcohol. Products available in parenteral form, such as diazepam and midazolam, must be administered with careful monitoring because of an increased risk for apnea and cardiac arrest.

Ophthalmic considerations The abuse potential of benzodiazepines is mild compared with that of drugs such as hydromorphone and cocaine. Nevertheless, long-term administration of these agents can cause physical dependence.

Ocular adverse effects can occur, although they tend to be dose related and transient. Decreased accommodation and diplopia from increased phorias have been reported. Transient allergic conjunctivitis with benzodiazepine use has also been observed.

Antidepressants

Psychotherapy, either alone or in combination with antidepressant medication, is the first line of intervention in mild to moderate depression. Prospective studies have found that major depression in older adults is associated with increased mortality. Collaborative care programs, which integrate depression care managers (usually nurses supervised by psychiatrists) into primary care practices, may decrease all-cause mortality. In patients with major depression, antidepressants can improve symptoms, increase the chances and rate of recovery, reduce the likelihood of suicide, and help social and occupational rehabilitation.

In general, antidepressants take 3–6 weeks to show significant effect. A summary of studies concluded that antidepressants are associated with a 50%–60% response rate among patients with major depression in the primary care setting. These drugs can result in mood elevation, improved appetite, better sleep, and increased mental and physical activity. Treatment is usually necessary for 3 to 6 months after recovery is apparent.

Table 11-3 shows the various classes of antidepressants. The SSRIs were developed in response to research that implicated specific monoamines such as serotonin in the etiology of depression. They are the most commonly prescribed agents, although a meta-analysis suggested that they are no more effective than older tricyclic or heterocyclic antidepressants. The most compelling reason for using the SSRIs is reduced severity of adverse effects because of these drugs' more targeted mechanism of action. The SSRIs are also less dangerous than other antidepressants if an overdose occurs. Common adverse effects include restlessness, insomnia, headache, gastrointestinal symptoms, mild sedation, and sexual dysfunction. The SSRIs may cause inhibition of platelet function that can increase the risk of gastrointestinal bleeding and possibly increase the risk for transfusions with major surgery. Whether this effect is clinically significant in ophthalmic surgery is unknown.

The SSRIs also cause nonspecific visual symptoms, such as blurred vision, in 2%–10% of patients. In addition, patients may report "tracking" difficulties, which are more common in younger than older patients and tend to occur upon withdrawal of the drug. The SSRIs can also cause mydriasis. Rare cases of angle-closure glaucoma have been reported, most commonly with paroxetine, which tends to have a stronger anticholinergic effect.

Table 11-3 Pharmacology of Antidepressants

Tricyclic and tetracyclic antidepressants	
Amitriptyline	Imipramine
Amoxapine	Maprotiline
Clomipramine	Nortriptyline
Desipramine	Protriptyline
Doxepin	Trimipramine
Selective serotonin reuptake inhibitors	
Citalopram	Fluvoxamine
Escitalopram	Paroxetine
Fluoxetine	Sertraline
Dopamine–norepinephrine reuptake inhibitor	
Bupropion	
Serotonin–norepinephrine reuptake inhibitors	
Duloxetine	Venlafaxine
Serotonin modulators	
Nefazodone	Trazodone
Noradrenergic and specific serotonergic antidepressant	
Mirtazapine	
Monoamine oxidase inhibitors	
Phenelzine	Tranylcypromine

There has been a concern that the SSRIs may initially increase the risk of suicide in some patients, especially in adolescents and children, although the data are controversial. Careful monitoring of patients is recommended when treatment is initiated. Abrupt cessation of SSRIs may result in a "discontinuation syndrome," characterized by dizziness, nausea, fatigue, muscle aches, chills, anxiety, and irritability. This syndrome may be problematic, but it is much more benign than the severe adverse effects that can occur if heterocyclic or monoamine oxidase inhibitor drugs (discussed later in this section) are abruptly discontinued.

The other major class of antidepressants comprises the *heterocyclics,* of which the tricyclic antidepressants were the first described. These drugs tend to have more pronounced adverse effects than those caused by the SSRIs, including anticholinergic symptoms such as dry eye and mouth, accommodative changes, constipation, urinary retention, tachycardia, and confusion or delirium. Sedation, weight gain, and orthostatic hypotension may also occur. Most concerning is the toxicity of these medications in overdose; they can be fatal in as little as 5 times the therapeutic dose. Mortality is usually due to arrhythmias, although anticholinergic toxicity and seizures can also occur. Sudden cessation may cause pronounced changes in affect, cognition, and cardiac dysrhythmias.

The *monoamine oxidase (MAO) inhibitors* have long been considered second-line drugs in the treatment of mood disorders. The significant risk of hypertensive crisis caused by interactions between MAO inhibitors and various drugs or foods with high tyramine content (including cheese, herring, chicken liver, yeast, yogurt, red wine, and beer) must be considered when these drugs are prescribed. Because MAO inhibitors prevent catabolism of catecholamines, patients taking these substances have exaggerated hypertensive responses to drugs containing vasopressors, such as cold remedies, nasal decongestants, and even topical or retrobulbar epinephrine.

Alternative nonpharmacologic treatments for depression are being evaluated. *Vagus nerve stimulation (VNS)* uses an implanted stimulator that sends electric impulses to the left vagus nerve in the neck via a lead wire implanted under the skin. In 2005, the US FDA approved the use of VNS for treatment-resistant depression, although there is some controversy about its effectiveness. Transcranial magnetic stimulation is a noninvasive method to excite neurons in the brain: weak electric currents are induced in the tissue by rapidly changing magnetic fields. Its efficacy is also controversial.

Mood stabilizers

Mood stabilizers are a heterogeneous group of medications that do not clearly share a common mechanism of action. They are the drugs of choice for treatment of mania, bipolar disorder, schizoaffective disorder, and cyclothymia. They may also be used to treat impulse control disorders, symptoms associated with intellectual disability (mental retardation), and aggressive behavior. This class consists essentially of lithium carbonate and various antiepileptic medications. Valproic acid, carbamazepine, and lamotrigine are the most commonly used antiepileptic drugs, but many others have been studied and prescribed. Notably, lamotrigine has been reported to cause a Stevens-Johnson reaction. The antiepileptic medications are discussed in the section Epilepsy, later in this chapter. The ocular adverse effects of lithium include blurred vision, irritation due to secretion in tears or changes in sodium transport, nystagmus (usually downbeat), and exophthalmos that is often associated with lithium-induced changes in thyroid function.

Ophthalmic considerations Although behavioral disorders do not directly affect the eye, several related issues are important for ophthalmologists. For example, awareness of the potential ocular adverse effects of the various psychiatric medications is important. Patient education and reassurance may be required because the underlying psychopathology may make anticholinergic adverse ophthalmic effects, such as dry eye and accommodative changes, much more frightening and less tolerable for patients with behavioral disorders than for those without such disorders. Failure to adhere to treatment is another common problem among patients with psychiatric illness, dementia, and depression. Malingering and functional vision loss require a high index of suspicion and special diagnostic skills on the part of the clinician. Some medications used to treat eye disease, including carbonic anhydrase inhibitors, brimonidine, oral corticosteroids, and possibly β-blockers, may induce or exacerbate depression.

Fraunfelder FT, Fraunfelder FW, Chambers WA. *Clinical Ocular Toxicology: Drug-Induced Ocular Side Effects.* Philadelphia: Elsevier/Saunders; 2008.

Richa S, Yazbek JC. Ocular adverse effects of common psychotropic agents: a review. *CNS Drugs.* 2010;24(6):501–526.

Neurologic Disorders

Parkinson Disease

Parkinson disease belongs to a group of conditions known as *bradykinetic movement disorders.* In addition to bradykinesia (slowed movements with reduced voluntary movement), patients can develop rigidity, postural instability, and resting tremor. Parkinson disease usually affects persons older than 50 years; the average age of onset is 60 years. However, the number of reported cases of "early-onset" Parkinson disease has increased; it is estimated that 5%–10% of patients are now younger than 40 years. Though rare, familial Parkinsonism can occur through a variety of genetic mutations and is also responsible for a juvenile form that presents before age 20 years. The differential diagnosis for Parkinson disease includes other neurodegenerative disorders such as dementia with Lewy bodies, corticobasal degeneration, multiple system atrophy, and progressive supranuclear palsy.

Etiology

The basal ganglia are a complex of deep gray-matter nuclei that includes the corpus striatum, globus pallidus, and substantia nigra. These structures regulate the initiation and control of movement. Patients with Parkinson disease have typically lost 80% or more of the dopamine-producing neurons in the substantia nigra. Depletion of dopamine in the complex nigrostriatal pathway produces an imbalance in inhibitory and excitatory neuronal signals, leading to the cardinal signs of Parkinson disease.

Although most cases are sporadic, genetic factors are implicated in the pathogenesis, especially in early-onset cases. At least 5 possible causative genes have been identified, and the number of Parkinson-like disorders associated with specific genetic defects is increasing. Many of these defects appear to be involved in cellular protein metabolism. Overall, Parkinson disease seems to have a multifactorial etiology that includes genetic predisposition, environmental factors, and age-related changes in neuron metabolism.

Symptoms

The first symptom of Parkinson disease is usually tremor of a limb at rest. Other common symptoms include bradykinesia, rigidity, a shuffling gait, postural instability, and stooped posture. Persons with Parkinson disease often have reduced facial expressions and speak in a soft voice. The disease is associated with nonmotor features such as depression, personality changes, sexual difficulties, hallucinations, autonomic dysfunction, and dementia. Parkinson disease is associated with depression in 40%–50% of cases.

Treatment

There is currently no cure for Parkinson disease. Dopamine replacement, with medications such as levodopa (L-dopa), is the main treatment. Dopamine itself cannot be given because it does not cross the blood–brain barrier. Although levodopa helps at least three-fourths of patients with Parkinson disease, not all symptoms respond equally to the drug. Bradykinesia and rigidity respond best; tremor may be only marginally reduced. Problems with balance and other symptoms may not be alleviated at all. Usually, patients are given levodopa combined with carbidopa, often as a combined pill. When added to levodopa, carbidopa delays the conversion of levodopa into dopamine until it reaches the brain, diminishing some of the adverse effects that often accompany levodopa therapy.

After years of therapy, patients can become acutely aware of a "wearing-off" effect that occurs about 4 hours after a dose of levodopa, when their symptoms return. Catechol-*O*-methyltransferase inhibitors such as entacapone extend the duration of the levodopa effect and reduce the "off" time by inhibiting the methylation of levodopa and dopamine.

Several additional therapies for Parkinson disease exist. Dopamine agonists (bromocriptine, pramipexole, ropinirole, rotigotine, and apomorphine) stimulate dopamine receptors in the brain and may delay the need for levodopa. The MAO B inhibitor selegiline may modestly improve symptoms of Parkinson disease. Anticholinergic drugs such as trihexyphenidyl and benztropine have a short-lived effect controlling tremor and rigidity. However, only about half of patients respond to anticholinergics, and typical anticholinergic adverse effects can be problematic.

Amantadine, an antiviral drug, may be used in the early stages of the disease, either alone or in combination with anticholinergics or levodopa. After several months, the effectiveness of amantadine wears off in one-third to one-half of patients taking the drug.

Modern surgical treatments consist primarily of deep-brain stimulation and pallidotomy or thalamotomy. The dopamine deficiency in Parkinson disease results in excitation of the globus pallidus, which in turn inhibits thalamic activity. Both surgical techniques serve to suppress this excessive globus pallidus activity. Deep-brain stimulation is safer than pallidotomy initially but requires intensive adjustments and lifelong maintenance, given the risk of hardware complications and infection. Pallidotomy carries the risk of complications such as stroke and hemorrhage, as well as the risk of irreversible adverse effects, and is seldom performed.

LeWitt PA, Dubow J, Singer C. Is levodopa toxic? Insights from a brain bank. *Neurology.* 2011;77(15):1414–1415.

Olanow CW, Kieburtz K, Rascol O, et al; Stalevo Reduction in Dyskinesia Evaluation in Parkinson's Disease (STRIDE-PD) Investigators. Factors predictive of the development of Levodopa-induced dyskinesia and wearing-off in Parkinson's disease. *Mov Disord.* 2013;28(8):1064–1071.

Rolinski M, Fox C, Maidment I, McShane R. Cholinesterase inhibitors for dementia with Lewy bodies, Parkinson's disease dementia and cognitive impairment in Parkinson's disease. *Cochrane Database Syst Rev.* 2012;3:CD006504.

Ophthalmic considerations There are numerous ophthalmologic findings in patients with Parkinson disease. These findings can be divided into eyelid disorders and ocular motor abnormalities. Eyelid disorders include seborrheic dermatitis and blepharitis, apraxia of eyelid opening, eyelid retraction, decreased blinking (with secondary dry eye), and blepharospasm. Ocular motor abnormalities include convergence insufficiency, limitation of upgaze, hypometric saccades, saccadic pursuit, square-wave jerks, and oculogyric crisis. Patients commonly report reading trouble, and ocular surface abnormalities and motor abnormalities may synergize with other ophthalmic and neurologic problems to increase visual difficulties.

Drug-related adverse effects may also be superimposed, especially for patients on anticholinergic medications, which may exacerbate dry eyes and cause accommodative changes or precipitate angle-closure glaucoma. Visual hallucinations may occur as a result of both the disease and its treatment; this adverse effect has been reported in particular with use of levodopa and anticholinergic agents. Amantadine has been reported to cause corneal infiltrates and edema, although these complications are rare.

Multiple Sclerosis

See BCSC Section 5, *Neuro-Ophthalmology.*

Epilepsy

Seizures result from synchronized electrical activity of neuronal networks in the cerebral cortex. Epilepsy is characterized by recurrent seizures due to a genetically determined or acquired brain disorder. More than 2 million persons in the United States—approximately 1 in 100—have experienced an unprovoked seizure or received a diagnosis of epilepsy. Patients with relatively controlled epilepsy may still have problems with depression, driving, employment, and insurance.

Etiology

Epilepsy has many possible causes. Any disturbance of normal neuronal activity, including injury, infection, and abnormal brain development, can lead to seizures. Approximately half of all seizures have no known cause. Seizures may develop because of an abnormality in brain wiring, an imbalance of neurotransmitters, or some combination of these factors. Epilepsy can result from brain damage that can be caused by numerous disorders; it can also be part of a set of symptoms of a variety of developmental and metabolic disorders, including cerebral palsy, neurofibromatosis, tuberous sclerosis, and autism. Epilepsy can be caused by mutations in specific genes; however, genetics probably plays an indirect role in the etiology of seizures.

Typically, seizures are divided into 2 major categories: partial seizures and generalized seizures. *Partial seizures* occur in only 1 part of the brain and are further divided into *simple* (without impairment of consciousness) and *complex* (with impairment of consciousness). Symptoms of simple partial seizures (also called *auras*) depend on the part of the brain from which the seizures originate and include motor symptoms, sensory symptoms, and even autonomic symptoms. Complex partial seizures are the most common type of seizures in adults with epilepsy. During the seizure, patients may appear to be awake but do not interact with others in their environment and do not respond normally to instructions or questions. They often stare into space and either remain motionless or engage in repetitive behaviors, called *automatisms,* such as facial grimacing or gesturing.

Generalized seizures cause impaired consciousness and abnormal activity in both hemispheres at the onset of the seizure. Generalized seizures may follow partial seizures. They may be nonconvulsive (absence, or "petit mal") or convulsive (tonic–clonic, or "grand mal"; or variations of tonic–clonic). Absence seizures almost always begin in childhood or adolescence and are frequently familial, suggesting a genetic cause. During seizures, some patients make purposeless movements, such as jerking an arm or rapidly blinking their eyes. Others have no noticeable symptoms except for brief periods of "absence." Childhood absence epilepsy usually stops when the child reaches puberty. A generalized tonic–clonic seizure is the most dramatic type of seizure. It begins with an abrupt alteration in consciousness, sometimes in association with a scream or shriek. All of the muscles then become stiff, and the patient may become cyanotic during the tonic phase. After approximately 1 minute, the muscles begin to jerk and twitch for an additional 1–2 minutes, and then the patient goes into a deep sleep.

The end of a seizure is referred to as the *postictal period* and signifies the recovery period for the brain. This period may last from several seconds up to a few days, though typically no more than a few hours. Postictal paresis (Todd paralysis) is a transient focal motor deficit that lasts for hours or, in rare cases, days after an epileptic convulsion. It is thought to be related either to neuronal exhaustion (from electrical overactivity during the seizure) or to active inhibition.

Diagnosis

The electroencephalogram (EEG) is the most common diagnostic test for epilepsy. In certain cases, a normal EEG result does not entirely rule out epilepsy. Computed tomography (CT), magnetic resonance imaging (MRI), positron emission tomography (PET), and single-photon emission computed tomography (SPECT) are useful tools for determining abnormalities in the brain that cause epilepsy.

Treatment

Currently available treatments control seizure activity at least some of the time in 80% of patients with epilepsy. The primary treatment for epilepsy is antiepileptic drugs; the choice of drug is determined by the type of epilepsy. Several new drugs have become available (Table 11-4). The drug dose is titrated up until the disease is controlled; a second agent may be added if necessary, but monotherapy is preferred, if possible, to minimize side effects.

There are 2 main categories of adverse effects for antiepileptic drugs: systemic and neurotoxic. Systemic adverse effects generally include problems such as nausea, rash, and anorexia. Neurotoxic adverse effects include somnolence, dizziness, and confusion. The neurotoxic effects seem to be an inevitable consequence of the mechanism of action of these drugs and often become the dose-limiting factor.

When medications inadequately control seizures, surgery is a potential option. The most commonly performed surgery for epilepsy is removal of a seizure focus by *lobectomy* or *lesionectomy.* Other, less common surgical procedures for epilepsy include multiple subpial transection, corpus callosotomy, and hemispherectomy. In patients with seizures

Table 11-4 Mechanisms of Action of Antiepileptic Drugs

Mechanism of Action	Drug
Affects voltage-dependent sodium channels	Carbamazepine, eslicarbazepine, lacosamide, lamotrigine, oxcarbazepine, phenytoin, rufinamide
Affects low-threshold T-type calcium currents	Ethosuximide
Affects GABA activity	Benzodiazepines, phenobarbital, tiagabine, vigabatrin
Affects glutamate receptors	Perampanel
Blocks NMDA receptor; potentiates GABA-mediated inhibition	Felbamate
Water-soluble prodrug of phenytoin	Fosphenytoin
Exact mechanism unknown; GABA analogue	Gabapentin
Exact mechanism unknown	Levetiracetam
Blocks voltage-dependent sodium channels; inhibits kainate/AMPA receptor; enhances GABA-mediated inhibition at GABA (A) receptors	Topiramate
Blocks voltage-dependent sodium channels; enhances postsynaptic GABA-mediated inhibition	Valproate
Blocks voltage-dependent sodium and T-type calcium channels	Zonisamide

AMPA = α-amino-3-hydroxy-5-methyl-4-isoxazolepropionic acid; GABA = gamma-aminobutyric acid; NMDA = *N*-methyl-D-aspartate.

that are poorly controlled by medications or surgery, VNS may be used. The device delivers short bursts of electrical energy to the brain via the vagus nerve.

Fountain NB, Van Ness PC, Swain-Eng R, Tonn S, Bever CT Jr; American Academy of Neurology Epilepsy Measure Development Panel and the American Medical Association-Convened Physician Consortium for Performance Improvement Independent Measure Development Process. Quality improvement in neurology: AAN epilepsy quality measures. Report of the Quality Measurement and Reporting Subcommittee of the American Academy of Neurology. *Neurology.* 2011;76(1):94–99.

Noe KH. Seizures: diagnosis and management in the outpatient setting. *Semin Neurol.* 2011; 31(1):54–64.

Ophthalmic considerations Transient unilateral or bilateral mydriasis can occur as an expression of seizure activity, during or after the event. This phenomenon is most common in children. In some patients, the dilated pupil reacts poorly to light. Horizontal or vertical gaze deviations are commonly associated with seizure activity. The gaze tends to be directed away from the side of the cortical seizure activity during the event and then toward the side of the prior activity after the seizure. Some patients experience conjugate, convergent, or monocular nystagmus during the clonic stage of a seizure. Clonic eyelid retraction has also been described in patients with absence or myoclonic seizures. It is unusual for patients with true seizures to shut their eyes during the episode, whereas patients who are feigning a seizure often keep their eyes closed.

Certain antiepileptic drugs have the potential for characteristic ocular adverse effects. Phenytoin can cause dose-related nystagmus, and maternal use of this medication can cause fetal hydantoin syndrome (which includes hypertelorism, epicanthal folds, glaucoma, optic nerve hypoplasia, and retinal colobomas). Carbamazepine has been reported to affect saccadic eye movements and has been associated with isolated cases of downbeat nystagmus and oscillopsia. Blurred vision, diplopia, and nystagmus may also occur with this medication. Topiramate has been associated with acute angle-closure glaucoma, anterior chamber shallowing, acute myopia, and choroidal effusions, usually within the first 2 weeks of therapy. These effects may be an idiopathic response related to the presence of sulfa in topiramate. Treatment of the glaucoma includes cessation of the drug and use of cycloplegics and topical hypotensives.

Vigabatrin has been approved in the United States for patients who are unresponsive to other medications. In as many as 30%–50% of patients with long-term exposure to vigabatrin, irreversible concentric visual field loss develops that is of varying severity and is often asymptomatic. Central vision can also be affected. A complete ophthalmic examination and visual field testing should be performed before starting therapy and repeated every 3 months. The onset and progression of vision loss from vigabatrin are unpredictable, and vision loss may occur or worsen precipitously between tests. Once detected, vision loss is irreversible, and it is expected that even with frequent monitoring, severe vision loss will develop in some patients. Because of this risk, the drug is available only through a special restricted distribution program.

Stroke

See Chapter 6, Cerebrovascular Disease.

Pain Syndromes

See BCSC Section 5, *Neuro-Ophthalmology.*

Alzheimer Disease and Dementia

Dementia is a disorder characterized by a persistent and general decrease in intellectual functioning that impairs daily activities. Dementia is not a specific disease. Although it is common in persons older than 80 years, dementia is not a normal part of the aging process. Dementia also differs from *delirium,* which is an acute but transient confusional state characterized by fluctuating awareness and attention. There are also frequent sensory misperceptions.

Alzheimer disease (AD) is the most common cause of dementia in people older than 65 years, but there are several other causes. Other major dementia syndromes include Lewy body dementia, vascular dementia, and frontotemporal dementia. On the basis of epidemiological data from the European Community Concerted Action Epidemiology of Dementia Group (EURODEM), most patients with dementia have AD (70%). The estimated cost of the disease in 2008 was €160 billion. Recent studies show that mortality associated with AD is significantly underestimated.

Vascular dementia is associated with findings on neurologic examination consistent with prior strokes; patients often show evidence of multiple infarcts on cerebral imaging. The incidence of vascular dementia is relatively high in persons of African descent, patients with hypertension, and patients with diabetes mellitus.

Lewy body dementia (LBD) is the second most common form of neurodegenerative dementia after AD. LBD is characterized pathologically by the presence of Lewy bodies in the brainstem and cortex. There may be considerable clinical and pathologic overlap between LBD, AD, and Parkinson disease. Ophthalmologists should be aware of LBD, however, because patients with this syndrome often present with complex (or formed) visual hallucinations. With treatment, patients with LBD can show marked improvements in cognition and behavioral symptoms, as well as fewer hallucinations. Referral to a neurologist or geriatric psychiatrist is warranted if this disease is suspected.

AD is an irreversible, progressive disorder that proceeds in stages, gradually destroying memory, reason, judgment, language, and eventually the ability to carry out even the simplest of tasks. AD is the most common neurodegenerative disorder in the United States, with a lifetime risk of 1 in 5 for women and 1 in 10 for men.

The pathologic hallmarks of AD are extraneuronal amyloid plaques (fragmented brain cells surrounded by amyloid-family proteins) and intraneuronal neurofibrillary tangles (tangles of filaments composed largely of proteins associated with the cytoskeleton). These 2 findings are associated with neuronal death and decreased levels of the neurotransmitter acetylcholine, as well as with abnormalities in other neurotransmitter systems. Signs of neuronal death appear first in the entorhinal cortex and eventually extend into the hippocampus (an area essential for memory storage). As the disease progresses, the basal forebrain and eventually the cerebral cortex become involved.

Etiology

The exact etiology of AD is unknown, but both genetic and environmental factors play a role.

Genetic factors There are 2 types of AD: *familial AD,* which follows a certain inheritance pattern, and *sporadic AD,* in which no inheritance pattern is obvious. AD is further described as *early onset* (occurring in persons younger than 65 years) and *late onset* (occurring in those older than 65 years). Early-onset AD is rare (10% of cases).

There does appear to be a genetic component in the more common form of late-onset AD. Patients who have a first-degree relative with dementia have a 10%–30%-increased risk of developing the disorder. A possible marker for the development of AD is the presence of the ε4 genotype of the protein apolipoprotein E. This protein has many functions, including participation in the transport of cholesterol throughout the body.

Diagnosis

Genetic tests are available for the early-onset, familial form of AD. There is no definitive antemortem diagnostic test for AD other than a brain biopsy. Physicians rely on a variety of methods, including history, physical examination, laboratory tests, brain scans, and assessments of memory, language skills, and other brain functions. Several imaging techniques are useful, and all may have specific uses in helping to diagnose AD or at least in eliminating other causes of dementia.

Treatment

Given the tremendous toll that AD takes on the patient, caregivers, and society, there is great interest in identifying factors that may prevent onset of this disease. Once it is diagnosed, psychosocial issues need to be addressed. Patients and family members must deal with matters such as driving and cooking safety, emotional lability, wandering, and falls. Resources are available to assist patients and their families with these issues, such as the Alzheimer's Association (www.alz.org).

Guidelines for the pharmacologic treatment of dementia have been released on the basis of a systematic review of the evidence for the efficacy of the cholinesterase inhibitors, such as donepezil, and the neuropeptide-modifying agent memantine. Treatment of dementia with these agents can result in benefits that are statistically significant but afford clinically marginal improvement in measures of cognition and global assessment of dementia. According to the guidelines, the current evidence does not support prescribing these medications to every patient with dementia. Clinical studies have not shown that other therapies used to treat dementia are effective, and these therapies remain controversial.

Because AD is associated with decreased brain acetylcholine, anticholinergic medications can make it worse. Worsening of the disease can occur with commonly used medications such as oxybutynin, tricyclic antidepressants, and even over-the-counter cold medications.

Ophthalmic considerations Patients with AD may report vague visual symptoms such as poor vision and reading difficulties. In general, AD does not seem to have any direct pathologic effect on the optic nerve and retina, and these vision problems are caused by disruption of central pathways. Specific findings include spatial contrast sensitivity disturbance, fixation instability, saccadic latency prolongation with hypometric saccades, and saccadic intrusions during smooth pursuit eye movements. Patients with AD can also manifest disorders of higher cortical function, such as visual agnosia and surface dyslexia. Defective motion perception (cerebral akinetopsia) has been described, as has Bálint syndrome (comprising simultanagnosia, which is the inability to recognize 2 or more things at the same time; acquired ocular apraxia; and optic ataxia).

James BD, Leurgans SE, Hebert LE, Scherr PA, Yaffe K, Bennett DA. Contribution of Alzheimer disease to mortality in the United States. *Neurology.* 2014;82(12): 1045–1050.

Pelak VS. Ocular motility of aging and dementia. *Curr Neurol Neurosci Rep.* 2010; 10(6):440–447.

UpToDate; www.uptodate.com.

The authors would like to thank Lindsey Delott, MD, and Kenneth Silk, MD, for their contributions to this chapter.

CHAPTER 12

Preventive Medicine

Recent Developments

- Multiple studies support the life-saving value of mammography in breast cancer screening. The frequency of mammography and other tests should be based on an assessment of the individual patient's risk of breast cancer.
- Screening for colorectal cancer can be accomplished with a number of procedures or through stool testing. Fecal immunochemical testing is more sensitive than guaiac-based fecal occult blood testing.
- More than 99% of all cervical cancers are positive for human papillomavirus (HPV). A vaccine against HPV is now available.
- Tdap (tetanus toxoid, diphtheria, and acellular pertussis vaccine) is recommended for all unvaccinated health care professionals as a means of preventing nosocomial outbreaks of pertussis.
- Hepatitis virus infection is the leading cause of liver disease in the world. Vaccines are available to prevent infection with the hepatitis A and hepatitis B viruses.
- The US Centers for Disease Control and Prevention (CDC) recommends one-time testing for hepatitis C for all persons born in the United States between 1945 and 1965. Many patients are unaware that they have a chronic, asymptomatic infection with the hepatitis C virus.

Screening Procedures

The goal of preventive medicine is not only to reduce premature morbidity and mortality but also to preserve function and quality of life.

Screening techniques can be used both for research and for practical disease prevention or treatment. Screening for nonresearch purposes is useful if the disease in question is

- detectable with some measurable degree of reliability
- treatable or preventable
- significant because of its impact (prevalence or severity)
- progressive
- generally asymptomatic (or has symptoms a patient might deny or might not recognize)

Screening techniques should not be applied to a certain population until the following concerns have been addressed:

- sensitivity and specificity of the test
- convenience and comfort of the test
- cost of finding a problem
- cost of not finding a problem

Cost can and should be measured in both economic and human terms, including the cost of discomfort, losing function, or dying.

The term *sensitivity* describes how often a test result is positive among persons with a target disease. *Specificity* measures the test's ability to exclude truly negative results. *Relative risk* is the probability of a disease based on a specific finding divided by the probability of that disease in the absence of that specific finding. (See Chapter 1 for additional discussion of these terms.)

Screening can be done as a one-time venture or by the sequential application of screening tests. Initially, a more sensitive test is administered; when appropriate, it is followed by a more specific test (which is often more costly or difficult to use). In judging the predictive value of the screens for an individual patient, the physician should account for the patient's clinical history, current medications, and physical examination.

Cardiovascular Diseases

Hypertension

Hypertension affects an estimated 73 million persons aged 20 years and older in the United States, about half of whom have been diagnosed and a third of whom are being treated. Hypertension currently afflicts approximately 1 billion people worldwide. The prevalence of hypertension in many developed countries is approximately 20% of the adult population, and it has reached as high as 29% in the United States. Hypertension in childhood is also becoming a more widely recognized problem.

The consequences of uncontrolled hypertension include significantly increased risk of thrombotic and hemorrhagic stroke, atherosclerotic heart disease, atrial fibrillation, congestive heart failure, left ventricular hypertrophy, aortic aneurysm and dissection, peripheral arterial disease, and renal failure. Approximately 30% of end-stage renal disease is related to hypertension.

Hypertension meets all 5 of the criteria mentioned previously for screening: it is detectable, treatable, highly prevalent, progressively damaging, and characteristically asymptomatic until late in its course. See Chapter 3 for discussion of the classification, evaluation, and pharmacologic treatment of hypertension.

Ram CV. The evolving definition of systemic hypertension. *Am J Cardiol.* 2007;99(8): 1168–1170.

Atherosclerotic cardiovascular disease

In the United States, atherosclerosis is responsible for approximately half of all deaths and for one-third of deaths between 35 and 65 years of age. Three-fourths of deaths related to atherosclerosis are from *coronary artery disease (CAD)*. Atherosclerosis is the leading cause of permanent disability and accounts for more hospital days than any other illness.

The rationale for early screening emerged when it was shown that reducing risk factors reduces the incidence of coronary disease events. For further discussion on identifying and modifying cardiovascular risk factors, see Chapter 4.

Screening for significant coronary artery atherosclerosis is more expensive and time-consuming than screening for associated reversible risk factors. In general, it is reasonable to screen for a history of cardiovascular symptoms and events (chest pain, dyspnea, syncope, arrhythmias, claudication, stroke) and reserve more specific testing (eg, exercise stress testing, cardiac computed tomography [CT] or magnetic resonance imaging [MRI]) for those in higher-risk categories.

Cancer

In women, the most common cancers are lung, breast, and colorectal. In men, they are lung, prostate, and colorectal. The types of cancer most amenable to screening are cervical cancer, breast cancer, urologic cancer, lung cancer, colorectal cancer, and melanoma. Table 12-1 shows a set of recommendations for early cancer detection. See also Chapter 13.

Siegel R, Naishadham D, Jemal A. Cancer statistics, 2013. *CA Cancer J Clin.* 2013;63(1):11–30.

Smith RA, Brooks D, Cokkinides V, Saslow D, Brawley OW. Cancer screening in the United States, 2013: a review of current American Cancer Society guidelines, current issues in cancer screening, and new guidance on cervical cancer screening and lung cancer screening. *CA Cancer J Clin.* 2013;63(2):88–105.

Cervical cancer

Cervical cancer is the most common gynecologic cancer in patients who are between 15 and 34 years of age. Overall, approximately 12,000 cases of invasive cancer of the cervix (about 4000 resulting in death) and 45,000 cases of carcinoma in situ occur each year in the United States. Approximately 86% of the 530,000 cervical cancer cases diagnosed worldwide each year occur in developing countries. Despite advances in the treatment of cervical cancer, approximately half the women with the disease will die. Cervical cancer is the eighth most common cause of cancer mortality in the United States. The incidence of cervical cancer in the nations of the European Union (EU) varies widely, with the highest incidence in Romania and the lowest in Finland. As of 2013, screening for cervical cancer is recommended in 15 EU countries.

The risk factors for cervical cancer are the number of lifetime sexual partners, the presence of high-risk serotypes of HPV, low socioeconomic status, positive smoking history, use of corticosteroid contraceptive hormones, and a history of other sexually transmitted diseases. More than 99% of all cervical cancers are positive for HPV. Early detection and appropriate treatment markedly reduce the morbidity and mortality from invasive cancer of the cervix. In many developed countries, mortality has been reduced by more than 50% by implementation of cytologic screening. Cervical cancer is asymptomatic when it occurs in situ, and the most effective screening technique remains the Papanicolaou test ("Pap smear"). HPV can be detected with polymerase chain reaction assay techniques, and patients aged 30–65 years should consider receiving HPV testing at the time of their

Table 12-1 American Cancer Society Recommendations for Early Cancer Detection in Asymptomatic Adult Patients, 2013

	Population		
Test or Procedure, by Cancer Type	**Sex**	**Age, Years**	**Frequency**
Colorectal			
Digital rectal examination	M, F	>50	Annually
Fecal immunochemical or DNA test	M, F	>50	Annually
AND one of the following:			
Colonoscopy	M, F	>50	Every 10 years if patient not high risk
CT colonography	M, F	>50	Every 5 years
Double-contrast barium enema	M, F	>50	Every 5 years
Sigmoidoscopy	M, F	>50	Every 5 years
Cervical			
Papanicolaou test	F	21–65; <20, if sexually active	Every 3 years; consider HPV testing every 5 years
Pelvic examination	F	20–40	Every 3 years
		>40	Annually
Endometrial			
Endometrial tissue sample	F	Women at high risk*	When indicated
Breast			
Breast self-examination	F	>20	Monthly (now considered optional)
Clinical breast examination	F	20–40	Every 3 years
		>40	Annually
Mammography	F	>40	Baseline, then annually
Prostate			
Serum PSA and rectal examination	M	>50	Discuss risks/benefits of testing
		Men at high risk†	Annually for high-risk patients
Lung			
Low-dose helical CT	M, F	55–74, smoker	Annually if patient identified as high risk
General			
Health counseling and cancer checkup‡	M, F	>20	At time of general checkup

CT = computed tomography; HPV = human papillomavirus; PSA = prostate specific antigen.
*History of infertility, obesity, failure to ovulate, abnormal uterine bleeding, or use of estrogen therapy.
†Positive family history of prostate cancer.
‡To include examination for cancers of the thyroid, testis, prostate, ovary, lymph nodes, oral region, and skin.

Papanicolaou test ("dual testing"). Vaccines to prevent HPV infection and its sequelae are discussed later in this chapter.

Cuzick J, Arbyn M, Sankaranarayanan R, et al. Overview of human papillomavirus-based and other novel options for cervical cancer screening in developed and developing countries. *Vaccine.* 2008;26(Suppl 10):K29–K41.

Moyer VA, US Preventive Services Task Force. Screening for cervical cancer: US Preventive Services Task Force recommendation statement. *Ann Intern Med.* 2012;156(12):880–891.

Breast cancer

Though now surpassed by lung cancer as the most common cause of death in women older than 40 years, breast cancer remains the most common malignancy in women. The overall prevalence of breast cancer in the United States is 10%–12%. The age-adjusted incidence of breast cancer declined by 6.7% in 2003 (12% decline in women older than 50 years). This decrease was mostly due to a 50% reduction in the use of hormone replacement therapy. Nevertheless, 235,000 new cases of breast cancer and more than 40,000 related deaths are projected for the United States alone for 2013. More than 75% of all breast cancers are cured with current therapy.

The importance of specific screening is increased by the presence of known risk factors, all of which are identifiable by history: (1) first-degree relative with breast cancer, (2) prior breast cancer, (3) nulliparity, (4) first pregnancy after age 30, and (5) early menarche or late menopause. Additional risk factors are high breast density, elevated serum estrogen or testosterone levels, high-fat diet, obesity, and sedentary lifestyle.

Hormone replacement therapy (HRT) with estrogen and progesterone was associated with an increased risk of invasive breast cancer and abnormal mammograms in the Women's Health Initiative, a US National Institutes of Health randomized trial. In the same trial, postmenopausal hormone therapy was also associated with an increased risk of venous thromboembolism, stroke, and coronary heart disease.

Approximately 42% of breast cancers detectable by mammography are not detectable by physical examination alone, and one-third of those found by mammographic screening are noninvasive or less than 1 cm in size if invasive. Because mammograms can yield false-negative results, the best detection strategy involves a physical examination plus mammography, with fine-needle aspiration or biopsy if either reveals an abnormality. Mammography has been shown to be safe as well as effective, and the current low-dose radiation associated with it does not increase the risk of radiation-induced cancer. Clinical breast examination and counseling are recommended every 3 years for women who are 20 through 40 years of age with an average risk of breast cancer, and annually after age 40 years. Mammographic screening, according to a recent recommendation by the US Preventive Services Task Force, should be performed every 2 years for average-risk women aged 50–75 years, and screening should be discussed with women from age 40 years. The American Cancer Society continues to recommend yearly mammography after age 40 years. In addition to general screening recommendations, assessment tools are available that estimate an individual patient's risk of breast cancer, an example of which is the Breast Cancer Risk Assessment Tool (www.cancer.gov/bcrisktool/). While the ideal mammographic screening interval is not clear, the American Cancer Society and US Preventive Services Task Force recommendations, as well as results of large studies done in the United Kingdom and Europe (EUROSCREEN), continue to support the life-saving value of mammography.

Other modalities available for breast cancer screening include ultrasonography, digital mammography, and MRI. Because MRI of the breast is more sensitive but less specific than other methods, it should be used primarily in high-risk younger patients. Women with known mutations in the breast cancer 1 gene *(BRCA1)* or *BRCA2* gene are at increased risk for breast and ovarian cancer and require more intensive counseling and surveillance, including yearly mammography and breast MRI.

Pace LE, He Y, Keating NL. Trends in mammography screening rates after publication of the 2009 US Preventive Services Task Force recommendations. *Cancer.* 2013;119(14): 2518–2523.

Urologic cancer

The prostate, bladder, kidney, and testes yield approximately 16% of new cancer cases per year in the United States, with most of the common malignancies in middle-aged and older men. Approximately 230,000 new cases of prostate cancer and nearly 40,000 related deaths occur each year in the United States. Prostate cancer can be detected early by digital examination of the prostate and by measurement of serum prostate-specific antigen (PSA). Serum PSA screening remains controversial, and data suggest that it does not affect mortality. The PSA false-negative rate varies between 15% and 38%, and only about 30% of patients with elevated PSA levels truly have prostate carcinoma. A trend of increasing PSA levels is a more sensitive indicator of prostate cancer than is an individual elevated PSA level. Because of the high rate of false-negatives, minimal disease identified by PSA screening, and the potentially significant adverse effects of treating minimal disease, the US Preventive Services Task Force has recommended individualized discussion of the risks and benefits of prostate cancer screening. Routine yearly serum PSA screening is no longer recommended except for higher-risk individuals, such as those with a positive family history of prostate cancer.

Although prostate cancer is a potentially lethal illness, many detectable prostate cancers are of little threat to life. Some men with low-grade prostate cancer receive curative treatment, even though their disease may not require treatment. Some studies suggest that more than 75% of men with screen-detected localized disease may not even need treatment. More specific screening methods are needed to allow differentiation between lethal and nonlethal cancers.

Moyer VA, US Preventive Services Task Force. Screening for prostate cancer: US Preventive Services Task Force recommendation statement. *Ann Intern Med.* 2012;157(2):120–134.

Lung cancer

Lung cancer is the leading cause of cancer-related deaths in adults in the United States. Worldwide, there were 1.4 million deaths due to lung cancer in 2008. Among male patients with lung cancer in the United States, 85% are smokers. The number and percentage of cases in women have risen with the increased incidence of smoking in women. The usefulness of chest radiography and sputum cytologic screening in the general population is generally considered to be low. In high-risk patient groups, screening protocols effect a higher yield and may include sputum cytology, low-dose helical chest CT (with possible fine-needle aspiration for suspicious lesions), and bronchoscopy with possible endobronchial biopsy. In the US National Lung Screening Trial, lung cancer mortality in high-risk patients decreased when these patients were screened annually with low-dose helical chest CT. Fluorescent bronchoscopy is a promising tool for identifying early malignant changes in the central airways; positron emission tomography may also be useful for this purpose. New molecular markers detected in sputum and serum show promise in the future of lung cancer screening. Prevention through smoking cessation remains the most effective way to decrease lung cancer mortality.

Bach PB, Mirkin JN, Oliver TK, et al. Benefits and harms of CT screening for lung cancer: a systematic review. *JAMA*. 2012;307(22):2418–2429.

Gastrointestinal cancer

The primary risk factors for squamous cell carcinoma of the esophagus are tobacco use and alcohol consumption, accounting for 80%–90% of cases of this type. The main risk factors for adenocarcinoma of the esophagus are gastroesophageal reflux disease (GERD), obesity, and history of Barrett esophagus. Treatment has poor results; thus, prevention or elimination of the risk factors is worthwhile. The incidence of adenocarcinoma of the esophagus is increasing in developed countries, but squamous cell carcinoma remains dominant in developing areas. Currently, no effective preventive screening programs are available, and most patients present with advanced or metastatic disease. Barrett esophagus is a complication of long-standing gastroesophageal reflux disease and is the premalignant condition for the majority of esophageal adenocarcinomas.

Gastric cancer appears to be associated with certain geographic areas (Japan, China, Central and South America, Eastern Europe, and parts of the Middle East), high ingestion of nitrates, loss of gastric acidity, lower socioeconomic status, and blood type A. It remains the second most frequent and lethal malignancy worldwide. Although routine endoscopic screening is not cost-effective, widespread screening for and treatment of *Helicobacter pylori* infection in high-incidence populations could be an effective strategy for reducing gastric cancer in these groups. Further testing is recommended only for high-risk groups.

Pancreatic cancer is 2–3 times more common in heavy smokers than in nonsmokers, and it has also been associated with chronic pancreatitis, diabetes mellitus, and obesity. Familial pancreatic cancer represents only about 5%–10% of all cases but carries a higher mortality than sporadic pancreatic cancer. Several genetic mutations have been identified that are responsible for a small percentage of familial cases.

Hepatocellular cancer is more common in persons with preexisting liver disease, especially cirrhosis and hepatitis C.

Colorectal cancer

Colorectal cancer is a major killer in developed countries, second only to lung cancer in incidence and mortality. The cumulative lifetime probability of developing colon cancer is roughly 6%, with a 3% probability of dying of this disease. The chance for survival 5 years after diagnosis remains only 40%, despite the optimistic theory that early detection would lead to curative surgery.

Most authorities accept the theory that colorectal cancer develops from an initially benign polyp in a mitotic process that occurs over 5–10 years. Colonoscopic removal or ablation of all polyps has become the standard of care where facilities and trained personnel are available. Factors associated with a higher risk of development of colon cancer include increased size and number of polyps, high-grade dysplasia or villous features on biomicroscopy, and sessile polyps only partially removed during a previous colonoscopy. Increased dietary fiber intake and reduced dietary fat intake have been associated with reduced risk of colorectal cancer. Also, calcium supplementation is associated with a moderate reduction in the risk of recurrent colorectal adenomas.

Detection must be improved with more widespread use of screening studies such as the fecal occult blood test (FOBT), fecal immunochemical test (FIT), flexible sigmoidoscopy, double-contrast barium enema, and colonoscopy, with aggressive follow-up of patients with positive test results. It is estimated that widespread adoption of these recommendations could reduce the mortality rate of colorectal cancer by more than 50%. Another stool-based method, fecal DNA testing, can detect molecular tumor markers associated with colorectal cancer. It is easier to use and more sensitive than FOBT, so patient adherence may be better. Unfortunately, no fecal DNA testing systems are currently approved by the Food and Drug Administration in the United States.

Flexible sigmoidoscopy (every 5 years) and home FOBT (annually) have been recommended in asymptomatic adults between 50 and 75 years of age. Recommendations remain controversial because of a lack of randomized trials. Sigmoidoscopy offers good specificity but misses proximal cancers. Home guaiac-based FOBT has been shown to decrease the mortality rate of colon cancer by up to 40%. For this test, 3 FOBT cards are completed at home; a single FOBT at the time of an annual physical examination is not sufficient. FIT appears to be more sensitive and more patient-friendly than guaiac-based FOBT and is now recommended by the American Cancer Society.

Colonoscopy as a screening test for asymptomatic patients older than 50 years has been increasingly used. When results are negative, the test is repeated every 10 years in low-risk patients. Many of the lesions discovered with colonoscopy would not be detected with sigmoidoscopy. Yearly colonoscopy has been advocated in populations at very high risk, such as patients with familial polyposis and first-degree relatives of patients with colon cancer. The disadvantages of colonoscopy are the increased cost, the number of trained personnel required, and the risks of intravenous sedation and colonic perforation (approximately 0.2%). CT colonography is also available as a screening tool. It may offer the ability to screen out patients without neoplasia, thus allowing colonoscopy to be reserved for patients with significant lesions, and may be preferable in patients not healthy enough for colonoscopy. For persons older than 50 years, current American Cancer Society guidelines recommend a combination of FIT or DNA testing and one of the following procedures: CT colonography, colonoscopy, double-contrast barium enema, or sigmoidoscopy. The European Council currently recommends only FOBT between the ages of 50 and 74 years, and 12 EU member states recommended this screening to their populace in 2013.

Deenadayalu VP, Rex DK. Fecal-based DNA assays: a new, noninvasive approach to colorectal cancer screening. *Cleve Clin J Med.* 2004;71(6):497–503.

Lansdorp-Vogelaar I, von Karsa L; International Agency for Research on Cancer. European guidelines for quality assurance in colorectal cancer screening and diagnosis. First Edition—Introduction. *Endoscopy.* 2012;44(Suppl 3):SE15–30.

Melanoma

Melanoma is the most deadly form of skin cancer, and its incidence is increasing faster than that of all other cancers. In the United States, about 1 in 75 persons will develop melanoma during his or her lifetime. According to the American Cancer Society, an estimated 76,690 new melanoma cases and 9480 related deaths were predicted in the United States in 2013.

Most melanomas probably arise from dysplastic nevi. Risk factors for melanoma include history of melanoma or atypical moles, presence of more than 75–100 moles, positive melanoma family history, history of previous nonmelanoma skin cancer, giant congenital nevus (>20 cm), xeroderma pigmentosum, treatment with UV-A and psoralens, frequent tanning with UV-A light, and a history of 3 or more severe (blistering) sunburns. Other, less significant risk factors are light complexion of the hair and eyes, freckles, inability to tan, indoor occupation with outdoor hobbies, and proximity to the equator.

UV damage probably causes most melanomas. Intense intermittent exposures are directly related to melanoma, whereas other skin cancers are more associated with cumulative exposure. UV radiation causes DNA damage, which is usually corrected by DNA repair enzymes; however, these DNA repair processes degrade with increasing age.

A pigmented lesion with any of the following characteristics, easily remembered by the *ABCDE* mnemonic, is suggestive of melanoma: *a*symmetrical lesions, *b*order (irregular), *c*olor (variable), *d*iameter (>6 mm), and *e*volving (change in size, shape, or color). Other characteristics suggestive of melanoma are pruritus, bleeding, changing morphology, and new lesions or scalp lesions. Everyone should perform self–skin examinations every 1 or 2 months; suspicious lesions require referral to a dermatologist and possible biopsy. Avoiding the sun during peak hours and using sunblock can reduce the risk of melanoma and other skin cancers. In addition to providing simple visualization, dermoscopy (epiluminescence microscopy) can increase the specificity of clinical examination for the detection of melanomas.

What are the key statistics about melanoma skin cancer? American Cancer Society website. Last medical review: 10/29/2013. www.cancer.org. Accessed August 24, 2014.

Infectious Diseases

The major public health screening efforts in the United States have been for tuberculosis and sexually transmitted diseases. Hepatitis screening is used primarily for blood donation, institutionalized populations, and health care workers rather than for the general population. These disorders are discussed in more detail in Chapter 14.

Tuberculosis

One-third of the world's population is infected with *Mycobacterium tuberculosis (TB)*. The prevalence of TB has recently increased in the United States, reversing decades of steady decline. Thus, TB skin testing should be performed in high-risk groups, and positive results should prompt chest radiography and consideration of chemoprophylaxis. Some experts advocate regular skin testing of all persons younger than 35 years at the time of routine health examination (for detection as well as for baseline data). The US Occupational Safety and Health Administration recommends that all health care facilities conduct a TB risk assessment, with testing performed if indicated; routine testing is no longer recommended. In addition to TB skin testing, an interferon-gamma release assay can be used to screen for TB exposure. This blood test may be more specific in some clinical situations. While acid-fast smears and histopathology remain the most common approach for confirming a diagnosis of TB, a number of nucleic acid amplification assays are also now available.

Several candidate vaccines for TB are currently being developed; they include subunit; DNA; microbial vector; and live, attenuated vaccines.

Hoft DF, Blazevic A, Abate G, et al. A new recombinant bacille Calmette-Guérin vaccine safely induces significantly enhanced tuberculosis-specific immunity in human volunteers. *J Infect Dis.* 2008;198(10):1491–1501.

Syphilis

Syphilis is almost always transmitted sexually; congenital disease transmitted in utero is now rare. In fact, the incidence of congenital syphilis has dropped 90% since the 1940s because of required premarital screening and pregnancy screening. Better prenatal care and increased syphilis screening during pregnancy improve the likelihood of detecting infants at risk for congenital syphilis, thus allowing early maternal treatment.

Latent, untreated cases of syphilis in which the primary or secondary mucocutaneous lesion is no longer present can be detected only by screening. It is important to detect early latent disease: in approximately 25% of cases, infectious mucocutaneous lesions reemerge spontaneously in the first 2 years. Late latent disease should be detected and treated because of the long-term destructive effects on the central nervous system, the aorta, and the skeletal system.

Screening is generally performed with the more sensitive, but less specific, nontreponemal antigen tests (VDRL, RPR, TRUST). Positive results are then confirmed with treponemal antigen tests (FTA-ABS, MHA-TP, TP-PA, TP-EIA), which are more expensive.

Miller R, Karras DJ. Commentary. Update on emerging infections: news from the Centers for Disease Control and Prevention. Congenital syphilis—United States 2003–2008. *Ann Emerg Med.* 2010;56(3):296–297.

Immunization

The development of immunization as a means of preventing the spread of infectious disease began in 1796, when Edward Jenner injected cowpox virus, which causes a mild disease, into a child to prevent smallpox, a severe, potentially fatal illness. Immunization today still relies on Jenner's inoculation methods to protect against disease. There are 2 types: active and passive.

In *active immunization,* the recipient develops an acquired immune response to inactivated or killed viruses, viral subtractions, bacterial toxoids or antigens, or synthetic vaccines. Once the immune response to a particular pathogen has developed, it protects the host against infection. The persistence of acquired immunity depends on the perpetuation of cell strains responsive to the target antigenic stimulus, and booster inoculations may be required for certain immunogens.

In general, live, attenuated vaccines produce longer-lasting immunity; however, they are contraindicated in immunocompromised persons or pregnant women because the pathogen can potentially replicate in the host. Ideally, active immunization should be completed before exposure; however, life-saving postexposure immunity can be developed through combining active and passive immunization.

The recommended US immunization schedules for the year 2012, developed by the Advisory Committee on Immunization Practices—including immunization schedules for persons aged 0–18 years, the catch-up schedule for ages 4 months–18 years, and the adult schedule—can be found on the CDC website (www.cdc.gov/vaccines/schedules/index.html). The catch-up protocols are for children who have missed some of the recommended immunization doses.

Passive immunization depends on the transfer of immunoglobulin in serum from a host with active immunity to a susceptible host. Passive immunity does not result in active immunity and sometimes even blocks the development of active immunity. Passive immunity is short-lived and without immune memory; however, it confers immediate protection on the recipient who has been exposed to the pathogen. Pooled human globulin, antitoxins, and human globulin with high antibody titers for specific diseases are the usual products available for passive immunization.

Immunization should be avoided in persons who have allergic reactions to the vaccine or its components. Idiopathic autoantibody or cross-reacting antibody development may occur after vaccination, resulting in systemic disease such as Guillain-Barré syndrome, a rare but devastating complication of vaccination. Immunization should be avoided during a febrile illness. Multidose immunization schedules that are interrupted can be resumed; however, doses given outside the schedule should not be counted toward completion of the vaccination sequence.

For patients who are pregnant, immunization against tetanus, diphtheria, and influenza is indicated; immunization against other diseases (hepatitis, pneumococcal or meningococcal disease) is indicated if a patient is at high risk of exposure. Additional immunizations may be considered but must be weighed against rare potential risks to the fetus.

The following sections are based on the more extensive recommended immunization schedules in the United States. In other parts of the world, immunizations are done based on World Health Organization (WHO) guidelines, national programs, or recommendations by multinational organizations such as the European Centre for Disease Prevention and Control (ECDC). As a general rule, national immunization schedules for children are quite similar, and recommended immunizations for adults vary widely between countries (see Table 12-2 for a sampling). For more information on the immunization schedules of EU nations, see the ECDC website (vaccine-schedule.ecdc.europa.eu/Pages/Scheduler.aspx).

ACIP Adult Immunization Work Group, Bridges CB, Woods L, Coyne-Beasley T; Centers for Disease Control and Prevention (CDC). Advisory committee on immunization practices (ACIP) recommended immunization schedule for adults aged 19 years and older—United States, 2013. *MMWR Surveill Summ.* 2013;62 Suppl 1:9–19.

ACIP Childhood/Adolescent Immunization Work Group, Akinsanya-Beysolow I, Jenkins R, Meissner HC; Centers for Disease Control and Prevention (CDC). Advisory Committee on Immunization Practices (ACIP) recommended immunization schedule for persons aged 0 through 18 years—United States, 2013. *MMWR Surveill Summ.* 2013;62 Suppl 1:2–8.

Chlibek R, Anca I, André F, et al. Adult vaccination in 11 Central European countries—calendars are not just for children. *Vaccine.* 2012;30(9):1529–1540.

McLean HQ, Fiebelkorn AP, Temte JL, Wallace GS; Centers for Disease Control and Prevention. Prevention of measles, rubella, congenital rubella syndrome, and mumps, 2013: summary recommendations of the Advisory Committee on Immunization Practices (ACIP). *MMWR Recomm Rep.* 2013;62(RR-04):1–34.

Table 12-2 National Adult Immunization Recommendations: A Sampling*

Vaccine	United States	United Kingdom	Finland	Germany	France	Spain
Influenza	Annually ≥18 years	Annually ≥65 years	Annually ≥65 years	Annually >60 years	Annually >65 years	Annually >65 years
Tetanus, diphtheria	Tdap once 19–64 years of age, then Td booster	Catch-up only	Tetanus and diphtheria boosters	Tetanus and diphtheria boosters	Tetanus and diphtheria boosters	Tetanus and diphtheria boosters
Pertussis	Pertussis as Tdap	Expectant mothers	Pertussis by age 15 years	Once as adult	Once as adult	–
Human papillomavirus (HPV)	Males and females, 3 doses	Females only	–	Females only	Females only	Females only
Zoster	1 dose, ≥60 years	1 dose, >70 years	–	–	–	–
Measles/mumps/rubella (MMR)	1–2 doses	Catch-up only	–	Catch-up only	Catch-up only	–
Pneumococcal	1 dose, >65 years	1 dose, >65 years	1 dose, >50 years	1 dose, >60 years	–	–

Td = tetanus and diphtheria toxoid vaccine; Tdap = tetanus toxoid, diphtheria, and acellular pertussis vaccine.

*Recommendations as of June 23, 2014.

Data from the European Centre for Disease Prevention and Control website, vaccine-schedule.ecdc.europa.eu/Pages/Scheduler.aspx. Accessed June 23, 2014.

Hepatitis

Infection with hepatitis A virus (HAV) is the leading cause of viral hepatitis in the United States. HAV is usually transmitted orally and may be acquired from contaminated water supplies and unwashed or undercooked foods. Vaccination against HAV infection is recommended for children aged 12–23 months and for persons at high risk of exposure to HAV (travelers to endemic areas, military personnel, drug abusers, family contacts of infected patients, laboratory workers exposed to the virus). Two preparations are available in the United States (Vaqta, Havrix), each consisting of viral antigens purified from human cell cultures.

Approximately 250,000 cases of hepatitis B occur annually in the United States. Between 6% and 10% of adult patients with hepatitis B become carriers, and chronic active hepatitis occurs in 25% of these carriers. Of the patients with chronic active disease, 20% will die of cirrhosis and 5% will die of hepatocellular carcinoma. Worldwide, 400 million persons are chronic carriers.

In the United States, the available recombinant vaccines based on hepatitis B virus (HBV) surface antigen are Engerix-B and Recombivax HB. In adults, HBV vaccine is usually administered in a series of 3 doses, with the second and third occurring 1 and 6 months after the initial injection. On this regimen, 90% of recipients develop protective antibody levels, which persist for at least 3 years. The recombinant vaccine can also be given on an accelerated dosing schedule, which requires vaccination at 0, 1, and 2 months followed by a booster dose at 12 months. Antibody levels that are greater than 10 milli-international units (mIU) per milliliter are considered to be adequate protection. Booster injections are advised for persons whose antibody levels are less than 10 mIU/mL. A second vaccination results in the development of protective antibodies in 50% of the nonresponders.

Vaccination before exposure to HBV is recommended and cost-effective for all infants and children and for certain high-risk groups: health care workers, hemodialysis patients, residents and staff of chronic care facilities, household and sexual contacts of chronic carriers of HBV, hemophiliacs, users of illicit injectable drugs, prison inmates, sexually active homosexual men, and HIV-seropositive patients. Vaccination can be combined with passive immunization for postexposure prophylaxis without affecting the development of active immunity. The incorporation of the vaccine into childhood immunization schedules has resulted in a decrease in the number of new hepatitis B cases reported annually, and there has also been a significant reduction in the number of hepatocellular carcinoma cases reported in children. Combination vaccines are available that protect against not only hepatitis B, but also hepatitis A, diphtheria, pertussis, tetanus, and polio.

Postexposure prophylaxis with hepatitis B immunoglobulin should be considered when there is accidental percutaneous or permucosal exposure to blood positive for HBV surface antigen, perinatal exposure of an infant born to a carrier, or sexual exposure (within 14 days) to a carrier of HBV. Hepatitis B immunoglobulin should be given as soon as possible after exposure in a single intramuscular dose of 0.06 mL/kg body weight; the recombinant HBV vaccine should be concurrently administered in an accelerated dosing schedule.

Lamivudine is a nucleoside analogue inhibitor of reverse transcriptase and was initially developed for the treatment of HIV infection. Interferon and lamivudine have been found to be very effective against HBV and are considered the drugs of choice for the treatment of patients with chronic HBV infection. Drugs such as adefovir, entecavir, telbivudine, and tenofovir are also effective, especially in cases of resistance to lamivudine.

Hepatitis C is the leading indication for liver transplantation in the United States. The CDC has recommended that all adults in the United States born between 1945 and 1965 have a one-time test for hepatitis C. Early intervention in chronically infected individuals, including treatment and alcohol counseling, can slow the progression of disease. Vaccines against hepatitis C and E are being developed. See Chapter 14 for additional discussion of hepatitis C and other forms of the hepatitis virus.

Smith BD, Morgan RL, Beckett GA, Falck-Ytter Y, Holtzman D, Ward JW. Hepatitis C virus testing of persons born during 1945–1965: recommendations from the Centers for Disease Control and Prevention. *Ann Intern Med.* 2012;157(11):817–822.

Influenza

Although influenza is usually a self-limited disease with rare sequelae, it can be associated with severe morbidity and mortality in older persons or those with chronic diseases. Influenza vaccines produce long-lasting immunity. However, antigenic shifts, primarily in type A rather than type B influenza virus, require yearly reformulation of the vaccine to contain the antigens of strains considered most likely to cause disease. Protection is correlated with the development of antihemagglutinin and antineuraminidase antibodies, which decrease the patient's susceptibility and the severity of the disease. The influenza vaccine is as effective in HIV-seropositive patients as it is in HIV-seronegative patients, regardless of $CD4^{+}$ T-cell counts. In the United States, annual vaccination is recommended for all adults and for children older than 6 months. The influenza vaccine is well tolerated, and there has been no increased risk of neurologic complications with the vaccines administered after 1991. Trivalent and quadrivalent *inactivated influenza vaccines (IIVs)* are available, as well as an intranasal *live, attenuated influenza vaccine (LAIV)* (FluMist). Pregnant women may safely receive the IIV. Health care workers working with severely immunocompromised patients should receive the IIV. Healthy nonpregnant persons younger than 50 years who have no other contraindications may receive the IIV or LAIV. These influenza vaccines should not be administered to persons with anaphylactic hypersensitivity to eggs, but new vaccines manufactured using cell culture (Flucelvax) or recombinant DNA technology (Flublok) may be used. A high-dose vaccine for patients older than 65 years (Fluzone high dose) is also available. Antiviral agents such as zanamivir and oseltamivir were initially very active against influenza types A and B, for prophylaxis as well as treatment. Unfortunately, significant resistance has emerged to these and other agents.

Varicella-Zoster

Varivax, an approved live, attenuated varicella-zoster vaccine, is recommended in the United States for immunocompetent pediatric patients older than 12 months with no history of previous infection with varicella-zoster virus (VZV). A second dose is given between 4 and 6 years of age. For patients older than 12 years, 2 doses of vaccine are given 4–8 weeks apart. Also, health care workers who have not been exposed to chickenpox (varicella) should be vaccinated. Varivax is safe and provides immunity for up to 20 years. Data from the CDC confirmed a dramatic decline in the incidence of varicella in the United States (87%) from 1995 to 2000.

Zostavax, a live, attenuated vaccine given as a single dose, is recommended for adults aged 60 years and older to reduce the risk of developing clinical zoster and postherpetic neuralgia. This vaccine reduces the risk of VZV infection by 50%–70%. Zostavax may not be used in place of Varivax in younger persons. Also see Chapter 14.

Measles

Vaccination has dramatically reduced the incidence of measles, along with associated encephalitis and mortality. Introduced in 1963, the initial vaccine was based on an inactivated virus that did not provide a long duration of protection. In 1967, a live, attenuated vaccine providing long-lasting immunity was introduced. Vaccination with the attenuated strain should be routine not only at age 15 months but also for persons born between 1957 and 1967 who were neither vaccinated nor infected and for persons who received the inactivated viral vaccine. Individuals born before 1957 are considered immune by virtue of natural infection. The vaccine is contraindicated for persons with allergy or previous anaphylactic reaction to gelatin or neomycin but is safe for patients with hypersensitivity to eggs. Measles-mumps-rubella (MMR) vaccination is recommended for all children and is usually given at about age 15 months and again between ages 4 and 6. The preservative thimerosal is no longer used in this vaccine, and multiple studies have refuted previous concerns about an association between MMR vaccines and autism. For nonimmunized persons exposed to measles, postexposure prophylaxis with immunoglobulin should be given within 72 hours if at all possible, or within 6 days.

Mumps

The number of reported cases of mumps in the United States has decreased steadily since the introduction of a live mumps vaccine in 1967. Although mumps is generally self-limited, meningeal signs may appear in up to 15% of cases and orchitis in up to 20% of clinical cases in postpubertal males. Other possible complications include permanent deafness and pancreatitis. Mumps vaccination is indicated for all children and susceptible adults, such as child care workers. Revaccination should be considered for patients who originally received only a single dose of the vaccine, particularly students entering college, health care workers, and those traveling to endemic areas.

Rubella

Rubella immunization is intended to prevent fetal infection and consequent congenital rubella syndrome, which can occur in up to 80% of fetuses of mothers infected during the first trimester of pregnancy. The number of reported cases of rubella in the United States has decreased steadily from more than 56,000 in 1969, the year rubella vaccine was licensed, to 10 cases in 2005. Rubella was declared eliminated from the United States in 2004, and from the Americas in 2010, although rare outbreaks still occur elsewhere in the world.

Rubella vaccine is recommended for adults, particularly women, unless proof of immunity is available (documented rubella vaccination on or after the first birthday or a positive serologic test result) or the vaccine is specifically contraindicated. A single subcutaneously administered dose of live, attenuated rubella vaccine provides long-term (probably lifetime) immunity in approximately 95% of persons vaccinated. Because of the theoretical risk to the fetus, women of childbearing age should receive the vaccine only if they are not pregnant.

Polio

Before the introduction of the first polio vaccine in 1955, polio (poliomyelitis) caused thousands of cases of paralysis. Despite widespread immunization with oral vaccine since 1962, polio persists in some nations in Asia and Africa. There are 2 forms of the vaccine: an oral form containing live, attenuated poliovirus (oral poliovirus vaccine [OPV], Sabin vaccine); and an injectable form containing killed virus (inactivated poliovirus vaccine [IPV], Salk vaccine), which is administered subcutaneously. To eliminate the risk of vaccine-associated paralytic poliomyelitis, a condition that has been associated more often with OPV than with IPV, IPV is used in the United States. Because OPV is cheaper and easier to distribute and because it transmits the virus to unimmunized contacts of those who are vaccinated, helping the former develop immunity, the WHO suggests that OPV be used for immunization in developing countries. OPV is contraindicated in pregnant women, who should receive only the inactivated virus vaccine.

Tetanus and Diphtheria

The combined tetanus and diphtheria toxoid vaccine (Td) is highly effective; it is used for both primary and booster immunization of adults. The pediatric vaccine, diphtheria-tetanus-pertussis (DTP), has been replaced with the newer pediatric vaccine, DTaP (diphtheria and tetanus toxoid with acellular pertussis). Tdap, which contains a lower concentration of diphtheria toxoid and acellular pertussis than does DTaP, is recommended in the United States as a one-time booster for all adults aged 19–64 years, and particularly for all health care professionals and anyone caring for infants younger than 12 months. Young adults should also receive a booster dose of Td every 10 years. If serious doubt exists about the completion of a primary series of immunization, 2 doses of 0.5 mL of the combined toxoids should be given intramuscularly at monthly intervals, followed by a third dose 6–10 months later. Thereafter, a booster dose of 0.5 mL should be given at 10-year intervals.

In wound management of tetanus, previously immunized persons with severe wounds should receive a booster if more than 5 years has elapsed since the last injection. The management of previously unimmunized patients with severe wounds should include tetanus immunoglobulin as well as Td. Although tetanus is uncommon, more than 60% of cases occur in persons older than 60 years. Therefore, older adults should be given a single booster at age 65.

Pneumococcal Pneumonia

Pneumococcal pneumonia is the most serious and prevalent of the community-acquired respiratory tract infections. Although pneumococcal disease affects children and adults, the incidence of pneumococcal pneumonia increases in persons older than 40 years. Pneumococci that are resistant to penicillin have emerged since 1974. The mortality rate from bacteremic pneumococcal infection exceeds 25% despite treatment with antibiotics.

The current unconjugated pneumococcal vaccine contains polysaccharide antigens from 23 of the types of *Streptococcus pneumoniae* most commonly found in bacteremic pneumococcal disease. The 23-valent pneumococcal polysaccharide vaccine (PPSV23) has been designed to induce a protective level of serum antibodies in immunocompetent adults and is highly effective in healthy young adults; however, its effectiveness in older persons and those in poor health has not been precisely determined. Nevertheless, the vaccine is well tolerated and is recommended in many countries for older adults, for patients with cardiac or respiratory disease, and for patients who are at high risk for pneumococcal infection, including those with sickle cell disease, splenic dysfunction, renal and hepatic disease, or immunodeficiency. The duration of protection afforded by primary vaccination with pneumococcal vaccine seems to be 9 years or more. Those who receive pneumococcal vaccine before age 65 years should be revaccinated at age 65 if more than 5 years has passed since the initial vaccination.

A pneumococcal conjugate vaccine (PCV) is recommended in the United States for all children younger than 5 years. It is administered in 4 intramuscular doses at 2, 4, 6, and 12–15 months of age. The vaccine provides coverage for approximately 80% of the invasive pneumococcal diseases in children in the United States. PCV is recommended for all infants and toddlers younger than 2 years and for all children between 2 and 5 years of age who have chronic cardiopulmonary disorders or immune suppression and for some adults older than 65 years. While immunization with PPSV23 or PCV appears to decrease the incidence of some pneumococcal disease, some studies question whether it decreases the incidence of pneumococcal pneumonia or mortality.

Haemophilus influenzae

A vaccine against *Haemophilus influenzae* type b (Hib) is recommended for all children before age 24 months. The vaccine has significantly reduced the number of infections caused by encapsulated Hib. In the past, approximately 60% of Hib infections were meningitis, amounting to about 10,000 cases each year in the United States. The type b capsule enhances the invasive potential of *H influenzae;* thus, the presence or absence of serum antibodies to these capsular antigens is a critical factor that determines an individual's susceptibility to systemic Hib infection.

The vaccine significantly reduces the risk of contracting Hib-related epiglottitis, meningitis, and orbital cellulitis. The vaccine is available as a conjugated protein between the capsular polysaccharide PRP and other agents that increase the immunologic response (PRP-OMP and PRP-T). It is also available in combination with other vaccines, such as DTaP, for increased patient convenience and adherence. The vaccine is administered in 2 or 3 doses, with the first dose given before age 7 months and the final dose after age 12 months. When the full series is given, the vaccine is more than 95% effective.

Centers for Disease Control and Prevention (CDC). Prevention and control of seasonal influenza with vaccines. Recommendations of the Advisory Committee on Immunization Practices—United States, 2013–2014. *MMWR Surveill Summ.* 2013;62(RR-07):1–43.

Meningococcus

A quadrivalent meningococcal polysaccharide vaccine (MPSV4) and a conjugate vaccine (MCV4) for the prevention of meningococcal meningitis are available and are recommended for use in military personnel, college students living in dormitories, travelers to endemic areas (such as sub-Saharan Africa), close contacts of infected patients, new outbreaks, and high-risk patients (especially splenectomized and complement-deficient patients). MCV is recommended for high-risk children aged 2–10 years. The vaccine is approximately 85% effective in preventing the spread of group C meningococcal infections but will not prevent infection from strains of meningococcus not represented in the vaccine. Immunity may wane over time, so revaccination may be required.

Cohn AC, MacNeil JR, Clark TA, et al; Centers for Disease Control and Prevention (CDC). Prevention and control of meningococcal disease: recommendations of the Advisory Committee on Immunization Practices (ACIP). *MMWR Recomm Rep.* 2013;62(RR-2):1–28.

Human Papillomavirus

The human papillomavirus (HPV) is a sexually transmitted virus that causes anal and genital warts (condylomata). More importantly, HPV is a leading cause of penile and anal cancer in men, and it is present in virtually all cervical cancers in women. It is hoped that preventing HPV infection will significantly reduce the incidence of cervical and other gynecologic cancers. HPV vaccines do not eradicate existing viral disease, so they are most effective if given before the patient becomes sexually active. Two vaccines are currently approved in the United States: a quadrivalent formulation (Gardasil) and a bivalent formulation (Cervarix). Either vaccine is given in a series of 3 doses over a 6-month period, beginning at age 11–12 years. Catch-up doses can be given up to age 21 years in men and age 26 in women.

Travel Immunizations

Precise travel vaccination recommendations depend on the geographic destinations, duration of travel, consumption of local food and untreated water, and likelihood of close contact with local populations. Routine childhood vaccinations should be reviewed in all travelers and updated as needed. Children older than 6 months should be immunized against measles (MMR) prior to travel abroad. Yellow fever vaccination may be required for anyone going to or through a yellow fever endemic area or, to prevent introduction of the disease, for travelers returning from an endemic area. Immunization against HBV should be considered in travelers who expect to have close contact with local populations known to have high rates of hepatitis B transmission. Japanese encephalitis vaccine should be offered to those whose travel plans include prolonged trips to rural areas in Southeast Asia or the Indian subcontinent during the endemic season. Typhoid fever and hepatitis A immunizations are recommended for travelers who may be exposed to potentially contaminated food and water sources. Preexposure rabies vaccination should be considered for travelers whose plans include a prolonged visit in a remote area or for those whose activities might involve working near animals. Travelers planning to visit areas endemic for malaria should consult the CDC or WHO websites to determine appropriate chemoprophylaxis for the region. The drugs used for malaria prevention include atovaquone/proguanil, chloroquine or hydroxychloroquine, doxycycline, mefloquine, and primaquine. All of these medications may cause serious adverse effects. Health information for travelers, including updated immunization and prevention recommendations for various regions of the world, can be found on the CDC website (wwwnc.cdc.gov/travel) and the WHO website (www.who.int/topics/travel/en).

Kotton CN. Vaccination and immunization against travel-related diseases in immunocompromised hosts. *Expert Rev Vaccines.* 2008;7(5):663–672.

New and Future Vaccines

New vaccines are now available for typhoid fever *(Salmonella typhi),* anthrax, yellow fever, and Japanese encephalitis. Vaccines undergoing investigation include those for HIV, cholera, dysentery, *Campylobacter,* rotavirus, *Clostridium difficile,* respiratory syncytial virus, Ebola virus, malaria, cytomegalovirus, rabies, viral encephalitis, herpes simplex type 2, Epstein-Barr virus, TB, *Pseudomonas aeruginosa, Helicobacter pylori, Staphylococcus, Streptococcus, Propionibacterium acnes,* parainfluenza virus, leishmaniasis, plague, and smallpox.

Passive immunization with human hyperimmunoglobulin is currently available to treat or prevent rabies, tetanus, respiratory syncytial virus, cytomegalovirus, hepatitis A, hepatitis B, hepatitis C, herpesvirus, and varicella-zoster infections.

Considering the worldwide impact of many other infectious diseases, there is great interest in developing new vaccines for the treatment of gonorrhea, syphilis, toxigenic *Escherichia coli* infection, leprosy, trachoma, and other infectious diseases. It is hoped that ongoing research will lead to the development of safe and effective vaccines for many or all of these illnesses.

Centers for Disease Control and Prevention website; www.cdc.gov/.

European Centre for Disease Prevention and Control website; www.ecdc.europa.eu/en/Pages/home.aspx.

Kanoi BN, Egwang TG. New concepts in vaccine development in malaria. *Curr Opin Infect Dis.* 2007;20(3):311–316.

World Health Organization website; www.who.int/topics/vaccines/en/.

CHAPTER **13**

Cancer

Recent Developments

- Biologic therapies continue to play a major role in the treatment of cancer.
- Advances in stem cell biology may alter therapeutic strategies for cancer.
- Genetic profiling of tumors and patients can contribute significantly to treatment and identify patients at risk for cancer.
- More precise molecular targets for cancer increase the effectiveness and reduce the toxicity of systemic therapies.

Introduction

Cancer is the second-leading cause of death in the United States, with approximately 23% of all US deaths due to cancer. In 2014, 1.6 million new cases were diagnosed in the United States, and some 580,000 deaths occurred. Currently, more than 13 million Americans have a history of cancer, and cancer will develop in 1 in 4 Americans during their lifetime. Worldwide, in 2012, there were 14 million new cases and 8.2 million deaths due to cancer. Developing countries are disproportionately affected, with 60% of all cases and 70% of all deaths due to cancer.

Cancer is actually many different diseases; questions of etiology, cancer prevention, and cancer cure must therefore address the specific types of tumors. Nonmelanotic skin cancers are the most common tumors, but these cancers are rarely a cause of death. After skin cancer, the most common forms of cancer in adult Americans (in decreasing order of incidence) are lung, breast, prostate, and colorectal. Approximately 80% of adult cancers arise from the epithelial tissues.

Cancer is the leading cause of death by disease in children younger than 15 years in the United States. Nevertheless, death rates have dropped and survival rates have risen sharply. The 5-year survival rate for all childhood cancers combined has improved in the United States, from approximately 51% in 1973 to over 90% today.

Etiology

Cancer is caused by mutations in genes that control cell division. Some of these genes, called *oncogenes,* stimulate cell division; others, called *tumor suppressor genes,* slow this process. In the normal state, both types of genes work together, enabling the body to replace dead cells and repair damaged ones. Mutations in these genes cause cells to proliferate out of control. Such mutations can be inherited or acquired through environmental insults. Cancer causes, therefore, are explained on the basis of chemical, radiation-related, or viral conditions that occur in a complex milieu, including host genetic composition and immunobiologic status.

Epidemiologic data suggest that as much as 80% of human cancer may be due to exogenous chemical exposure. If these chemicals could be properly identified, a major proportion of human cancers could be prevented by reducing host exposure or by protecting the host. Science is looking at a number of issues that need to be resolved before causation is established.

Cancer arises from genetic mutations that cause a cell to grow and divide without regard for cell death. The cell cycle is regulated biochemically, with 2 important groups of enzymes involved in this process, cyclin-dependent kinases (CDKs) and cyclin-dependent phosphatases. An example of CDK function involves the p53 tumor suppressor gene, which upregulates the p21 inhibitor of CDK function.

The general population is exposed to both naturally occurring ionizing radiation and man-made ionizing radiation. Man-made sources deliver an average of 106 millirems per year to each person. These sources include medical diagnostic equipment and technologically altered natural sources (such as phosphate fertilizers and building materials containing small amounts of radioactivity). The carcinogenic effects of radiation exposure result from molecular lesions caused by random interactions of radiation with atoms and molecules. Most molecular lesions induced in this way are of little consequence to the affected cell. However, DNA is not repaired with 100% efficiency, and mutations and chromosomal aberrations accrue with increasing radiation doses. Parameters that influence the response of the target tissue include the total radiation dose, the dose rate, the quality of the radiation source, the characteristics of certain internal emitters (such as radioiodine), and individual host factors.

The role of viruses in the etiology of cancer has been studied extensively. For example, researchers have inoculated laboratory animals with specific viruses to see whether tumor development is induced. Several human cancers show a definite correlation with viral infection and the presence and retention of specific virus nucleic acid sequences and virus proteins in the tumor cells (Burkitt lymphoma, nasopharyngeal carcinoma, carcinoma of the cervix, and hepatocellular carcinoma).

All of the DNA virus groups except the parvovirus family have been associated with cancer. This is notable because all the DNA viruses associated with cancer contain double-stranded DNA, whereas the parvoviruses contain only single-stranded DNA. There are 9 RNA virus groups, but only 1, the retrovirus group, is associated with oncogenicity. The papillomavirus of the papovavirus group has been associated with squamous cell carcinoma, cervical cancer, and laryngeal papilloma in humans. A vaccine against human papillomavirus (HPV) is now available. Immunization against HPV may prevent most cases of cervical cancer in women; see Chapter 12 for additional discussion. Infection with the hepatitis B virus has been associated with primary hepatocellular carcinoma in humans.

The Epstein-Barr virus, also known as human herpesvirus 4, causes infectious mononucleosis and has been associated with Burkitt lymphoma and nasopharyngeal carcinoma.

Herpes simplex virus type 1, which causes gingivostomatitis, encephalitis, keratoconjunctivitis, neuralgia, and labialis, has been associated with carcinoma of the lip and oropharynx. Herpes simplex virus type 2, which causes genital herpes, disseminated neonatal herpes, encephalitis, and neuralgia, has been associated with cancer of the uterine cervix, vulva, kidneys, and nasopharynx. The cytomegalovirus, which causes cytomegalovirus disease, transfusion mononucleosis, interstitial pneumonia, and congenital defects, has been associated with prostate cancer, Kaposi sarcoma, and carcinoma of the bladder and uterine cervix. The varicella-zoster virus, which causes chickenpox, shingles, and varicella pneumonia, is to date unassociated with any specific human cancers.

Finally, cancers may aggregate in a nonrandom manner in certain families. These cancers may be of the same type or dissimilar. Such cancer-cluster families may have several children with soft tissue sarcoma and relatives with a variety of cancers, especially of the breast in young women. Multiple endocrine neoplasia types 1 and 2 are yet other examples of hereditary cancer syndromes. The recognition of familial cancer syndromes permits early detection that may be life-saving.

Radiation Therapy

For many patients with cancer, radiation therapy, which uses ionizing radiation to kill cancer cells and shrink tumors, is part of the treatment plan. Ionizing radiation interacts with tissues by an energy transfer and a chemical reaction, with the release of free radicals and the decomposition of water into hydrogen, hydroxyl, and perhydroxyl ionic forms. These ionic forms probably react with DNA and RNA in vital enzymes, producing biologic injury. The injuries noted to date include mitotic-linked death and chromosomal aberrations such as breakage, sticking, and cross-bridging. Consequent cell death occurs in both normal tissue and malignant lesions. In radiotherapy, biochemical recovery and biologic repair occur in the normal host, maintaining the integrity of vital systems.

The poorly differentiated lymphoid cells, intestinal epithelium, and reproductive cells are more readily damaged and recover more quickly than the highly differentiated cells of the body. Lymphocytes are damaged by 1 gray (Gy) of radiation and central nervous system tissue by 50 Gy. Surface irradiation of approximately 10 Gy produces skin erythema. The most serious damage is the late development of postradiation malignant changes, manifesting as squamous cell carcinoma and basal cell carcinoma. Radiation absorption in bone can produce osteogenic sarcomas and fibrosarcomas as well.

Radiation can be delivered through external beam radiotherapy (EBRT; most common) or internal placement (brachytherapy); radiation can also be administered systemically (eg, radioactive substance bound to a monoclonal antibody). In EBRT, high-energy X-ray beams generated either by linear accelerators, which produce photons or electrons, or by cobalt machines, which use radioactive decay of an element such as cobalt 60, are aimed at the tumor site. Planning for EBRT involves not only localizing the tumor, but also determining the proper dose, one that will kill the malignant cells while minimizing damage to the surrounding noncancerous tissue. There are many other methods of EBRT, including particle therapy and stereotactic radiosurgery.

In brachytherapy (also called *internal radiation therapy*), radioactive material is implanted within or adjacent to the tumor, delivering radiation while minimizing damage to the surrounding normal tissue. The term *brachytherapy* refers to various types of procedures, one example of which is seed implantation, used in the treatment of prostate cancer and some uveal melanomas.

For some conditions, monoclonal antibodies are available as a vector to deliver radiation directly to the target tissue; these antibodies are discussed later in this chapter.

Guerrero Urbano MT, Nutting CM. Clinical use of intensity-modulated radiotherapy: part I. *Br J Radiol.* 2004;77(914):88–96.

Ophthalmic considerations Ocular manifestations of fetal irradiation in the first trimester include microphthalmos, congenital cataracts, and retinal dysplasia. A 0.5-Gy dose of radiation may cause congenital anomalies in a fetus. Fetal exposure to approximately 0.30–0.80 Gy doubles the incidence of congenital defects; 5 Gy (the median lethal dose [LD_{50}] for a human fetus) generally induces an abortion.

The ocular effects of irradiation depend not only on total dose, fractionation, and treatment portal size but also on associated systemic diseases such as diabetes mellitus and hypertension. Concomitant chemotherapy has an additive effect.

The lens is the most radiosensitive structure in the eye, followed by the cornea, the retina, and the optic nerve. The orbit is completely included in the treatment portal in diseases such as large retinoblastomas; it is partially included in tumors of adjacent structures, such as the maxillary antrum, nasopharynx, ethmoid sinus, and nasal cavity. Usual doses range from 20 to 100 Gy. The total dose is usually fractionated during the treatment. In brachytherapy, a low-energy isotope such as radioactive iodine delivers a high dose of radiation within a few millimeters of the tumor but does not penetrate deep into it. This allows for radioactive episcleral implants to deliver a dose of 100 Gy to the apex of a tumor but much less to the rest of the eye. The sclera can tolerate doses up to 400–800 Gy.

Doses to the lens as low as 2 Gy in 1 fraction may cause cataract formation. However, cataracts caused by low doses may be asymptomatic and may not progress. Cataracts due to higher doses (7–8 Gy) may continue to progress, resulting in considerable vision loss. The average latent period for the development of radiation-induced cataracts is 2–3 years.

The clinical picture of radiation retinopathy resembles that of diabetic retinopathy. Development of radiation retinopathy is very rare with a fractionated dose of less than 50 Gy over 5–6 weeks. At higher fractionated doses (70–80 Gy), however, radiation retinopathy develops in most patients. The usual interval between radiation therapy and the development of radiation-induced retinopathy is 2–3 years. Radiation retinopathy may develop earlier in patients with diabetes or those undergoing chemotherapy.

The earliest clinical manifestation of radiation retinopathy is usually cotton-wool spots. After several months, these spots fade away, leaving areas of capillary nonperfusion. Telangiectatic vessels grow from the retina into these areas. Microaneurysms may also develop. These ischemic changes may cause rubeosis iridis, which in turn may lead to neovascular glaucoma. The capillary endothelial cell is the first type of cell to be damaged, followed closely by the pericytes and then the endothelial cells of the larger vessels. The new intraretinal telangiectatic vessels have thick collagenous walls. There may be spotty occlusion of the choriocapillaris.

Doses to the optic nerve in the range of 60–70 Gy cause some injury in a small number of patients. Damage to the optic nerve is called *radiation optic neuropathy.* Clinically, these patients have disc pallor with splinter hemorrhages. Injury to the more proximal part of the optic nerve resembles retrobulbar optic neuropathy. Affected patients may report unilateral headaches and ocular pain; the disc may not reveal edema or hemorrhage. With doses of 60–70 Gy, a dry eye syndrome sometimes develops. This syndrome usually develops within a year and occasionally progresses to corneal ulceration and severe pain.

Chemotherapy

The goal of cancer chemotherapy is to damage or destroy cancer cells without killing normal cells. The first candidate drugs to selectively target rapidly dividing cells were sulfur and nitrogen mustards that were noted to suppress bone marrow when used in warfare. These compounds bound covalently to DNA, and therefore DNA was the first molecular target of chemotherapy. In the 1950s, attention was directed to the precursors of DNA, and drugs such as methotrexate were found effective. The recognition that some tumors were hormonally dependent led to hormonal therapy or suppression as a treatment for cancer. Since the 1970s, many drugs have been developed that inhibit mitotic spindle formation.

Natural Products

Natural products, either naturally occurring or synthetically modified, have played a significant role in cancer chemotherapy and include a variety of agents, the most common of which are vinca alkaloids, podophyllin derivatives, paclitaxel, antitumor antibiotics, and related drugs (Table 13-1). *Vinca alkaloids* are derived from the periwinkle plant; they include vincristine, vinblastine, and several investigational agents. These agents block incorporation of orotic acid and thymidine into DNA and cause arrest and inhibition of mitosis.

Podophyllin derivatives and semisynthetic plant derivatives arrest cells in the G_2 phase. Etoposide and teniposide are gaining acceptance in many treatment protocols.

Paclitaxel is a compound originally isolated from the bark of the Pacific yew tree. It was approved by the US Food and Drug Administration (FDA) to treat breast, ovarian, and lung cancers as well as AIDS-related Kaposi sarcoma. Paclitaxel stops microtubules

Table 13-1 Antineoplastic Drugs

Drugs by Class	Mechanism of Action	Tumors Commonly Responsive	Toxicity and Comments
Alkylating agents			
Chlorambucil Cyclophosphamide Ifosfamide Mechlorethamine (nitrogen mustard) Melphalan	Alkylation of DNA with restriction of strands' uncoiling and replication	Hodgkin, malignant lymphoma, small cell lung Ca, Ca of breast and testis, CLL	Alopecia with high IV dose; nausea and vomiting; myelosuppression; hemorrhagic cystitis (especially with ifosfamide), which can be ameliorated with mesna; muto- and leukemogenic; aspermia; permanent sterility possible
Antimetabolites			
Folate antagonist methotrexate (MTX)	Folate antagonist with binding to dihydrofolate reductase and interference with (pyrimidine) thymidylate synthesis	Choriocarcinoma (female), Ca of head and neck, ALL, Ca of ovary, malignant lymphoma, osteogenic sarcoma	Mucosal ulceration; bone marrow suppression; toxicity increased with renal function impairment or ascitic fluid (with pooling of drug). Leucovorin rescue can reverse toxicity at 24 h (10–20 mg q 6 h × 10 doses).
Cytarabine (Ara-C)	DNA polymerase inhibition	Acute leukemia (especially nonlymphocytic), malignant lymphoma	Myelosuppression, nausea and vomiting, cerebellar and conjunctival toxicities at high doses, rash
Purine antagonist 6-mercaptopurine (6-MP)	Blocks de novo purine synthesis	Acute leukemia	Myelosuppression, alopecia
Pyrimidine antagonist 5-fluorouracil (5-FU)	Interferes with thymidylate synthase to reduce thymidine production	GI neoplasms, Ca of breast	Mucositis, alopecia, myelosuppression, diarrhea and vomiting, hyperpigmentation. When given after MTX, synergistic effect is significant.

Drugs by Class	Mechanism of Action	Tumors Commonly Responsive	Toxicity and Comments
Plant alkaloids			
Vincas			
Vinblastine	Mitotic arrest by alteration of microtubular proteins	Lymphomas, leukemias, Ca of breast, Ewing sarcoma, Ca of testis	Alopecia, myelosuppression, peripheral neuropathy, ileus
Vincristine	As above	As above	Peripheral neuropathy, SIADH. Dose commonly "capped" at total of 2 mg in adults.
Paclitaxel	Promotes assembly of microtubules	Ca of breast, lung, ovary, head, neck, and bladder	Myelosuppression, alopecia, myalgia, arthralgia, neuropathy
Podophyllotoxins Etoposide Teniposide	Inhibition of mitosis by unknown mechanisms	Lymphoma, Hodgkin, Ca of testis, Ca of lung (especially small cell), acute leukemia	Nausea, vomiting, myelosuppression, peripheral neuropathy. Etoposide cleared by liver (teniposide by kidney); increased toxicity in renal failure.
Antibiotics			
Actinomycin D (dactinomycin)	Inhibits DNA-directed RNA synthesis	Gestational trophoblastic neoplasm, Wilms tumor, rhabdomyosarcoma, Ewing sarcoma, malignant hydatidiform mole	Bone marrow suppression, fatigue, hair loss, mouth ulcers, loss of appetite, diarrhea
Bleomycin	Incision of DNA strands	Squamous cell Ca, lymphoma, Ca of testis, Ca of lung	Anaphylaxis, chills and fever, rash; pulmonary fibrosis at doses >200 mg/m^2; requires renal excretion
Doxorubicin	Intercalation between DNA strands inhibits uncoiling of DNA	Acute leukemia, Hodgkin, other lymphomas, Ca of breast, Ca of lung	Nausea and vomiting, myelosuppression, alopecia. Cardiac toxicity at cumulative dose >500 mg/m^2. Higher dose tolerated when given by continuous IV.
Mitomycin	Inhibits DNA synthesis by acting as a bifunctional alkylator	Gastric adenocarcinoma; Ca of the colon, breast, and lung; transitional cell Ca of the bladder	Local extravasation causes tissue necrosis; myelosuppression, with leukopenia and thrombocytopenia 4–6 wk after treatment; alopecia; lethargy; fever; hemolytic uremic syndrome

(Continued)

Table 13-1 *(continued)*

Drugs by Class	Mechanism of Action	Tumors Commonly Responsive	Toxicity and Comments
Nitrosoureas			
Carmustine	Alkylation of DNA with restriction of strands' uncoiling and replication	Brain tumors, lymphoma	Myelosuppression, pulmonary toxicity (fibrosis), renal toxicity
Lomustine	Carbamoylation of amino acids in proteins	As above	As above
Inorganic ions			
Cisplatin	Intercalation and intracalation between DNA strands inhibits uncoiling of DNA	Ca of lung (especially small cell), testis, breast, and stomach; lymphoma	Anemia, ototoxicity, peripheral neuropathy, myelosuppression, nausea, vomiting
Angiogenesis inhibitors			
Aflibercept	Inhibition of tumor endothelial proliferation	Colorectal Ca	Severe bleeding, DVT, hypertension, GI perforation
Bevacizumab	Inhibition of tumor endothelial proliferation	Colorectal Ca, Ca of cervix, glioblastoma	DVT, hypertension, ovarian failure, severe bleeding
Enzymes			
Asparaginase	Depletion of asparagine, on which leukemic cells depend	ALL	Acute anaphylaxis, hyperthermia, pancreatitis, hyperglycemia, hypofibrinogenemia
Hormones			
Flutamide	Binding of androgen receptor	Ca of prostate	Decreased libido, hot flushes, gynecomastia
Tamoxifen	Places cells at rest: binding of estrogen receptor	Ca of breast	Hot flushes, hypercalcemia, DVT

ALL = acute lymphocytic leukemia; Ca = cancer; CLL = chronic lymphocytic leukemia; DVT = deep venous thrombosis; GI = gastrointestinal; IV = intravenous; SIADH = syndrome of inappropriate antidiuretic hormone secretion.

Data from Modalities of cancer therapy. *The Merck Manual* [online medical library]. http://www.merck.com/mmpe/sec11.html. Accessed September 1, 2014.

from breaking down. In normal cell growth, microtubules are formed when a cell starts dividing. Once the cell stops dividing, the microtubules are broken down or destroyed. With paclitaxel, cancer cells become clogged with microtubules and cannot grow and divide.

Antitumor antibiotics are compounds produced by species of *Streptomyces* in culture. These agents interfere with the synthesis of nucleic acid. They include

- *anthracyclines* (doxorubicin and derivatives), which interfere with template function of DNA
- *bleomycin,* which causes DNA-strand scission
- *actinomycin D* (dactinomycin), which inhibits DNA-directed RNA synthesis
- *mitomycin,* which impairs replication by causing cross-linking between DNA strands

A unique adverse effect of anthracyclines is cardiac muscle degeneration that leads to cardiomyopathy. The major dose-limiting toxicity of mitomycin is myelosuppression. Mitomycin has also been implicated as a cause of the hemolytic uremic syndrome.

Angiogenesis Inhibitors

Angiogenesis is important to the growth and spread of cancers, as new blood vessels are critical to the formation of tumors. In animal studies, angiogenesis inhibitors have successfully stopped the formation of new blood vessels, causing tumors to shrink and die. Various angiogenesis inhibitors have been evaluated in human clinical trials. These studies include patients with cancers of the breast, prostate, brain, pancreas, lung, stomach, ovary, and cervix; patients with certain leukemias and lymphomas; and those with AIDS-related Kaposi sarcoma.

Antibodies against vascular endothelial growth factor (VEGF), which promotes vascular proliferation, have proven effective in cancer therapy. Bevacizumab, a humanized monoclonal antibody directed against VEGF-A, was the first angiogenesis inhibitor approved for the treatment of cancer in the United States. It has demonstrated clinical efficacy in the treatment of colorectal and other solid tumors and, on an off-label basis, in the treatment of neovascular ("wet") age-related macular degeneration (AMD). Bevacizumab is also effective in the treatment of optic nerve gliomas in children. Tyrosine kinase inhibitors (TKIs), including pazopanib, have also shown promising antitumor activity. Aflibercept is a recombinant fusion protein that functions as a decoy receptor for VEGF. This agent inactivates VEGF-A, VEGF-B, and placental growth factor and is effective in the treatment of colorectal cancer and wet AMD.

Avery RA, Hwang EI, Jakacki RI, Packer RJ. Marked recovery of vision in children with optic pathway gliomas treated with bevacizumab. *JAMA Ophthalmol.* 2014;132(1):111–114.

Biologic Therapies

Biologic therapies (sometimes called *immunotherapy, biotherapy,* or *biologic response modifier therapy*) use the immune system, either directly or indirectly, to fight cancer or to lessen the side effects that may be caused by some cancer treatments. Further, cancer may develop when the immune system breaks down or is not functioning adequately. Biologic therapies are designed to repair, stimulate, or enhance the immune system's responses.

Cells in the immune system secrete 2 types of proteins: antibodies and cytokines. Cytokines are nonantibody proteins produced by some immune system cells to communicate with other cells. Types of cytokines include lymphokines, interferons, interleukins, and colony-stimulating factors. Some antibodies and cytokines, called *biologic response modifiers,* can be used in the treatment of cancer. Other biologic response modifiers include monoclonal antibodies, which can also be used to treat cancer, and vaccines.

Interleukins occur naturally in the body and can be made in the laboratory. Many interleukins have been identified; interleukin-2 has been the most widely studied in cancer treatment. Interleukin-2 stimulates the growth and activity of many immune cells, such as lymphocytes, that can destroy cancer cells. The FDA has approved interleukin-2 for the treatment of metastatic kidney cancer and metastatic melanoma.

Colony-stimulating factors (sometimes called *hematopoietic growth factors*) usually do not directly affect tumor cells but instead stimulate bone marrow production. Colony-stimulating factors allow doses of anticancer drugs to be increased without increasing the risk of infection or need for transfusion.

Monoclonal antibodies (mAbs) are produced by a single type of cell and are specific for a particular antigen. Researchers continue to examine ways to create mAbs that are specific for the antigens found on the surface of cancer cells being treated. Some examples of mAbs currently used in cancer treatment are rituximab and trastuzumab.

Therapeutic mAbs are made by injecting human cancer cells into mice, which stimulates an antibody response. The cells producing antibodies are then removed and fused with laboratory-grown cells to create hybrid cells called *hybridomas.* Hybridomas can produce large quantities of these mAbs indefinitely.

Monoclonal antibodies have many potential uses in cancer treatment, such as linking them to anticancer drugs, radioisotopes, other biologic response modifiers, or other toxins. When the antibodies attach to cancer cells, they can deliver these poisons directly to the cells. For example, ado-trastuzumab emtansine uses trastuzumab to deliver a cytotoxic microtubule inhibitor. Another example is tositumomab radioconjugate, which delivers specifically targeted radiotherapy to tumors. Monoclonal antibodies carrying radioisotopes may also prove useful in diagnosing certain cancers, such as colorectal, ovarian, and prostate cancer.

Cancer vaccines are being developed to help the immune system recognize cancer cells. These vaccines are designed to be injected after the disease is diagnosed rather than before it develops. They may help the body reject tumors and prevent cancer from recurring. Vaccines are being studied in the treatment of melanomas, lymphomas, and cancers of the kidney, breast, ovaries, prostate, colon, and rectum.

Other biologic approaches to cancer therapy include *genetic profiling* of certain tumors. Current management of lung cancer and melanoma is based on such profiling. Further, genetic profiling may prove more helpful and effective than classifying tumors by their organ of origin. An example of this is the differentiation between those tumors with a normal and those with an abnormal tumor suppressor gene p53. Tumor cells with normal p53 genes are far more sensitive to chemotherapy than those with mutant p53.

Vose JM, Wahl RL, Saleh M, et al. Multicenter phase II study of iodine-131 tositumomab for chemotherapy-relapsed/refractory low-grade and transformed low-grade B-cell non-Hodgkin's lymphomas. *J Clin Oncol.* 2000;18(6):1316–1323.

Ophthalmic considerations The eye and its adnexa are frequently involved in systemic malignancies as well as in extraocular malignancies that extend into ocular structures (including local malignancies of skin, bone, and sinuses). Breast and lung cancers frequently metastasize to the eye and are the most common intraocular tumors in adults. Acute myelogenous and lymphocytic leukemias often have uveal and posterior choroidal infiltrates as part of their generalized disease. In children, these manifestations are often signs of central nervous system involvement and suggest a poor prognosis. Although malignant lymphomas do not usually involve the uveal tract, histiocytic lymphoma is one type that often involves the vitreous and presents as uveitis. The retina and choroid may also be involved.

Tumors of the eye and adnexa are discussed in several other BCSC volumes, including Section 4, *Ophthalmic Pathology and Intraocular Tumors;* Section 6, *Pediatric Ophthalmology and Strabismus;* Section 7, *Orbit, Eyelids, and Lacrimal System;* and Section 8, *External Disease and Cornea.*

American Cancer Society website; www.cancer.org.
European Society for Medical Oncology website; www.esmo.org.
UpToDate; www.uptodate.com.

CHAPTER 14

Infectious Diseases

Recent Developments

- Vancomycin-resistant strains of enterococci and staphylococci have recently emerged as a cause of life-threatening infection in hospitalized patients.
- DNA probes using polymerase chain reaction (PCR) provide more sensitive diagnostic tools for detecting gonorrhea; syphilis; Lyme disease; and infections caused by *Chlamydia,* mycobacteria, fungi, and many viruses.
- The early treatment of HIV infections has improved, and it is now recommended that all individuals between the ages of 15 and 65 years be screened for HIV.
- The treatment of cytomegalovirus (CMV) retinitis has evolved from placement of ganciclovir implants to use of intravitreal ganciclovir or foscarnet and oral valganciclovir.
- Newer antibiotics such as meropenem, cefepime, linezolid, quinupristin-dalfopristin, evernimicin, telithromycin, daptomycin, grepafloxacin, and teicoplanin provide expanded antimicrobial coverage and offer treatment options for multidrug-resistant infections.

General Microbiology

Despite formidable immune and mechanical defense systems, the human body harbors an extensive, well-adapted population of microorganisms on the skin and in the gastrointestinal, vaginal, and upper respiratory tracts. The organisms maintain their foothold on these epithelial surfaces chiefly by adherence, and they indirectly benefit the host by excluding pathogenic bacterial colonization and by priming the immune system. If antimicrobial agents alter this host–microbe interplay by eliminating the normal flora, the host's susceptibility to normally excluded pathogenic microorganisms is increased. When the mechanical defenses of the epithelial layers are breached so as to expose normally sterile areas, or if a critical component of the immune system that usually prevents microbial invasion fails, severe infections can result from the normal microbial flora.

Components of the immune system of multicellular organisms are categorized into innate and adaptive immunity. *Innate immunity* is present in nearly all multicellular organisms and includes humoral and cellular immune receptors that have broad specificity. These receptors recognize many related molecular structures called PAMPs (*p*athogen-*a*ssociated *m*olecular *p*atterns). PAMPs are polysaccharides and polynucleotides that differ very little among pathogens but are not found in the host. The innate immune response is usually immediate; there is no immune memory of prior exposure.

Adaptive immunity is found only in vertebrates and does involve immune memory of prior exposure. Pathogens are recognized by many randomly generated B-lymphocyte and T-lymphocyte receptors, each of which has a very narrow specificity, that can recognize a particular antigen (epitope). Most epitopes are derived from polypeptides and reflect the individuality of each pathogen. Adaptive immune response is initially slower (days), because the clones of responding immune cells take time to proliferate. After the first encounter, the adaptive immune response is faster and stronger, because of immunologic memory.

However, even when both the mechanical and immune defense systems are intact, pathogenic microbes can cause infections by means of specific virulent characteristics that allow the microbes to invade and multiply. These virulent traits vary among different species.

Following are several mechanisms of virulence:

- *Attachment. Neisseria gonorrhoeae* and *Neisseria meningitidis* breach epithelial barriers by adhering to host epithelial cell–surface receptors by means of a ligand on the bacteria's pili. Presence of the cell-surface receptors is genetically determined.
- *Polysaccharide encapsulation. Streptococcus pneumoniae, N meningitidis,* and *Haemophilus* and *Bacteroides* species evade phagocytosis in the absence of antibody and complement because of their polysaccharide coating.
- *Blocking of lysosomal fusion.* Intracellular existence, as well as protection from humoral immune mechanisms, is a characteristic of *Chlamydia, Toxoplasma, Legionella,* and *Mycobacterium* species.
- *Antigenic surface variation.* Antigenic shifts in the cell wall of *Borrelia recurrentis* incapacitate the humoral immune system, which has a lag time in antibody production. Similar antigenic shifts are found in *Chlamydia* and influenza viruses.
- *Immunoglobulin A (IgA) protease. Haemophilus influenzae, N gonorrhoeae,* and *N meningitidis* eliminate the IgA antibody normally found on mucosal surfaces, which would otherwise prevent the microbes' adherence.
- *Endotoxin.* A normal constituent of the gram-negative bacterial cell wall, endotoxin produces dramatic systemic physiologic responses ranging from fever and leukocyte margination to disseminated intravascular coagulation and septic shock.
- *Exotoxins.* Exotoxins are a diverse set of proteins with specific actions on target tissues that can cause severe systemic effects in such diseases as cholera and tetanus.
- *Biofilm formation.* Staphylococci can develop biofilms on various biomaterials, such as catheters and prosthetic heart valves.
- *Multiple mechanisms.* Some organisms, such as coagulase-positive *Staphylococcus aureus,* may possess multiple mechanisms of virulence. Also, it appears that nearly any *S aureus* genotype carried by humans can transform into a life-threatening pathogen, but certain clones are more virulent than others.

The immune system, which makes possible the host's adaptive response to colonization and infection, is classically divided into the humoral and cellular immune systems. The *humoral immune system,* composed of cells derived from the B lymphocytes, is responsible for antibody-mediated opsonization, complement-mediated bacterial killing, antitoxin, and mediation of intracellular infections. The *cellular immune system,* determined by the T lymphocytes, is responsible for interaction with and stimulation of the humoral immune system, direct cytotoxicity, release of chemical messengers, and control of chronic infections. The successful interplay between the humoral and cellular immune systems mitigates and usually eradicates infections, allowing for repair and healing. Also see Part I, Immunology, in BCSC Section 9, *Intraocular Inflammation and Uveitis.*

Staphylococcus

Staphylococcus aureus colonizes the anterior nares and other skin sites in 15% of community isolates. Of the tertiary care hospital isolates, more than 25% are resistant to all β-lactam antibiotics. Transmission of organisms is usually by direct contact. Resistance of organisms to antimicrobials is usually plasmid determined and varies by institution. The increasing prevalence of methicillin-resistant *S aureus* (MRSA) in tertiary referral hospitals appears to be related to the population of high-risk patients at such centers. Unfortunately, MRSA is now an increasingly common cause of serious infection in primary care settings as well. The natural history of staphylococcal infections indicates that immunity is brief and incomplete. Delayed hypersensitivity reactions to staphylococcal products may be responsible for chronic staphylococcal disease. Conditions caused by staphylococcal infections include furuncle, acne, bullous impetigo, paronychia, osteomyelitis, septic arthritis, deep-tissue abscesses, bacteremia, endocarditis, enterocolitis, pneumonia, wound infections, scalded skin syndrome, toxic shock syndrome, and food poisoning.

Acute serious staphylococcal infections require immediate intravenous antibiotic therapy. A penicillinase-resistant penicillin or first-generation cephalosporin is normally used, pending the results of susceptibility tests. With the emergence of methicillin-resistant staphylococci, vancomycin has become the drug of choice for treating life-threatening infections, pending susceptibility studies. The increasing emergence of vancomycin-resistant enterococci (VRE) has led to concern about cases of vancomycin-resistant *S aureus* (VRSA) infection, mediated through plasmid transfer.

Since 1997, infections due to strains of *S aureus* with reduced susceptibility to vancomycin (glycopeptide-intermediate *S aureus*) have been identified, and their frequency is increasing throughout the world. Many of the cases occurred after prolonged inpatient treatment with intravenous vancomycin. Some reported cases have been successfully treated with various forms of combination therapy, including rifampin and trimethoprim-sulfamethoxazole; vancomycin, gentamicin, and rifampin; and vancomycin and nafcillin. Other agents with activity against vancomycin-intermediate *S aureus* (VISA) are ampicillin-sulbactam and some newer antibiotics, such as daptomycin, evernimicin, linezolid, ceftaroline, and quinupristin-dalfopristin. The first case of true VRSA was reported in July 2002, and since then 5 additional van-A mutation–positive cases have been confirmed in the United States. Exposure to vancomycin-intermediate and vancomycin-resistant isolates of *S aureus* increases the organism's resistance to vancomycin and other agents, such as teicoplanin. Most VISA and nearly all VRSA isolates reported to date have arisen from endemic MRSA and, in the case of VRSA, have acquired genes from VRE.

Accordingly, the emergence of VISA and VRSA provides strong motivation for containing MRSA and VRE transmission.

Staphylococcus epidermidis is an almost universal inhabitant of the skin, present in up to 90% of skin cultures. It can cause infection when local defenses are compromised. Its characteristic adherence to prosthetic devices makes it the most common cause of prosthetic heart valve infections, and it is a common infectious organism of intravenous catheters and cerebrospinal fluid shunts.

Most isolates are resistant to methicillin and cephalosporins; therefore, the drug of choice is vancomycin, occasionally in combination with rifampin or gentamicin. Unfortunately, there have also been reports of vancomycin-resistant infections caused by coagulase-negative *Staphylococcus.* In addition to antibiotic therapy, management usually involves removal of the infected prosthetic device or vascular catheter.

Gould IM. Treatment of bacteraemia: meticillin-resistant *Staphylococcus aureus* (MRSA) to vancomycin-resistant *S. aureus* (VRSA). *Int J Antimicrob Agents.* 2013;42(Suppl):S17–21.

Holmes RL, Jorgensen JH. Inhibitory activities of 11 antimicrobial agents and bactericidal activities of vancomycin and daptomycin against invasive methicillin-resistant *Staphylococcus aureus* isolates obtained from 1999 through 2006. *Antimicrob Agents Chemother.* 2008;52(2):757–760.

Streptococcus

Group A β-hemolytic streptococci *(Streptococcus pyogenes)* cause a variety of acute suppurative infections through droplet transmission. The infection is modulated by an opsonizing antibody, which provides a type-specific immunity that lasts for years and is directed against the protein in the cell-wall pili. Suppurative streptococcal infections in humans include pharyngitis, impetigo, pneumonia, erysipelas, wound and burn infections, puerperal infections, and scarlet fever. Genetically mediated humoral and cellular responses to certain strains of group A streptococci play a role in the development of the postinfectious syndromes of glomerulonephritis, rheumatic fever, and necrotizing soft-tissue infection (flesh-eating bacterial infection), all of which represent delayed, nonsuppurative, noninfectious complications of group A streptococcal infections. Rapid identification with antigen detection tests allows prompt treatment of patients with pharyngitis due to this strain of *Streptococcus* and can reduce the risk of spread of infection.

Streptococcus pyogenes remains highly susceptible to penicillin G; however, in the presence of allergy, erythromycin or (if no cross-allergy exists) a cephalosporin is substituted. Macrolide-resistant and clindamycin-resistant strains of group A β-hemolytic streptococci have been reported. Antibiotic prophylaxis against bacterial endocarditis is administered for procedures that may result in transient bacteremia. However, such prophylaxis may not prevent acute glomerulonephritis.

Streptococcus pneumoniae are lancet-shaped diplococci that cause α-hemolysis on blood agar. Although 10%–30% of the normal population carry 1 or more serologic types of pneumococci in the throat, the incidence of and mortality from pneumococcal pneumonia increase sharply after 50 years of age, with a fatality rate approaching 25%. Pneumococcal virulence is determined by its complex polysaccharide capsule, of which there are more than 80 distinct serotypes.

Besides pneumonia, conditions caused by *S pneumoniae* include sinusitis, meningitis, otitis media, and peritonitis. Pneumococci are usually highly susceptible to penicillin, other β-lactams, erythromycin, or the newer fluoroquinolones. Routine susceptibility testing should be performed on patients with meningitis, bacteremia, or other life-threatening infections. Penicillin-resistant strains of *S pneumoniae* have been reported with increasing frequency. In several regions of the world, more than 25% of isolates are penicillin resistant; many of these are also resistant to cephalosporins and macrolides. Recently, some cases of ketolide and fluoroquinolone resistance have been reported as well. Treatment of highly resistant strains may require vancomycin or meropenem. Prophylaxis is available through use of the 23-valent pneumococcal conjugate vaccine for adults and the 7- or 13-valent vaccine for children (see Chapter 12). Interestingly, new drug-resistant strains have evolved in pediatric pneumococcal infections because of the widespread use of the 7-valent vaccine.

α-Hemolytic streptococci and staphylococci cause 55% and 30% of cases of subacute bacterial endocarditis (SBE), respectively. Other pathogens that cause SBE include *Enterococcus* and *Haemophilus* species and fungi. The SBE prophylaxis recommendations changed dramatically in 2007. Prophylaxis is no longer recommended following routine gastrointestinal or genitourinary surgical procedures. It is usually not considered necessary for routine ocular surgery in a patient without infection but can be considered for surgery involving the nasolacrimal drainage system or sinuses or for surgical repair of orbital trauma, if the patient has a high-risk cardiac congenital or valvular condition (Table 14-1).

Table 14-1 SBE Prophylaxis Regimens for Dental and Incisional Nasolacrimal Procedures

		Regimen: Single Dose 30 to 60 min Before Procedure	
Situation	**Agent**	**Adults**	**Children**
Oral	Amoxicillin	2 g	50 mg/kg
Unable to take oral medication	Ampicillin **OR** Cefazolin or ceftriaxone	2 g IM or IV 1 g IM or IV	50 mg/kg IM or IV 50 mg/kg IM or IV
Allergic to penicillins or ampicillin—oral	Cephalexin*† **OR** Clindamycin **OR** Azithromycin or clarithromycin	2 g 600 mg 500 mg	50 mg/kg 20 mg/kg 15 mg/kg
Allergic to penicillins or ampicillin and unable to take oral medication	Cefazolin or ceftriaxone† **OR** Clindamycin	1 g IM or IV 600 mg IM or IV	50 mg/kg IM or IV 20 mg/kg IM or IV

IM = intramuscular; IV = intravenous; SBE = subacute bacterial endocarditis.
*Or other first- or second-generation oral cephalosporin in equivalent adult or pediatric dosage.
†Cephalosporins should not be used in an individual with a history of anaphylaxis, angioedema, or urticaria with penicillins or ampicillin.

Modified with permission from Wilson W, Taubert KA, Gewitz M, et al. Prevention of infective endocarditis. Guidelines from the American Heart Association: a guideline from the American Heart Association Rheumatic Fever, Endocarditis, and Kawasaki Disease Committee; Council on Cardiovascular Disease in the Young; and the Council on Clinical Cardiology; Council on Cardiovascular Surgery and Anesthesia; and the Quality of Care and Outcomes Research Interdisciplinary Working Group. *Circulation.* 2007;116(15):1736–1754, Table 5. Full online text available at: http://circ.ahajournals.org/cgi/content/full/116/15/1736.

Duesberg CB, Malhotra-Kumar S, Goossens H, et al. Interspecies recombination occurs frequently in quinolone resistance-determining regions of clinical isolates of *Streptococcus pyogenes*. *Antimicrob Agents Chemother.* 2008;52(11):4191–4193.

Grabenstein JD, Musey LK. Differences in serious clinical outcomes of infection caused by specific pneumococcal serotypes among adults. *Vaccine.* 2014;32(21):2399–2405.

Nishimura RA, Carabello BA, Faxon DP, et al; American College of Cardiology/American Heart Association Task Force. ACC/AHA 2008 guideline update on valvular heart disease: focused update on infective endocarditis: a report of the American College of Cardiology/American Heart Association Task Force on Practice Guidelines: endorsed by the Society of Cardiovascular Anesthesiologists, Society for Cardiovascular Angiography and Interventions, and Society of Thoracic Surgeons. *Circulation.* 2008;118(8):887–896.

Wilson W, Taubert KA, Gewitz M, et al. Prevention of infective endocarditis. Guidelines from the American Heart Association: a guideline from the American Heart Association Rheumatic Fever, Endocarditis, and Kawasaki Disease Committee, Council on Cardiovascular Disease in the Young, and the Council on Clinical Cardiology, Council on Cardiovascular Surgery and Anesthesia, and the Quality of Care and Outcomes Research Interdisciplinary Working Group. *Circulation.* 2007;116(15):1736–1754.

Clostridium difficile

Clostridium difficile is an endemic anaerobic gram-positive bacillus that is part of the normal gastrointestinal flora. It has acquired importance because of its role in the development of pseudomembranous enterocolitis following the use of antibiotics. Typically, fever and diarrhea develop 1–14 days after the start of antibiotic therapy. The diarrhea occasionally becomes bloody and typically contains a cytopathic toxin that is elaborated by *C difficile.*

In the past, a tissue-culture assay for the toxin was the best diagnostic test. Newer enzyme immunoassay and PCR tests allow more rapid detection. The most frequently implicated antibiotics include clindamycin, ampicillin, chloramphenicol, tetracycline, erythromycin, and the cephalosporins. New, hypervirulent strains of *C difficile* have recently emerged in the United States, Europe, and Japan. Initial treatment includes discontinuing the causative antibiotic and administering metronidazole for 10 days. Vancomycin is also effective, but its use should be limited to minimize the development of vancomycin-resistant organisms such as enterococci and staphylococci. It is also much more expensive than metronidazole. Vancomycin should be used only in patients who cannot tolerate or have not responded to metronidazole, or in situations in which metronidazole use is contraindicated, such as during the first trimester of pregnancy. Rifampin, fusidic acid, nitazoxanide, ramoplanin, rifaximin, intravenous immunoglobulin, and a new toxin-binding polymer have been evaluated as potential alternative therapies, and trials evaluating a new toxoid vaccine are ongoing. Corticosteroids have been proven to reduce the diarrhea associated with *C difficile* infection.

Khanna S, Pardi DS. *Clostridium difficile* infections: management strategies for a difficult disease. *Therap Adv Gastroenterol.* 2014;7(2):72–86.

Persson S, Torpdahl M, Olsen KE. New multiplex PCR method for the detection of *Clostridium difficile* toxin A (tcdA) and toxin B (tcdB) and the binary toxin (cdtA/cdtB) genes applied to a Danish strain collection. *Clin Microbiol Infect.* 2008;14(11):1057–1064.

Haemophilus influenzae

Haemophilus influenzae is a common inhabitant of the upper respiratory tract in 20%–50% of healthy adults and 80% of children. *H influenzae* is divided into 6 serotypes on the basis of differing capsular polysaccharide antigens. Both encapsulated and unencapsulated species cause disease, but systemic spread is typical of the encapsulated strain, whose capsule protects it against phagocytosis. Infants are usually protected for a few months by passively acquired maternal antibodies. Thereafter, active antibody levels increase with age, as they are inversely related to the risk of infection. *H influenzae* is 1 of 3 organisms responsible for most cases of bacterial meningitis. Of the patients with meningitis, roughly 14% develop significant neurologic damage. Other infections caused by this organism include epiglottitis, orbital cellulitis, arthritis, otitis media, bronchitis, pericarditis, sinusitis, and pneumonia. A DNA PCR probe assay is available for rapid diagnosis of *H influenzae* type b (Hib) infections.

Treatment of acute *H influenzae* infections has been complicated by the emergence of ampicillin-resistant strains, with an incidence approaching 50% in some geographic areas. Current recommendations are to start empirical therapy with amoxicillin-clavulanate, trimethoprim-sulfamethoxazole, a quinolone such as ciprofloxacin, or a third-generation cephalosporin, pending susceptibility testing of the organism. Nearly all isolates of *H influenzae* are now resistant to macrolides. Serious or life-threatening infections should be treated with an intravenous third-generation cephalosporin with known activity against *H influenzae,* such as ceftriaxone or cefotaxime, pending results of sensitivity testing. Recent reports note an increase in the number of isolates with reduced sensitivity to cephalosporins and quinolones, especially in patients with chronic pulmonary disease.

Haemophilus influenzae type b conjugate vaccines are available for use in infants and have shown their effectiveness in protecting infants and older children against meningitis and other invasive diseases caused by Hib infection. In studies of fully immunized populations, Hib infection has been nearly eradicated since these vaccines were introduced. Also, the incidence of meningitis, orbital cellulitis, and other infections caused by Hib has been reduced significantly since Hib conjugate vaccines became available. However, it is important to remember that immunized patients are still susceptible to infections caused by strains of *H influenzae* other than type b.

Davis S, Feikin D, Johnson HL. The effect of *Haemophilus influenzae* type B and pneumococcal conjugate vaccines on childhood meningitis mortality: a systematic review. *BMC Public Health.* 2013;13(Suppl 3):S21.

Schmitt HJ, Maechler G, Habermehl P, et al. Immunogenicity, reactogenicity, and immune memory after primary vaccination with a novel *Haemophilus influenzae-Neisseria meningitidis* serogroup C conjugate vaccine. *Clin Vaccine Immunol.* 2007;14(4):426–434.

Neisseria

Most *Neisseria* organisms are normal inhabitants of the upper respiratory and alimentary tracts; the commonly recognized pathogenic species are the meningococci and the gonococci. Meningococci can be cultured in up to 15% of healthy persons in nonepidemic periods. Virulence is determined by the polysaccharide capsule and the potent endotoxic activity of the cell wall, which can cause cardiovascular collapse, shock, and disseminated intravascular coagulation. Persons who are complement deficient or asplenic are at risk for serious clinical infections. Diagnostic testing may include Gram stain, blood and cerebrospinal fluid cultures, enzyme-linked immunosorbent assay (ELISA), and PCR. An automated fluorescent multiplex PCR assay that can simultaneously detect *N meningitidis, H influenzae,* and *S pneumoniae* can be used to evaluate patients with suspected meningitis. This test provides extremely high sensitivity and a specificity of 100% for each organism.

The range of meningococcal infections includes meningitis; mild to severe upper respiratory tract infections; and, less often, endocarditis, arthritis, pericarditis, pneumonia, endophthalmitis, and purpura fulminans. *Neisseria meningitidis* serogroup B is the most common cause of bacterial meningitis in children and young adults. Meningitis with a petechial or pupuric exanthem is the classic presentation, although each may occur in isolation.

Historically, the treatment of choice for meningococcal meningitis has been high-dose penicillin or, in the case of allergy, chloramphenicol or a third-generation cephalosporin. However, in one European study, 39% of asymptomatic carriers and approximately 55% of infected patients had isolates with decreased susceptibility to penicillin. Rifampin or minocycline is used as chemoprophylaxis for family members and intimate personal contacts of the infected individual. Polysaccharide vaccines are most effective in older children and adults. The routine administration of meningococcal vaccines is not recommended, except in patients who have undergone splenectomy, patients who are complement deficient, military personnel, travelers to endemic regions, and close contacts of infected patients.

Gonococci are not normal inhabitants of the respiratory or genital flora, and their major reservoir is the asymptomatic patient. Among women with gonococcal infections, 50% are asymptomatic, whereas 95% of men with these infections have symptoms. Asymptomatic patients are infectious for several months, with a transmissibility rate of 20%–50%. Nonsexual transmission is rare. The key to prevention is identification and treatment of asymptomatic carriers and their sexual contacts.

Chlamydia trachomatis coexists with gonorrhea in 25%–50% of women with endocervical gonorrhea and 20%–33% of men with gonococcal urethritis. Diagnosis of gonococcal infections, as well as infections caused by many other bacteria, mycobacteria, viruses, and *Mycoplasma,* has been enhanced with the development of highly sensitive DNA probes that use PCR techniques. The range of gonococcal infections includes cervicitis; urethritis; pelvic inflammatory disease; pharyngitis; conjunctivitis; ophthalmia neonatorum; and disseminated gonococcal disease with fever, polyarthralgias, and rash.

Because penicillin-resistant and tetracycline-resistant gonococcal strains have become common in many areas of the United States, treatment should be tailored to their local prevalence. Tetracycline is effective for patients who are infected by susceptible strains, are allergic to penicillin, or have concurrent chlamydial infections. Ceftriaxone (via intramuscular injection) is the drug of choice for penicillinase-resistant strains; thus far, reduced susceptibility to this antibiotic has been extremely rare. Other alternatives include oral cefixime, cefuroxime, azithromycin, and the fluoroquinolones. The macrolides and fluoroquinolones have the added benefit of excellent activity against concomitant *C trachomatis* infection. However, gonococcal isolates with reduced sensitivity to macrolides and fluoroquinolones have been reported with increasing frequency, and the US Centers for Disease Control and Prevention (CDC) recently recommended that clinicians no longer use fluoroquinolones as a first-line treatment for gonorrhea in one high-risk group, men who have sex with men.

Matsumoto T. Trends of sexually transmitted diseases and antimicrobial resistance in *Neisseria gonorrhoeae. Int J Antimicrob Agents.* 2008;31(Suppl 1):S35–S39.

Workowski KA, Berman SM, Douglas JM Jr. Emerging antimicrobial resistance in *Neisseria gonorrhoeae:* urgent need to strengthen prevention strategies. *Ann Intern Med.* 2008; 148(8):606–613.

Pseudomonas aeruginosa

Pseudomonas aeruginosa is a gram-negative bacillus found free-living in moist environments. Together with *Serratia marcescens, P aeruginosa* is 1 of the 2 most consistently antimicrobial-resistant pathogenic bacteria. Infection usually requires either a break in the first-line defenses or altered immunity resulting in a local pyogenic response. The virulence of this organism is related to extracellular toxins, endotoxin, and a polysaccharide protection from phagocytosis. Systemic spread can result in disseminated intravascular coagulation, shock, and death.

Usual sites of infection include the respiratory system, skin, eye, urinary tract, bone, and wounds. Systemic infections caused by a resistant organism carry a high mortality rate and are usually associated with depressed immunity, often in a hospital setting.

More than half of *P aeruginosa* isolates are now resistant to aminoglycosides. Therefore, treatment of serious infections relies on combined antimicrobial coverage with either a semisynthetic penicillin or a third-generation cephalosporin with an aminoglycoside. Ceftazidime has been the most effective cephalosporin for treatment of pseudomonal infections. Piperacillin-tazobactam, imipenem, and meropenem also remain highly effective against most isolates, but resistance to the carbapenems and fluoroquinolones has been increasing gradually. The initial choice of antimicrobials depends on local susceptibility prevalence and should be guided by susceptibility testing. Multidrug-resistant *P aeruginosa* arises in a stepwise manner following prolonged exposure to antipseudomonal antibiotics and results in adverse outcomes, with high mortality.

The use of vaccines incorporating multiple *P aeruginosa* serotypes is under investigation for the treatment of patients with severe burns, cystic fibrosis, or immunosuppression. Oral fluoroquinolones, as well as macrolides such as azithromycin, have been useful as prophylactic agents in patients with cystic fibrosis.

Hocquet D, Berthelot P, Roussel-Delvallez M, et al. *Pseudomonas aeruginosa* may accumulate drug resistance mechanisms without losing its ability to cause bloodstream infections. *Antimicrob Agents Chemother.* 2007;51(10):3531–3536.

Tam VH, Chang KT, LaRocco MT, et al. Prevalence, mechanisms, and risk factors of carbapenem resistance in bloodstream isolates of *Pseudomonas aeruginosa. Diagn Microbiol Infect Dis.* 2007;58(3):309–314.

Treponema pallidum

The spirochete *Treponema pallidum* (syphilis) is exclusively a human pathogen. Infection usually follows sexual contact. Transplacental transmission from an untreated pregnant woman to her fetus before 16 weeks' gestation results in *congenital syphilis.*

Stages

The course of the disease is divided into 4 stages: primary, secondary, latent, and tertiary (late). Initial inoculation occurs through intact mucous membranes or abraded skin and, within 6 weeks, results in a broad, ulcerated, painless papule called a *chancre.* The spirochetes readily enter the lymphatic system and bloodstream. The ulcer heals spontaneously, and signs of dissemination appear after a variable quiescent period of several weeks to months.

The secondary stage is heralded by fever, malaise, adenopathy, and patchy loss of hair. Meningitis, uveitis, optic neuritis, and hepatitis are less common. Maculopapular lesions may develop into wartlike condylomata in moist areas, and oral mucosal patches sometimes appear. All of these lesions are highly infectious. The secondary lesions usually resolve in 2–6 weeks, although up to 25% of patients may experience relapse in the first 2–4 years. Without treatment, the disease enters the latent stage.

Latent syphilis, characterized by positive serologic results without clinical signs, is divided into 2 stages. The *early latent stage* occurs within 1 year of infection. During this time, the disease is potentially transmissible, because relapses associated with spirochetemia are possible. The *late latent stage* is associated with immunity to relapse and resistance to infectious lesions.

Tertiary manifestations can occur from 2 to 20 years after infection, and one-third of untreated cases of latent disease progress to this stage. The remaining two-thirds of cases either are subclinical or resolve spontaneously. *Tertiary disease* is characterized by destructive granulomatous lesions with a typical endarteritis that can affect the skin, bones, joints, oral and nasal cavities, parenchymal organs, cardiovascular system, eyes, meninges, and central nervous system (CNS). Few spirochetes are found in lesions outside the CNS.

Pathologically, obliterative endarteritis with a perivascular infiltrate of lymphocytes, monocytes, and plasma cells is a feature of all active stages of syphilis. Gummata of tertiary syphilis are evidenced by a central area of caseating necrosis with a surrounding granulomatous response.

Diagnosis

Most cases of syphilis are diagnosed serologically. *Nontreponemal tests* such as the VDRL test or rapid plasma reagin (RPR) test are usually positive during the early stages of the primary lesion, uniformly positive during the secondary stage, and progressively nonreactive in the later stages. In patients with neurosyphilis, the serum VDRL test result may be negative and the cerebrospinal fluid VDRL test result may be positive. These patients require careful evaluation and aggressive treatment with close follow-up. Nontreponemal test results become predictably negative after successful therapy and can be used to assess the efficacy of treatment; however, they can be falsely positive in a variety of autoimmune diseases, especially systemic lupus erythematosus and the antiphospholipid antibody syndrome (see Chapter 9). Fewer than 50% of patients with the antiphospholipid antibody syndrome have lupus. False-positive VDRL test results can also occur in liver disease, diseases with a substantial amount of tissue destruction, pregnancy, or infections caused by other treponemae.

The *fluorescent treponemal antibody absorption (FTA-ABS) test* involves specific detection of antibody to *T pallidum* after the patient's serum is treated with nonpathogenic treponemal antigens to avoid nonspecific reactions. Hemagglutination tests specific for treponemal antibodies also have high sensitivity and specificity for detecting syphilis. These tests include the hemagglutination treponemal test for syphilis (HATTS), the *T pallidum* hemagglutination assay (TPHA), and the microhemagglutination test for *T pallidum* (MHA-TP). Treponemal antibody detection tests are more specific than nontreponemal tests, but the titers do not decrease with successful treatment; thus, such tests should be considered confirmatory, especially in later stages of disease. Results of treponemal tests can be falsely positive in 15% of patients with systemic lupus erythematosus; in patients with other treponemal infections or Lyme disease; and, in rare instances, in patients who have lymphosarcoma or who are pregnant, although the fluorescent staining is typically weak.

Newer, more sensitive diagnostic tests for syphilis are ELISA, Western blot, and DNA PCR techniques. These methods may also improve the diagnosis of congenital syphilis and neurosyphilis. Currently, it is recommended that treponemal enzyme immunoassays (EIAs) be used in conjunction with other screening tests.

Management

Treatment of syphilis is determined by stage and by CNS involvement. *Treponema pallidum* is exquisitely sensitive to penicillin, which remains the antimicrobial of choice. In infected individuals younger than 1 year, the treatment of choice is an intramuscular injection of penicillin G, 2.4 million U. Patients older than 1 year should be treated with an intramuscular injection of penicillin G, 2.4 million U weekly for 3 weeks, and those with neurosyphilis should receive intravenous penicillin G, 2–4 million U, every 4 hours for 10 days. Treatment of ocular syphilis is the same as for neurosyphilis. Erythromycin, azithromycin, chloramphenicol, tetracycline, doxycycline, and the cephalosporins are acceptable alternatives to penicillin. Lumbar puncture should be performed to determine cerebrospinal fluid involvement in a number of circumstances, namely latent syphilis of more than 1 year's duration, suspected neurosyphilis, treatment failure, HIV coinfection, high RPR titers (>1:32), and evidence of other late manifestations (cardiac involvement, gummata). Either penicillin G or a single oral dose of azithromycin has been recommended for treatment of patients who were recently exposed to a sexual partner with infectious syphilis. There have been reports of syphilis treatment failures with use of azithromycin, but the cure rate is still higher than that of penicillin G.

Many reports have described an accelerated clinical course of syphilis in HIV-infected patients; furthermore, such patients may experience an incomplete response to standard therapy. A patient coinfected with HIV and syphilis often requires a longer and more intensive treatment regimen, ongoing follow-up to assess for recurrence, and a complete neurologic workup with an aggressive cerebrospinal fluid investigation for evidence of neurosyphilis. Ceftriaxone compares favorably with intravenous penicillin for the treatment of neurosyphilis in HIV-coinfected patients. Patients with any stage of clinical syphilis should be tested for HIV serostatus.

Bai ZG, Yang KH, Liu YL, et al. Azithromycin vs. benzathine penicillin G for early syphilis: a meta-analysis of randomized clinical trials. *Int J STD AIDS.* 2008;19(4):217–221.

Bosshard PP. Usefulness of IgM-specific enzyme immunoassays for serodiagnosis of syphilis: comparative evaluation of three different assays. *J Infect.* 2013;67(1):35–42.

Gottlieb SL, Pope V, Sternberg MR, et al. Prevalence of syphilis seroreactivity in the United States: data from the National Health and Nutrition Examination Surveys (NHANES) 2001–2004. *Sex Transm Dis.* 2008;35(5):507–511.

Pialoux G, Vimont S, Moulignier A, Buteux M, Abraham B, Bonnard P. Effect of HIV infection on the course of syphilis. *AIDS Rev.* 2008;10(2):85–92.

Borrelia burgdorferi

Borrelia burgdorferi is a large, microaerophilic, plasmid-containing spirochete. When transmitted to humans and domestic animals through the bite of the *Ixodes* genus of ticks, this organism can cause both acute and chronic illness, now known as *Lyme disease.* First recognized in 1975, Lyme disease is the most common vector-borne infection in the United States. Although cases have been reported in nearly all states, clusters are apparent in the northeast Atlantic, the upper Midwest, and the Pacific southwest areas, corresponding to the distribution of the *Ixodes* tick population. The range of the disease extends throughout Europe and Asia.

The life cycle of the spirochete depends on its horizontal transmission through a mouse. Early in the summer, an infected *Ixodes* tick nymph (juvenile) bites a mouse, which becomes infected; then, in late summer, the infection is transmitted to an immature uninfected larva after it bites the infected mouse. This immature larva then molts to become a nymph, and the cycle is repeated. Once a nymph matures to an adult, its favorite host is the white-tailed deer, although it can survive in other hosts. Recently, scientists discovered that 2 other tick-borne zoonoses (babesiosis and human granulocytic ehrlichiosis) can be cotransmitted with Lyme disease.

Stages

Lyme disease usually occurs in 3 stages following a tick bite: *localized (stage 1), disseminated (stage 2),* and *persistent (stage 3).* Localized disease (stage 1), present in 86% of infected patients, is characterized by skin involvement, initially a red macule or papule, which later expands in a circular manner, usually with a bright red border and a central clear indurated area, known as *erythema chronicum migrans.* Hematogenous dissemination (stage 2) can occur within days to weeks and is manifested as a flulike illness with headaches, fatigue, and musculoskeletal aches.

More profound symptoms occur as the infection localizes to the nervous, cardiovascular, and musculoskeletal systems (stage 3). Neurologic complications such as meningitis, encephalitis, cranial neuritis (including Bell palsy), radiculopathy, and neuropathy occur in 10%–15% of patients. A study from Boston revealed that Lyme disease was responsible for 34% of pediatric cases of acute facial nerve palsy. Cardiac manifestations include myopericarditis and variable heart block in 5% of patients. Unilateral asymmetric arthritis occurs in up to 80% of untreated patients.

Late persistent manifestations are usually confined to the nervous system, skin, and joints. Late neurologic signs include encephalomyelitis as well as demyelinating and psychiatric syndromes. Joint involvement includes asymmetric pauciarticular arthritis; skin involvement is characterized by acrodermatitis chronica atrophicans or localized lesions resembling those of systemic sclerosis.

Other systemic manifestations during the initial dissemination or the late persistent state include lymphadenopathy, conjunctivitis, keratitis, neuritis, uveitis, orbital myositis, hematuria, and orchitis. In some studies, serologic testing of patients with chronic fatigue syndrome has shown an increased incidence of positive results for *B burgdorferi* antibodies.

Diagnosis

During the early stages of infection, the immune response is minimal, with little cellular reactivity to *B burgdorferi* antigens and nonspecific elevation of IgM. During the disseminated phase, the cellular antigenic response is markedly increased and specific IgM is followed by a polyclonal B-lymphocyte activation; specific IgG antibody develops within weeks of the initial infection. Histopathology shows lymphocytic tissue infiltration, often in a perivascular distribution. Late manifestations may be either human leukocyte antigen (HLA)-mediated autoimmune damage or prolonged latency followed by persistent infection.

Laboratory diagnosis of *B burgdorferi* infection depends on serodiagnosis. However, there is a poor recovery rate of positive serology from blood, cerebrospinal fluid, and synovial fluid during the early stages of infection. Skin biopsy specimens with monoclonal antibody staining have demonstrated good sensitivity in identifying the organism. Although serodiagnosis remains the practical solution for establishing the diagnosis, laboratory methodology is not standardized.

The most commonly used serologic tests are the immunofluorescence antibody assay or the more sensitive ELISA. The ELISA is 50% sensitive during the early stages of the disease, and almost all symptomatic patients test seropositive during the later disseminated and persistent phases of the infection. These tests should be used only to support a clinical diagnosis of Lyme disease, not as the primary basis for making diagnostic or treatment decisions. Positive IgG and IgM ELISA results are usually confirmed with Western immunoblot testing. Serologic testing is not useful early in the course of Lyme disease because of the low sensitivity of tests in early disease. Serologic testing is more helpful in later disease, when the sensitivity and specificity are greater. False-positive results can occur in patients with syphilis, Rocky Mountain spotted fever, yaws, pinta, *B recurrentis* infection, and various rheumatologic disorders. PCR has been used to detect *B burgdorferi* DNA in serum and cerebrospinal fluid, but its sensitivity in neuroborreliosis is no better than that of the ELISA methods. Although patients with Lyme disease may test positive on the FTA-ABS test for syphilis, their VDRL test result should be nonreactive.

Management

Treatment of *B burgdorferi* infection depends on the stage and severity of the infection. Early Lyme disease is typically treated with oral doxycycline, amoxicillin, cefuroxime, or erythromycin. Mild disseminated disease is treated with oral doxycycline or amoxicillin. Serious disease (with cardiac or neurologic manifestations) is typically treated with ceftriaxone or high-dose penicillin G for up to 6 weeks. Infections that do not respond to the initial regimen may require alternate or combination therapy. In up to 15% of patients, a *Jarisch-Herxheimer reaction* (symptoms worsen during the first day of treatment) may occur.

Bacon RM, Kugeler KJ, Mead PS; Centers for Disease Control and Prevention (CDC). Surveillance for Lyme disease—United States, 1992–2006. *MMWR Surveill Summ.* 2008; 57(10):1–9.

Klempner MS, Baker PJ, Shapiro ED, et al. Treatment trials for post-Lyme disease symptoms revisited. *Am J Med.* 2013;126(8):665–669.

Marques A. Chronic Lyme disease: a review. *Infect Dis Clin North Am.* 2008;22(2):341–360.

Chlamydia trachomatis

Chlamydia trachomatis is a small, obligate, intracellular parasite that contains DNA and RNA and has a unique biphasic life cycle. These prokaryotes use the host cell's energy-generating capacity for their own reproduction. The bacterium can survive only briefly outside the body. Transmitted by close contact, *C trachomatis* is the causative agent of the most common sexually transmitted infection, with 4 million new cases per year in the United States. More than 15% of pregnant women and 10% of men with chlamydial infections are asymptomatic.

Infection is initiated by local inoculation and ingestion of the organism by phagocytes, followed by intracellular reproduction and eventual spread to other cells. The mechanism for immunologic eradication of *Chlamydia* is uncertain but appears to involve cell-mediated immunity. Infections in humans include trachoma, inclusion conjunctivitis, nongonococcal urethritis, epididymitis, mucopurulent cervicitis, proctitis, salpingitis, infant pneumonia syndrome, and lymphogranuloma venereum. Genital *C trachomatis* infection can cause pelvic inflammatory disease, tubal infertility, and ectopic pregnancy. In one study, 80% of ocular adnexal lymphoma samples carried DNA of a related organism, *Chlamydophila psittaci*, suggesting that this species plays an etiologic role in some cases of lymphoma. Diagnostic techniques include culture, direct immunofluorescence antibody testing of exudates, enzyme immunoassay, and DNA probes using PCR.

Chlamydial infections are readily treated with tetracycline, erythromycin, or one of the quinolones or macrolides. Although single-dose azithromycin or sparfloxacin therapy for urethritis and cervicitis has proven effective in some studies, it is usually recommended that patients continue treatment for at least 7 days to ensure complete eradication. Sexual partners of patients with chlamydial infections, as well as other sexually transmitted diseases, should be examined and counseled for consideration of antibiotic treatment as well. See BCSC Section 8, *External Disease and Cornea,* for more information.

Gaydos CA, Ferrero DV, Papp J. Laboratory aspects of screening men for *Chlamydia trachomatis* in the new millennium. *Sex Transm Dis.* 2008;35(11 Suppl):S45–S50.

Karunakaran KP, Rey-Ladino J, Stoynov N, et al. Immunoproteomic discovery of novel T cell antigens from the obligate intracellular pathogen *Chlamydia. J Immunol.* 2008;180(4):2459–2465.

Mycoplasma pneumoniae

Mycoplasma pneumoniae is a unique bacterium that may cause multiple disorders—including pharyngitis, otitis media, tracheobronchitis, pneumonia, endocarditis, nephritis, encephalitis, meningitis, optic neuritis, and facial nerve palsy—and has been implicated in some cases of chronic fatigue and fibromyalgia syndromes. Serious *M pneumoniae* infections requiring hospital admission occur in both adults and children and may involve multiple organ systems. Extrapulmonary complications involving all the major organ systems can occur in association with *M pneumoniae* infection as a result of direct invasion or autoimmune response. Recent evidence suggests that *M pneumoniae* may play a contributory role in chronic lung disorders such as asthma.

PCR assays have been adapted for the direct detection of *M pneumoniae* organisms, but in clinical practice, sensitive serologic tests are usually used initially to detect antibodies. Initial treatment of *M pneumoniae* infections typically involves use of a macrolide, tetracycline, or fluoroquinolone.

Atkinson TP, Balish MF, Waites KB. Epidemiology, clinical manifestations, pathogenesis and laboratory detection of *Mycoplasma pneumoniae* infections. *FEMS Microbiol Rev.* 2008;32(6):956–973.

Nilsson AC, Björkman P, Persson K. Polymerase chain reaction is superior to serology for the diagnosis of acute *Mycoplasma pneumoniae* infection and reveals a high rate of persistent infection. *BMC Microbiol.* 2008;8:93.

Nomanpour B, Ghodousi A, Babaei T, Jafari S, Feizabadi MM. Single tube real time PCR for detection of *Streptococcus pneumoniae, Mycoplasma pneumoniae, Chlamydophila pneumoniae* and *Legionella pneumophila* for clinical samples of CAP. *Acta Microbiol Immunol Hung.* 2012;59(2):171–184.

Mycobacteria

Mycobacteria include a range of pathogenic and nonpathogenic species distributed widely in the environment. *Mycobacterium tuberculosis* is the most significant human pathogenic species. This bacterium infects an estimated 2 billion persons worldwide (33% global prevalence) and causes approximately 1.4 million deaths each year. There are at least

8 million new cases of tuberculosis each year, most of which occur in Africa and Southeast Asia. Nontuberculous mycobacteria may be responsible for up to 5% of all clinical mycobacterial infections. Atypical mycobacterial infections are more prevalent in immunosuppressed patients, including those with AIDS. Infections caused by nontuberculous mycobacteria include lymphadenitis, pulmonary infections, skin granulomas, prosthetic valve infections, and bacteremia. Despite their low virulence, atypical mycobacterial infections are difficult to treat because of their resistance to standard antituberculous regimens.

Tuberculosis

Infection with *M tuberculosis* usually occurs through inhalation of infective droplets and, in rare cases, by way of the skin or gastrointestinal tract. Cell-mediated hypersensitivity to tuberculoprotein develops 3–9 weeks after infection, with a typical granulomatous response that slows or contains bacterial multiplication. Most organisms die during the fibrotic phase of the response. Reactivation is usually associated with depressed immunity and aging. Systemic spread occurs with reactivation and results in a granulomatous response to the infected foci. Acquired immunity is cell mediated but incomplete, and the role of delayed hypersensitivity is complex: high degrees of sensitivity to tuberculoprotein can cause caseous necrosis, which leads to spread of the disease. Infections include pulmonary involvement, which can lead to systemic spread with involvement of any organ system.

Laboratory diagnosis involves culture of infective material on Löwenstein-Jensen medium for 6–8 weeks and use of the acid-fast type of Ziehl-Neelsen stain or fluorescent antibody staining of infected material. In addition, DNA probes using PCR techniques for *M tuberculosis* and other mycobacteria are available. Newer PCR assays can identify resistant strains of TB by detecting isoniazid- and rifampin-resistance mutations in organisms from cultures or from smear-positive specimens.

The tuberculin skin test measures delayed hypersensitivity to tuberculoprotein. Purified protein derivative (PPD) produced from a culture filtrate of *M tuberculosis* is standardized and its activity expressed as tuberculin units (TU). A positive PPD reaction is defined as a 10 mm or greater area of induration in the area of intradermal injection of 0.1 mL of PPD read 48–72 hours later. For children, the tine test is an easily administered alternative to the PPD. In 2005, the first interferon-gamma release assay received approval from the US Food and Drug Administration (FDA) as an alternative to the PPD skin test. This test detects the release of interferon-γ from sensitized patients. Its specificity is higher than, but the sensitivity is similar to, that of the PPD skin test. It also appears to be less affected by previous BCG vaccination, which causes false-positive reactions to the PPD skin test and thus interferes with the efficacy of the test as a diagnostic and epidemiologic tool. The false-positive effect of BCG decreases over time, so PPD may still be useful in patients who have previously received the BCG vaccine.

Among patients in whom skin testing yields positive results, the overall risk of disease reactivation is 3%–5%. A positive PPD test result should be considered in light of the individual patient's radiologic and clinical data, as well as age, to determine the need for prophylactic treatment. Administration of isoniazid daily for 1 year reduces the risk of reactivation by 80%; however, the risk of isoniazid hepatotoxicity increases with age and alcohol use. Nevertheless, patients with a positive tuberculin skin test result who require long-term high-dose corticosteroids or other immunosuppressive agents should be treated prophylactically with isoniazid for the duration of their immunosuppressive therapy in order to prevent reactivation.

Treatment of active infection involves the use of 2 or 3 drugs because of the emergence of *M tuberculosis* resistance to certain drugs and because of delay in receiving the results of culture susceptibility studies. Standard regimens employ multiple drugs for 18–24 months, but with the addition of newer agents, treatment for 6–9 months has been found equally effective. Currently used drugs include isoniazid, rifampin, rifabutin, ethambutol, streptomycin, pyrazinamide, aminosalicylic acid, ethionamide, and cycloserine. All currently used agents have toxic adverse effects, especially hepatic and neurologic, which should be carefully monitored during the course of therapy. Isoniazid and ethambutol can cause optic neuritis in a small percentage of patients, and rifampin may cause pink-tinged tears and blepharoconjunctivitis.

Outbreaks of nosocomial and community-acquired multidrug-resistant TB (MDRTB) have increased, particularly in the presence of concurrent HIV infection. MDRTB in HIV-infected patients is associated with widely disseminated disease, poor treatment response, and substantial mortality. MDRTB infection has also been documented in health care workers exposed to these patients. MDRTB represents a serious public health threat that will require an aggressive governmental and medical response to limit its spread. Newer fluoroquinolones and some of the newer classes of broad-spectrum antibiotics, such as linezolid, are effective against many isolates of MDRTB, as well as against atypical mycobacteria, and have been recommended as potential therapeutic alternatives.

Dover LG, Bhatt A, Bhowruth V, Willcox BE, Besra GS. New drugs and vaccines for drug-resistant *Mycobacterium tuberculosis* infections. *Expert Rev Vaccines.* 2008;7(4):481–497.

Sollai S, Galli L, de Martino M, Chiappini E. Systematic review and meta-analysis on the utility of Interferon-gamma release assays for the diagnosis of *Mycobacterium tuberculosis* infection in children: a 2013 update. *BMC Infect Dis.* 2014;14(Suppl 1):S6.

Zumla AI, Gillespie SH, Hoelscher M, et al. New antituberculosis drugs, regimens, and adjunct therapies: needs, advances, and future prospects. *Lancet Infect Dis.* 2014;14(4): 327–340.

Fungal Infections

Candida albicans is a yeast that is normally present in the oral cavity, lower gastrointestinal tract, and female genital tract. Under conditions of disrupted local defenses or depressed immunity, overgrowth and parenchymal invasion occur, with the potential for systemic spread. Increased virulence of *Candida* is related to its mycelial phase, when it is more resistant to the host's cellular immune system, which acts as the primary modulator of infection. Infections include oral lesions (thrush) and vaginal, skin, esophageal, and urinary tract involvement. Chronic mucocutaneous lesions may occur in persons with specific T-lymphocyte defects. Disseminated disease can involve any organ system, most commonly the kidneys, brain, heart, and eyes, and is more common in immunocompromised patients and those with indwelling vascular catheters.

Other important invasive fungal infections are cryptococcosis, histoplasmosis, blastomycosis, aspergillosis, and coccidioidomycosis. Invasive fungal infections have become a major problem in immunocompromised patients. Fungal PCR assays allow more rapid diagnosis of serious fungal infections and offer higher sensitivity compared with fungal cultures.

Treatment of serious systemic infections has traditionally involved the use of intravenous amphotericin B, sometimes combined with flucytosine or an imidazole. Lipid complex and liposome-encapsulated formulations of amphotericin B were developed to reduce the nephrotoxic and myelosuppressive effects of this drug. A controlled study revealed that intravenous amphotericin B prophylaxis reduced the incidence of systemic fungal infections in immunocompromised patients with leukemia. Imidazoles, such as fluconazole, itraconazole, and voriconazole, are less toxic and better-tolerated alternatives. In fact, itraconazole has replaced ketoconazole as the treatment of choice for nonmeningeal, non–life-threatening cases of histoplasmosis, blastomycosis, and paracoccidioidomycosis. Itraconazole is also effective in treating patients with cryptococcosis and coccidioidomycosis, including those with meningitis.

Lehmann LE, Hunfeld KP, Emrich T, et al. A multiplex real-time PCR assay for rapid detection and differentiation of 25 bacterial and fungal pathogens from whole blood samples. *Med Microbiol Immunol.* 2008;197(3):313–324.

Prasad PA, Coffin SE, Leckerman KH, Walsh TJ, Zaoutis TE. Pediatric antifungal utilization: new drugs, new trends. *Pediatr Infect Dis J.* 2008;27(12):1083–1088.

Toxoplasma

Toxoplasmosis is caused by infection with the protozoan parasite *Toxoplasma gondii,* which infects up to one-third of the world's population. Acute infections may be asymptomatic in pregnant women; however, the infection can be transmitted to the fetus and cause severe complications, including cognitive impairment, blindness, and epilepsy. As many as 4000 new cases of congenital toxoplasmosis occur each year in the United States. Of the nearly 750 US deaths attributed to toxoplasmosis each year, approximately half are believed to be caused by eating contaminated undercooked or raw meat. *Toxoplasma gondii* can also be transmitted to humans by ingestion of oocysts, an environmentally resistant form of the organism, through exposure to cat feces, water, or soil containing the parasite or from eating unwashed contaminated fruits or vegetables.

Infection can be prevented in large part by cooking meat to a safe temperature, peeling or thoroughly washing fruits and vegetables before eating, and cleaning cooking surfaces and utensils after they have contacted raw meat. Pregnant women should avoid changing cat litter and handling raw or undercooked meat. Also, pet owners should keep cats indoors, where they are less likely to eat infected prey and subsequently acquire *T gondii.*

Primary infection is usually subclinical, but in some patients cervical lymphadenopathy or ocular disease can be present. The ocular manifestations include uveitis and chorioretinitis with macular scarring. The clinical picture and histopathology of toxoplasmosis are a reflection of the immune response, which includes an early humoral response, followed by the cellular response. The latter response varies from low-grade mononuclear infiltrate to total tissue destruction. In immunocompromised patients, reactivation of latent disease can cause life-threatening encephalitis.

Diagnosis of toxoplasmosis can be established by direct detection of the parasite or by serologic techniques. Real-time PCR is a very sensitive technique for diagnosing infection caused by *T gondii* and for determining the precise genotype of the organism. The most commonly used therapeutic regimen, and probably the most effective, comprises pyrimethamine combined with sulfadiazine and folinic acid. Recently, sulfadiazine has been replaced by sulfadoxine, which has a longer half-life and provides a dosing schedule resulting in improved adherence to treatment. Newer drugs with activity against *T gondii* include azithromycin, atovaquone, and clindamycin. See BCSC Section 12, *Retina and Vitreous,* for more details on the treatment of toxoplasmosis.

Alfonso Y, Fraga J, Cox R, et al. Comparison of four DNA extraction methods from cerebrospinal fluid for the detection of *Toxoplasma gondii* by polymerase chain reaction in AIDS patients. *Med Sci Monit.* 2008;14(3):MT1–MT6.

Fricker-Hidalgo H, Bulabois CE, Brenier-Pinchart MP, et al. Diagnosis of toxoplasmosis after allogeneic stem cell transplantation: results of DNA detection and serological techniques. *Clin Infect Dis.* 2009;48(2):e9–e15.

Herpesvirus

As a class, viruses are strictly intracellular parasites, relying on the host cell for their replication. Herpesviruses, which are large-enveloped, double-stranded DNA viruses, are some of the most common human infectious agents and are responsible for a wide spectrum of acute and chronic diseases. Herpesviruses of particular interest to the ophthalmologist are the herpes simplex viruses (HSV-1 and HSV-2), varicella-zoster virus (VZV), cytomegalovirus (CMV), and Epstein-Barr virus (EBV). There are 8 recognized types of human herpesviruses. Type 1 is HSV-1; type 2 is HSV-2; type 3 is VZV; type 4 is EBV; and type 5 is CMV; types 6 and 7, members of the genus *Roseolovirus,* cause roseola infantum and encephalitis; and type 8 is associated with Kaposi sarcoma and HIV-related lymphomas.

Herpes Simplex

Herpes simplex virus has 2 antigenic types, each of which has numerous antigenic strains. Each type has different epidemiologic patterns of infection. Seroepidemiologic studies show a high prevalence of HSV-1 antibodies and a lower prevalence of HSV-2 antibodies. Many persons with HSV antibodies are asymptomatic. Infection is modulated by a predominantly cellular response. The presence of high titers of neutralizing antibodies to HSV does not seem to retard the cell-to-cell transmission of the virus, which can spread within nerves and cause a latent infection of sensory and autonomic ganglia. Reactivation of HSV from the trigeminal ganglia may be associated with asymptomatic excretion or with the development of mucosal herpetic ulceration. Serologic testing, DNA PCR testing, and viral culture can help diagnose difficult cases, particularly CNS infections.

HSV-1 is associated with mucocutaneous infections of the pharynx, skin, oral cavity, vagina, eye, and brain. Ophthalmic infection most often manifests as corneal dendritic or stromal disease but may present as acute retinal necrosis. (The ocular manifestations of HSV infection are discussed in more detail in BCSC Section 8, *External Disease and Cornea,* and Section 9, *Intraocular Inflammation and Uveitis.*) Herpes encephalitis carries a 15% mortality rate. *HSV-2* infection is an important sexually transmitted disease that is associated with genital infections, aseptic meningitis, and congenital infection. *Neonatal herpes infection* involves multiple systems and, if untreated, has a mortality rate as high as 80%.

The drug of choice for treating acute systemic infections is acyclovir. Localized disease can be treated with oral acyclovir. Topical treatment of skin or mucocutaneous lesions with acyclovir ointment decreases the healing time. Oral acyclovir can also be used prophylactically for severe and recurrent genital herpes. Long-term suppressive oral acyclovir (400 mg twice a day) also reduces the recurrence of herpes simplex epithelial keratitis and stromal keratitis. Intravenous acyclovir is used to treat herpes encephalitis.

Two additional antiviral agents, famciclovir and valacyclovir, have been approved in the United States for the treatment of herpes zoster and herpes simplex infections. Compared with acyclovir, these agents have better bioavailability and achieve higher blood levels. In Europe, valacyclovir is used mostly for the treatment and prophylaxis of localized herpes zoster and herpes simplex infections. HSV is also sensitive to vidarabine. Cidofovir, an antiviral drug used to treat CMV infections, is also very effective against acyclovir-resistant herpes simplex.

Varicella-Zoster

Varicella-zoster virus, also sometimes referred to as *herpes zoster,* produces infection in a manner similar to that of HSV. After a primary infection, VZV remains latent in dorsal root ganglia; host cellular immune interaction inhibits reactivation. Primary infection usually occurs in childhood in the form of *chickenpox (varicella),* a generalized vesicular rash accompanied by mild constitutional symptoms. Reactivation may be heralded by pain in a sensory nerve distribution, followed by a unilateral vesicular eruption occurring over 1 to 3 dermatomic areas. New crops of lesions appear in the same area within 7 days. Resolution of the lesions may be followed by postherpetic neuralgia. Other neurologic sequelae following VZV reactivation include segmental myelitis, Guillain-Barré syndrome, and Ramsay Hunt syndrome. The incidence of VZV is 2 to 3 times higher in patients older than 60 years. Postherpetic neuralgia occurs after VZV infection in approximately 50% of patients older than 50 years. The pain of postherpetic neuralgia can be severe and debilitating and may persist for months or even years. Immunosuppressed persons experience recurrent lesions and an increased incidence of disseminated disease.

For immunocompetent adults with cutaneous VZV infection, recommended 7-day treatment regimens include famciclovir (500 mg twice a day), valacyclovir (1000 mg 3 times a day), and acyclovir 800 mg (5 times a day). Treatment of acute infection in immunocompromised patients or those with visceral involvement may include acyclovir, famciclovir, or valacyclovir. Newer drugs being evaluated for resistant VZV strains or concomitant HIV infection include sorivudine, brivudine, fialuridine, fiacitabine, netivudine, lobucavir, foscarnet, and cidofovir. Varivax, a live attenuated varicella-zoster vaccine, is available for prevention of primary disease. This vaccine is recommended in the United States for immunocompetent persons 12 months of age and older. Zostavax, a live attenuated vaccine given as a single dose, is recommended for immunocompetent adults aged 60 years and older to reduce the risk of developing clinical zoster and postherpetic neuralgia.

In some patients, tricyclic antidepressants, pregabalin, carbamazepine, gabapentin, and topical capsaicin cream reduce the pain of postherpetic neuralgia. For refractory cases, transcutaneous electronic nerve stimulation or nerve blocks are sometimes helpful.

Engelmann I, Petzold DR, Kosinska A, Hepkema BG, Schulz TF, Heim A. Rapid quantitative PCR assays for the simultaneous detection of herpes simplex virus, varicella zoster virus, cytomegalovirus, Epstein-Barr virus, and human herpesvirus 6 DNA in blood and other clinical specimens. *J Med Virol.* 2008;80(3):467–477.

Plentz A, Jilg W, Kochanowski B, Ibach B, Knöll A. Detection of herpesvirus DNA in cerebrospinal fluid and correlation with clinical symptoms. *Infection.* 2008;36(2):158–162.

Cytomegalovirus

Cytomegalovirus is a ubiquitous human virus: 50% of adults in developed countries harbor antibodies, which are usually acquired during the first 5 years of life. The virus can be isolated from all body fluids, even in the presence of circulating neutralizing antibodies, for up to several years after infection. Serologic and PCR testing is available to assist in the diagnosis of CMV infection. Presence of the pp65 antigen, as detected by PCR, indicates the need for preemptive therapy against CMV.

Congenital CMV disease carries a 20% incidence of hearing loss or cognitive impairment and a 0.1% incidence of various other severe congenital disorders, including jaundice, hepatosplenomegaly, anemia, microcephaly, and chorioretinitis. Infections in adults include heterophile-negative mononucleosis, pneumonia, hepatitis, and Guillain-Barré syndrome. In immunocompromised patients, CMV interstitial pneumonia carries a 90% mortality rate. Disseminated spread to the gastrointestinal tract, CNS, and eyes is common in patients with AIDS. Latent infection within leukocytes accounts for transfusion-associated disease. Recent cases of CMV retinitis have been reported following intravitreal corticosteroid injections. CMV replication itself can further suppress cell-mediated immunity, with resultant depressed lymphocyte response and development of severe opportunistic infections.

Allice T, Cerutti F, Pittaluga F, et al. Evaluation of a novel real-time PCR system for cytomegalovirus DNA quantitation on whole blood and correlation with pp65-antigen test in guiding pre-emptive antiviral treatment. *J Virol Methods.* 2008;148(1–2):9–16.

Lazzarotto T, Guerra B, Lanari M, Gabrielli L, Landini MP. New advances in the diagnosis of congenital cytomegalovirus infection. *J Clin Virol.* 2008;41(3):192–197.

Ophthalmic considerations The FDA has approved several systemic treatments for CMV retinitis: intravenous or oral ganciclovir, intravenous foscarnet, and intravenous cidofovir. Because comparative trials have demonstrated similar efficacy for all of these systemic medications, the use of oral valganciclovir, a prodrug of ganciclovir, has largely surpassed the use of the other systemic medications, as it achieves greater bioavailability than does either intravenous or oral ganciclovir. All of these medications are administered at high doses for 3 weeks and then at maintenance doses to prevent relapse of retinitis. Intravitreal injections of ganciclovir or foscarnet are commonly used to supplement treatment.

Epstein-Barr Virus

Epstein-Barr virus antibodies are found in 90%–95% of all adults. Childhood infections are usually asymptomatic, while EBV infection in young adults is symptomatic. Infectious mononucleosis is the usual clinical disease in most symptomatic adults. Lymphoproliferative disorders may develop in transplant recipients taking cyclosporine and in patients with AIDS. EBV is epidemiologically associated with Burkitt lymphoma and nasopharyngeal carcinoma and has been reported in EBV-associated hemophagocytic lymphohistiocytosis (EBV-HLH), also known as *EBV-associated hemophagocytic syndrome.* This disease develops mostly in children and young adults and may be fatal. EBV has also been reported as a cause of pediatric acute renal failure. A highly sensitive PCR assay is available for detecting primary EBV infection and infectious mononucleosis.

Treatment of acute disease is largely supportive, although the EBV DNA polymerase is sensitive to acyclovir and ganciclovir, which decrease viral replication in tissue culture. No vaccine is currently available against EBV, but research is ongoing toward developing a cytotoxic T-lymphocyte–based vaccine.

Paramita DK, Fachiroh J, Haryana SM, Middeldorp JM. Evaluation of commercial EBV RecombLine assay for diagnosis of nasopharyngeal carcinoma. *J Clin Virol.* 2008;42(4): 343–352.

Rey J, Xerri L, Bouabdallah R, Keuppens M, Brousset P, Meggetto F. Detection of different clonal EBV strains in Hodgkin lymphoma and nasopharyngeal carcinoma tissues from the same patient. *Br J Haematol.* 2008;142(1):79–81.

Influenza

See Chapter 12 for a discussion of influenza and immunization.

Hepatitis

Hepatitis A and B

See Chapter 12 for discussion of hepatitis A and B and immunization.

Hepatitis C and Other Forms of Hepatitis

Approximately 20%–40% of acute viral hepatitis cases reported in the United States are of the non-A, non-B type; of this group, most cases are caused by the hepatitis C virus (HCV). Worldwide prevalence is approximately 1%. Current estimates suggest that 170,000 new cases of HCV infection occur annually in the United States; in 50%–80% of these patients, there is evidence of chronic hepatitis, and cirrhosis develops in 20% of those patients. Only 6% of reported cases of hepatitis C are transfusion related. Other recognized risk factors for the transmission of HCV include parenteral drug use, hemodialysis, and occupational exposure to HCV-infected blood. Although the role of sexual activity in the transmission of HCV remains to be fully elucidated, this mode is clearly not a predominant source of transmission. Of all the hepatitis viruses, HCV causes the most damage in immunocompetent hosts because of direct hepatocyte cytotoxicity, and it may cause cirrhosis, fulminant hepatitis, and hepatocellular carcinoma. At present, hepatitis C is the most common indication for liver transplantation in the United States.

A sensitive enzyme immunoassay has been developed for the detection and quantification of total HCV core antigen in anti-HCV-positive or anti-HCV-negative sera. Also, a 1-step PCR assay is available to detect HCV RNA and provide HCV genotyping.

Treatment of acute HCV infection with interferon-α_{2a} reduces the rate of acute infections converting to chronic HCV infections. The current treatment of choice for chronic active hepatitis C is combination therapy with peginterferon-α_{2a} or peginterferon-α_{2b} and the antiviral agent ribavirin. This combination can achieve up to 80% response rates for hepatitis C genotypes 2 and 3 and approximately a 50% response rate for patients with genotype 1, cirrhosis, or nonresponse to previous treatments. Management of chronic persistent hepatitis C is largely supportive, but some studies advocate prolonged therapy with peginterferon. A vaccine against HCV is being investigated.

Chronic delta hepatitis is a severe form of chronic liver disease caused by hepatitis delta virus (hepatitis D virus) infection superimposed on chronic hepatitis B. Both interferon-α_{2a} and lamivudine have been found to be beneficial in treating chronic hepatitis D infection.

Hepatitis E virus is a small, nonenveloped RNA virus that is transmitted enterically and causes sporadic as well as epidemic acute viral hepatitis in many developing countries. As a superinfection in patients with preexisting chronic liver disease, hepatitis E may cause severe liver decompensation, often complicated by hepatic encephalopathy and renal failure. Acute hepatitis E in these patients has a protracted course, with high morbidity and mortality.

Hepatitis G virus often occurs in the setting of coinfection with hepatitis B virus or HCV but usually does not increase their pathogenicity. GB virus C and the hepatitis G virus are variants of the same RNA flavivirus, a lymphotropic virus that replicates primarily in the spleen and bone marrow.

Transfusion-transmitted virus (TTV) is a virus identified in a small percentage of patients with non-A, G posttransfusion hepatitis. In some patients, the virus causes coinfection with HCV. TTV DNA is common in high-risk populations, such as patients with hemophilia, those on hemodialysis, and intravenous drug users. TTV has recently been implicated alone, as well as in coinfection with EBV, as a potential cause of 30%–50% of cases of lymphoma and Hodgkin disease.

Aitken CK, Lewis J, Tracy SL, et al. High incidence of hepatitis C virus reinfection in a cohort of injecting drug users. *Hepatology.* 2008;48(6):1746–1752.

Brant LJ, Ramsay ME, Balogun MA, et al. Diagnosis of acute hepatitis C virus infection and estimated incidence in low- and high-risk English populations. *J Viral Hepat.* 2008;15(12): 871–877.

Human Papillomavirus

Human papillomavirus (HPV) infection is highly prevalent and is closely associated with condylomata (genital warts), cervical intraepithelial neoplasia, cervical cancer (>99% of all cervical cancers are positive for HPV), conjunctival intraepithelial neoplasia, and some cases of head and neck squamous cell carcinoma. A recent review suggests that HPV has a possible etiologic role in some cases of lung adenocarcinoma as well. More than 50% of all persons are infected with HPV during their lifetimes, via either intrauterine or sexually transmitted infection. HPV can be detected with PCR assay techniques, and women at high risk for HPV should receive HPV testing at the time of the Papanicolaou (Pap) test. Vaccines to prevent HPV infection and its sequelae have recently become available. HPV in association with cervical cancer is discussed further in Chapter 12.

Cuzick J, Arbyn M, Sankaranarayanan R, et al. Overview of human papillomavirus-based and other novel options for cervical cancer screening in developed and developing countries. *Vaccine.* 2008;26(Suppl 10):K29–K41.

Acquired Immunodeficiency Syndrome

During the 1980s, AIDS emerged as a major public health problem. AIDS was originally described in 1981, when *Pneumocystis jirovecii* (formerly, *Pneumocystis carinii*) pneumonia and Kaposi sarcoma were noted to occur in men who had sex with men and intravenous drug users. Since then, the number of cases has increased exponentially. In 1983, researchers discovered that AIDS is caused by infection with the retrovirus HIV (human immunodeficiency virus). Subsequently, it became evident that HIV caused a spectrum of diseases, including an asymptomatic carrier state, early symptomatic HIV infection (formerly known as the AIDS-related complex, or ARC), and AIDS itself.

Currently, it is estimated that more than 1.1 million persons in the United States are infected with HIV and that 15% are unaware of their infection. Each year, 50,000 new cases of HIV infection are identified. In 2011, 1.1 million US adults were reported to have AIDS, and the total cumulative number of deaths of persons with AIDS was 636,000. On the positive side, improved combination antiretroviral therapy has led to a significant decline in the number of AIDS cases in the United States and a 70% reduction in deaths due to AIDS since 1995. Furthermore, AIDS is no longer the leading cause of death in young adults in the United States.

Worldwide, 35.3 million individuals are living with AIDS or HIV infection, and 3.34 million children are infected with HIV; most of these children were infected by their HIV-seropositive mothers during childbirth or through breast-feeding. In Europe, 131,202 new HIV infections were diagnosed in 2012, and the number of persons living with HIV infection continues to increase. AIDS continues to take a devastating toll, particularly in sub-Saharan Africa and in Asian nations with large, impoverished populations. However, the number of cases per year has actually decreased recently, because of increasing awareness and funding of HIV prevention and treatment programs.

Etiology and Pathogenesis

AIDS is caused by infection with HIV, which has 2 subtypes, HIV-1 and HIV-2. HIV-1 (previously known as the human T-lymphotropic retrovirus type 3 [HTLV-3], lymphadenopathy-associated virus, and AIDS-related virus) is further classified into several groups, including M, N, and O. Thus far, there are 9 known serotypes of HIV-1 group M, and 1 each of HIV-1 groups N and O. In the United States, HIV-1 group M, serotype B is the most common form of HIV. HIV-2, another human T-lymphotropic retrovirus, has been isolated from West Africans and is closely related to simian immunodeficiency virus.

HIV belongs to a family of viruses known as *retroviruses.* A retrovirus encodes its genetic information in RNA and uses a unique viral enzyme named *reverse transcriptase* to copy its genome into DNA. Other members of this retrovirus family include the human T-lymphotropic retrovirus type 1 (HTLV-1), which can cause adult T-lymphocyte leukemia and chronic progressive myelopathy with atrophy of the spinal cord. The human T-lymphotropic retrovirus type 2 (HTLV-2) is associated with hairy-cell leukemia.

HIV preferentially infects T lymphocytes, especially helper T ($CD4^+$) lymphocytes. The virus infects mature T lymphocytes in vitro, although other cells can serve as targets. CD4 is the phenotypic marker for this subset and is identified by monoclonal antibodies OKT4 and Leu3.

The hallmark of the immunodeficiency in AIDS is a depletion of the $CD4^+$ helper-inducer T lymphocytes. HIV selectively infects these lymphocytes as well as macrophages; with HIV replication, the helper T lymphocytes are killed. Because the helper T lymphocytes are central to the immune response, loss of this subset results in a profound immune deficiency, leading to the life-threatening opportunistic infections indicative of AIDS. This selective depletion of $CD4^+$ helper T lymphocytes leads to the characteristic inverted $CD4^+/CD8^+$ ratio (also known as the *T4/T8 ratio*). A normal $CD4^+/CD8^+$ ratio is 2. Years may pass between the initial HIV infection and the development of these immune abnormalities.

In addition to cellular immunodeficiency, patients with AIDS have abnormalities of B-lymphocyte function. These patients are unable to mount an antibody response to novel T lymphocyte–dependent B-lymphocyte challenges, although they have B-lymphocyte hyperfunction with polyclonal B-lymphocyte activation, hypergammaglobulinemia, and circulating immune complexes. This B-lymphocyte hyperfunction may be a direct consequence of HIV infection: studies have demonstrated that polyclonal activation can be induced in vitro by adding HIV to B lymphocytes.

HIV has also been documented to infect the brains of patients with AIDS. It is thought that HIV infection of the brain is responsible for the HIV encephalopathy syndrome. HIV-infected cells in the brain have generally been identified as macrophages.

Clinical Syndromes

A variety of symptoms and signs can be associated with an acute HIV infection, known as the *acute retroviral syndrome.* The most common are fever, lymphadenopathy, sore throat, rash, myalgia/arthralgia, and headache. Painful mucocutaneous ulceration is a classic manifestation of acute HIV infection. Some patients with early HIV infection may be asymptomatic or have only very mild symptoms. In early HIV infection, the viral RNA level is typically very high (eg, >100,000 copies/mL) and the CD4 cell count can drop transiently. HIV-1 infection is divided into the following stages:

- primary HIV infection (also called *acute HIV infection* or *acute seroconversion syndrome*)
- seroconversion
- clinical latent period with or without persistent generalized lymphadenopathy (PGL)
- early symptomatic HIV infection, previously known as AIDS-related complex, or ARC, and also referred to as category B according to the 1993 CDC classification
- AIDS, as defined in the 1987 CDC criteria and revised 1993 CDC criteria that include a CD4 cell count below 200/μL, regardless of the presence or absence of symptoms
- advanced HIV infection characterized by a CD4 cell count below 50/μL

Diagnosis

When acute or early HIV infection is suspected, the most sensitive immunoassay available (a combination antigen/antibody immunoassay) should be performed, along with an HIV viral load test. A positive immunoassay should be followed by a confirmatory Western blot test. Acute or early HIV infection is diagnosed by a negative result on immunoassay in the presence of a positive viral load or by a negative or indeterminate result on a Western blot test in the presence of a positive immunoassay result and a positive viral load. For a patient with a negative serologic test result, a viral RNA level below 10,000 copies/mL may indicate a false-positive viral load test result, as patients with acute or early HIV infection typically have very high levels of viremia. The virologic test should be immediately repeated on a new blood specimen. A second positive viral load test result suggests HIV infection, which can be confirmed by a second serologic test performed several weeks later to evaluate for seroconversion.

Newly diagnosed patients should be referred promptly to an appropriate specialist to discuss treatment options. Drug-resistance testing should be performed after the initial diagnosis of HIV infection, as infection with a virus that harbors at least 1 drug-resistance mutation is estimated to occur in up to 20% of newly infected patients. Current screening recommendations for HIV testing include routine testing of all persons, including pregnant women, between the ages of 15 and 65 years. Some even advocate routine testing of all patients in all clinical settings. Persons at high risk for HIV infection should be screened for HIV at least annually. Specific signed consent for HIV testing should not be required. General informed consent for medical care should be considered sufficient to include informed consent for HIV testing. However, patients must not be tested without their knowledge. Perinatal transmission rates can be reduced to less than 2% with universal screening of pregnant women, prophylactic treatment with antiretroviral drugs, scheduled cesarean delivery when appropriate, and avoidance of breast-feeding.

Panlilio AL, Cardo DM, Grohskopf LA, Heneine W, Ross CS; US Public Health Service. Updated U.S. Public Health Service guidelines for the management of occupational exposures to HIV and recommendations for postexposure prophylaxis. *MMWR Recomm Rep.* 2005;54(RR09):1–17.

Schneider E, Whitmore S, Glynn MK, Dominguez K, Mitsch A, McKenna MT; Centers for Disease Control and Prevention (CDC). Revised surveillance case definitions for HIV infection among adults, adolescents, and children aged <18 months and for HIV infection and AIDS among children aged 18 months to <13 years—United States, 2008. *MMWR Recomm Rep.* 2008;57(RR10):1–8.

Modes of Transmission

The modes of transmission of HIV infection are

- sexual contact
- intravenous drug use
- transfusion
- perinatal transmission from an infected mother to her child

There have been no documented cases of transmission by casual contact. Furthermore, although HIV infection may be transmitted via blood or blood products, the risk of transmission by accidental needle-stick injury appears quite low (<0.5%). Studies have revealed that nonsexual household contacts of patients with HIV infection are at minimal or possibly no risk of infection with HIV.

At the beginning of the AIDS epidemic, almost all cases in the United States were found in men who had sex with men, but that proportion has been steadily decreasing, with corresponding increases in the number of cases in intravenous drug users and in persons infected through heterosexual contact. Furthermore, in Africa the male to female ratio is 1 to 1, and epidemiologic data have suggested that the disease is transmitted predominantly by heterosexual activity, perinatal exposure from infected mothers to their newborns, and parenteral exposure to blood transfusion and unsterilized needles.

Prognosis and Treatment

AIDS is still considered an incurable and potentially fatal disease. Nevertheless, HIV-infected patients are living much longer and have had better quality of life than infected patients in previous years because of significant improvements in antiretroviral therapy. For that reason, HIV infection is now managed more as a chronic illness than as a terminal disease. The risk factors that are most closely associated with decreased survival in HIV-infected patients are reduced $CD4^+$ levels, length of time since diagnosis, previous opportunistic infections, high viral load, and new "clinical progression" events. $CD4^+$ cell counts are good predictors of risk of opportunistic coinfection. Plasma HIV RNA levels are even better predictors of disease progression and are the best single predictors of response to therapy.

It is now well established that superinfection with a second strain, or clade, of HIV-1 occurs in humans, often following a period of immunologic stability. Detection of increasing viral DNA, which results from infection of a cell by 2 or more HIV clades, suggests that superinfection occurs more frequently than previously thought. The second virus (usually from a different clade) can superinfect cells well after the initial infection, and this superinfection is associated with rapid viral rebound and immunologic decline. Primary infection with a specific HIV clade appears to provide inadequate immune protection against superinfection with a different clade.

Recommended laboratory studies for a newly diagnosed case of HIV infection include complete blood count with differential; $CD4^+$ cell count; HIV viral load (RNA level) determination; measures of electrolyte levels; renal and liver function tests; urinalysis; PPD (TB test); and serologic tests for syphilis, hepatitis B virus, HCV, *T gondii,* CMV, and VZV. Female patients should undergo a Papanicolaou test because of the high risk of invasive cervical cancer in HIV-infected persons. The recommended vaccinations for HIV-seropositive patients are those against *Pneumococcus* (every 5 years), hepatitis B virus, hepatitis A virus (especially if the patient is HCV positive), influenza virus (yearly), diphtheria/tetanus (every 10 years), and measles (contraindicated in severe immunosuppression). Immunizations that are contraindicated and should not be administered in HIV-infected patients include live, attenuated influenza; VZV; oral polio; smallpox; typhoid; and yellow fever vaccines.

It is recommended that all patients with early HIV infection begin antiretroviral therapy (ART) because initiation of ART soon after initial HIV infection may be associated with a greater chance of immune reconstitution to normal or near-normal CD4 cell levels. The goals of ART include durable suppression of HIV viral load to less than 50 copies/mL, restoration of immune function (as indicated by the $CD4^+$ cell count), prevention of HIV transmission, prevention of drug resistance, and improvement in quality of life. ART regimens for treatment-naive patients are composed of a "base" medication and a "backbone" regimen. The base is either an integrase strand transfer inhibitor (dolutegravir, elvitegravir, or raltegravir), a nonnucleoside reverse transcriptase inhibitor (NNRTI; efavirenz or rilpivirine), or a boosted protease inhibitor (PI) (darunavir or atazanavir). The backbone typically consists of 2 nucleoside reverse transcriptase inhibitors (NRTIs; abacavir and lamivudine or tenofovir disoproxil fumarate and emtricitabine). The particular choice of agents may depend on adverse-effect profiles, comorbidities, potential drug interactions, results of resistance testing, allergy history, pregnancy status, and/or patient convenience; alternatives are available.

A small percentage of the population appears to be naturally immune to HIV infection. These persons have defective genes for CCR5, a surface receptor that HIV requires to attach to T lymphocytes. Also, approximately 50% of long-term survivors of HIV infection are heterozygous for the CCR5 defect. This finding has led to speculation concerning the possibilities for genetic therapy, in which anti-HIV genes could be "injected" into a patient's chromosomes with a harmless viral vector. In one study, recombinant lentiviral vectors were used to deliver the *CCR5-delta32* gene into human cell lines, and resistance to HIV was transmitted to most of these cells. This procedure may become useful for stem cell–based or T-lymphocyte–based gene therapy for HIV-1 infection. Several small-molecule CCR5 receptor inhibitors are being evaluated in clinical trials.

ART has been shown to dramatically reduce the HIV viral load, increase $CD4^+$ cell counts, delay disease progression, reduce the number of opportunistic infections, decrease the number of hospitalizations, and prolong survival. Some statistics show up to an 82% decline in the number of opportunistic infections in patients on ART. These advantages are translating into improved survival and enhanced quality of life for HIV-infected patients.

Although no highly successful HIV vaccines have been developed, pre-exposure prophylaxis with tenofovir-emtricitabine can be considered in high-risk patients. Condoms are highly effective at preventing HIV transmission.

Günthard HF, Aberg JA, Eron JJ, et al. Antiretroviral treatment of adult HIV infection. 2014 Recommendations of the International Antiviral Society–USA Panel. *JAMA*. 2014;312(4): 410–425.

Hulgan T, Shepherd BE, Raffanti SP, et al. Absolute count and percentage of $CD4^+$ lymphocytes are independent predictors of disease progression in HIV-infected persons initiating highly active antiretroviral therapy. *J Infect Dis*. 2007;195(3):425–431.

Opportunistic Infections (Table 14-2)

Treatment of Pneumocystis jirovecii *pneumonia*

Pneumocystis jirovecii pneumonia (PCP; formerly, *Pneumocystis carinii*) continues to affect a significant percentage of patients with AIDS and is a major cause of mortality in these patients. However, recent advances in diagnosis and management, appropriately targeting chemoprophylaxis to HIV-infected patients at high clinical risk for PCP, and the introduction of ART have contributed to a dramatic reduction in the incidence of PCP. Nevertheless, PCP remains the most common opportunistic pneumonia and the most common life-threatening infectious complication in HIV-infected patients.

PCP is generally treated with oral or, if necessary, intravenous trimethoprim-sulfamethoxazole (TMP-SMX). Inhaled pentamidine prevents the recurrence of PCP (secondary prophylaxis) and appears to be efficacious for primary prophylaxis when used in patients with HIV infection and $CD4^+$ cell counts below 200/μL. The regimen for inhaled pentamidine is generally 300 mg every 4 weeks by use of a nebulizer. This form of therapy avoids the toxicity of systemically administered pentamidine.

Several studies show that oral TMP-SMX prophylaxis is more effective than aerosolized pentamidine for PCP prophylaxis in those patients who can tolerate it. This regimen may also be used to provide systemic prophylaxis against toxoplasmosis infection. However, adverse reactions are frequent in HIV-infected patients. Dapsone, alone or in combination with pyrimethamine, is effective for primary and secondary prophylaxis against PCP and is tolerated by most patients who develop rashes with use of TMP-SMX. Primaquine, clindamycin, and atovaquone have been successfully used to treat PCP, but these

Table 14-2 AIDS-Defining Conditions

- Bacterial infections, multiple or recurrent*
- Candidiasis of bronchi, trachea, or lungs
- Candidiasis of esophagus[†]
- Cervical cancer, invasive[§]
- Coccidioidomycosis, disseminated or extrapulmonary
- Cryptococcosis, extrapulmonary
- Cryptosporidiosis, chronic intestinal (>1 month's duration)
- Cytomegalovirus disease (other than liver, spleen, or nodes), onset at age >1 month
- Cytomegalovirus retinitis (with loss of vision)[†]
- Encephalopathy, HIV related
- Herpes simplex: chronic ulcers (>1 month's duration) or bronchitis, pneumonitis, or esophagitis (onset at age >1 month)
- Histoplasmosis, disseminated or extrapulmonary
- Isosporiasis, chronic intestinal (>1 month's duration)
- Kaposi sarcoma[†]
- Lymphoid interstitial pneumonia or pulmonary lymphoid hyperplasia complex*[†]
- Lymphoma, Burkitt (or equivalent term)
- Lymphoma, immunoblastic (or equivalent term)
- Lymphoma, primary, of brain
- *Mycobacterium avium* complex or *Mycobacterium kansasii*, disseminated or extrapulmonary[†]
- *Mycobacterium tuberculosis* of any site, pulmonary,[†§] disseminated,[†] or extrapulmonary[†]
- *Mycobacterium*, other species or unidentified species, disseminated[†] or extrapulmonary[†]
- *Pneumocystis jirovecii* pneumonia[†]
- Pneumonia, recurrent[†§]
- Progressive multifocal leukoencephalopathy
- *Salmonella* septicemia, recurrent
- Toxoplasmosis of brain, onset at age >1 month[†]
- Wasting syndrome attributed to HIV infection

*Only among children aged <13 years.
[†]Condition that might be diagnosed presumptively.
[§]Only among adults and adolescents aged ≥13 years.

drugs are reserved for use in patients who cannot tolerate TMP-SMX or pentamidine, or for those with resistant infections. Judicious use of corticosteroids may help reduce morbidity in patients with severe pulmonary inflammation caused by PCP.

Treatment of cytomegalovirus infections

Oral valganciclovir and intravitreal ganciclovir or foscarnet injections are the most common treatment for CMV retinitis. The treatment of CMV retinitis is discussed in further detail in BCSC Section 9, *Intraocular Inflammation and Uveitis,* and Section 12, *Retina and Vitreous.*

Barrett L, Walmsley S. CMV retinopathy in the antiretroviral therapy era: prevention, diagnosis, and management. *Curr Infect Dis Rep.* 2012;14(4):435–444.

Kempen JH, Min YI, Freeman WR, et al; Studies of Ocular Complications of AIDS Research Group. Risk of immune recovery uveitis in patients with AIDS and cytomegalovirus retinitis. *Ophthalmology.* 2006;113(4):684–694.

Treatment of spore-forming intestinal protozoa

Spore-forming intestinal protozoa are a frequent cause of gastrointestinal tract infections in patients with AIDS. This group of infections includes cryptosporidiosis (caused by

Cryptosporidium parvum), microsporidiosis (Microsporidia), isosporiasis *(Isospora belli),* and cyclosporiasis *(Cyclospora cayetanensis).*

Cryptosporidiosis can be treated with clarithromycin; azithromycin; rifabutin; albendazole; metronidazole; or a newer, more effective agent, nitazoxanide. HIV-infected patients on ART have a dramatically lower incidence of cryptosporidiosis, which is attributable to the effects of intestinal immune reconstitution.

Isosporiasis and cyclosporiasis have been successfully treated with TMP-SMX. There are no curative drugs for invasive microsporidiosis, but recent studies have revealed that albendazole or fumagillin may control disease symptoms. Importantly, chronic diarrhea in HIV-infected patients may also be caused by many nonprotozoan pathogens, particularly *Salmonella, Shigella, Campylobacter, C difficile, Vibrio parahaemolyticus, Escherichia coli, Mycobacterium avium* complex (MAC), and CMV.

Treatment of tuberculosis and Mycobacterium avium *complex*

The incidence of TB is increasing in HIV-infected patients in Africa and Asia. HIV-induced immunosuppression alters the typical clinical presentation of TB, causing atypical signs and symptoms and more frequent extrapulmonary disease dissemination. Also, the treatment of TB is more difficult to manage in HIV-infected patients because of drug interactions between PIs and rifampicin or rifabutin. In addition, increased use of ART in developed countries may be responsible for a paradoxical worsening of TB clinical manifestations, due to immune restoration and the subsequent inflammatory responses against TB.

Multidrug resistance has become an increasing problem—particularly in Africa and Asia—in patients with AIDS who have TB or atypical mycobacterial *(M avium, Mycobacterium kansasii)* infections. Delay in diagnosis and multidrug resistance are strong risk factors for mortality.

The standard treatment of TB in a patient with HIV infection consists of isoniazid, a rifamycin, ethambutol, and pyrazinamide. The treatment of MAC in an HIV-infected patient consists of clarithromycin and ethambutol. Prophylactic therapy with azithromycin, clarithromycin, rifabutin, or combination therapy may help prevent disseminated MAC in patients with AIDS. However, a significant reduction in the incidence of disseminated atypical mycobacterial infections as a consequence of antiretroviral therapy has been documented. Also, the clinical picture of atypical mycobacterial infections in patients treated with ART has shifted from one of primarily disseminated disease with bacteremia to one of localized infections. Data from several controlled trials led to the current practice of discontinuing prophylaxis against disseminated MAC infections when the $CD4^+$ cell counts remain stable at more than 100 cells/μL. Furthermore, because of the potential drug interactions and adverse effects of antimycobacterial therapy, some authors suggest that routine prophylaxis should not be recommended, even in patients with low $CD4^+$ cell counts, unless these patients do not respond to ART.

Lange CG, Woolley IJ, Brodt RH. Disseminated Mycobacterium avium-intracellulare complex (MAC) infection in the era of effective antiretroviral therapy: is prophylaxis still indicated? *Drugs.* 2004;64(7):679–692.

Treatment of other opportunistic infections

Other opportunistic infections encountered in patients with AIDS include CNS toxoplasmosis; disseminated fungal infections; and coinfection with viral hepatitis, herpes simplex, or herpes zoster. Although toxoplasmosis has traditionally been treated with sulfadiazine, pyrimethamine, or clindamycin, more recent data suggest that TMP-SMX may be equally effective, with far fewer adverse effects. Also, TMP-SMX has been used as prophylactic therapy against PCP as well as toxoplasmosis.

Hepatitis B or C coinfection has been encountered more frequently in HIV-infected patients. Recent guidelines for screening and prevention of opportunistic infections suggest that all HIV-infected patients should be tested for hepatitis B and C. HIV coinfection accelerates HCV-related liver disease, causing more rapid progression to cirrhosis, end-stage liver disease, and hepatocellular carcinoma. Although some antiretroviral agents, such as PIs, have significant anti–hepatitis B virus activity, they have little direct impact on HCV infection. Valacyclovir and famciclovir, as well as other antiviral agents such as cidofovir, offer alternatives to acyclovir in treating AIDS patients with refractory or disseminated herpes simplex or herpes zoster infections.

Treatment of disseminated fungal infections is evolving with the availability of the newer imidazoles, namely fluconazole and itraconazole. Amphotericin B remains important in the treatment of advanced invasive fungal disease, and new formulations of the drug in lipid complexes or liposomes reduce systemic toxicity. In addition to the commonly recognized benefits of ART for opportunistic infections (such as reestablishing immune competency), a recent study has proven that the PI indinavir directly inhibits the growth rate of the opportunistic fungal pathogen *Cryptococcus neoformans.*

Treatment of AIDS- and HIV-associated malignancies

Kaposi sarcoma is usually a localized disease that can be treated with radiotherapy, but metastatic or disseminated disease may require combined chemotherapy. In addition, immunotherapy with interferon-β has been used to treat some patients with Kaposi sarcoma. B-lymphocyte lymphomas in patients with AIDS often involve the lymph nodes, CNS, and lungs and may require treatment with multidrug chemotherapy and sometimes with regional radiotherapy. Since the advent of potent combination ART, the incidence of Kaposi sarcoma in HIV-infected patients has declined dramatically—as much as 87%, according to one review.

Hodgkin lymphoma is the most common non–AIDS-defining tumor in HIV-infected patients. Although the introduction of ART led to a decreased incidence of several malignancies among HIV-infected patients, the incidence of HIV-associated Hodgkin lymphoma has been persistent. This disease's highly aggressive behavior is related to an increased frequency of unfavorable histologic types, higher tumor stages, and extranodal involvement by the time of presentation, as well as poorer therapeutic outcome, when compared with Hodgkin lymphoma in non–HIV-infected patients. Treatment of HIV-associated Hodgkin lymphoma is challenging because of the underlying immunodeficiency caused by HIV itself, and it may increase the risk of opportunistic infections by inducing further immunosuppression. Consequently, less aggressive treatment regimens have been developed to achieve tumor control in HIV-infected patients with Hodgkin lymphoma.

Several other malignancies appear to be associated with HIV infection. These include cervical carcinoma in situ, anogenital neoplasms, leiomyosarcoma, and conjunctival squamous cell carcinoma.

Immune reconstitution syndromes

Some patients starting ART develop new or worsening opportunistic infections or malignancies despite improvements in the clinical markers of HIV infection. These examples of paradoxical clinical worsening, also called *immune reconstitution syndromes (IRSs),* are increased in patients with previous opportunistic infections or low $CD4^+$ T-lymphocyte levels. IRSs are thought to result from an inflammatory response to reemergence of the immune system's ability to recognize pathogens or tumor antigens that were previously present but asymptomatic. With the increased availability of ART, more cases and more new forms of IRSs are likely to be recognized. Immune recovery uveitis (IRU) occurs in nearly 10% of HIV-infected patients with immune recovery and a history of CMV retinitis. Of these IRU patients, 46% develop significant cystoid macular edema and 49% develop epiretinal membrane.

Ophthalmic considerations The ocular manifestations of HIV infection and AIDS are discussed in BCSC Section 9, *Intraocular Inflammation and Uveitis.* HIV has been found in tears, conjunctival epithelial cells, corneal epithelial cells, aqueous, retinal vascular endothelium, and retina. Although transmission of HIV infection via ophthalmic examinations or ophthalmic equipment has not been documented, several precautions are recommended.

Health care professionals performing eye examinations or other procedures involving contact with tears should wash their hands immediately after the procedure and between patients. Hand washing alone should be sufficient, but when practical and convenient, disposable gloves may be worn. The use of gloves is advisable when the hands have cuts, scratches, or dermatologic lesions.

Any instrument that comes into direct contact with external surfaces of the eyes should be wiped clean and disinfected by a 5- to 10-minute exposure to one of the following:

- a fresh solution of 3% hydrogen peroxide
- a fresh solution containing 5000 parts per million (ppm) free available chlorine—a one-tenth dilution of common household bleach (sodium hypochlorite)
- 70% ethanol
- 70% isopropanol

The device should be thoroughly rinsed in tap water and dried before use.

Contact lenses used in trial fittings should be disinfected between fittings with a commercially available hydrogen peroxide contact lens–disinfecting system or with the standard heat disinfection regimen (78°–80°C for 10 minutes). The demonstration of HIV in corneal epithelium has led to the recommendation that all corneal donors be screened for antibodies to HIV and that all potential donor corneas from HIV antibody–positive persons be discarded.

For more specific recommendations, see the American Academy of Ophthalmology's Information Statement titled "Infection Prevention in Eye Care Services and Operating Areas and Operating Rooms—2012," available at http://one.aao.org/clinical-statement/infection-prevention-in-eye-care-services-operatin.

Centers for Disease Control and Prevention website; www.cdc.gov.

Chu PL, Nieves-Rivera I, Grinsdale J, et al. A public health framework for developing local preventive services guidelines. *Public Health Rep.* 2014;129(Suppl 1):70–78.

European Centre for Disease Prevention and Control website; www.ecdc.europa.eu/en/Pages/home.aspx.

Thompson MA, Aberg JA, Cahn P, et al. Antiretroviral treatment of adult HIV infection: 2010 recommendations of the International AIDS Society-USA panel. *JAMA.* 2010;304(3):321–333.

UpToDate; www.uptodate.com.

Update on Antibiotics

For more than 60 years, the main trends in the management of infectious diseases have been the evolution and refinement of antibiotic therapy. Factors that have stimulated the development of new antibiotics include the continuous emergence of resistant bacteria, economics, and the desire to eliminate adverse effects. During the past 25 years, emphasis has gradually shifted from aminoglycosides to β-lactams and the development of new classes of antibiotics such as carbapenems and monobactams. In addition, vancomycin, TMP-SMX, erythromycin, and rifampin have enjoyed a popular resurgence and new applications. Quinolones offer the possibility of treating serious infections on an outpatient basis.

For the characteristics of selected antibiotics, see Tables 14-3 and 14-4. Antiretroviral agents are discussed in detail earlier in this chapter.

Antibacterial Agents

Antibacterial agents can be separated into groups according to their specific targets on or within bacteria:

- β-Lactams and glycopeptides inhibit cell-wall synthesis.
- Polymyxins distort cytoplasmic membrane function.
- Quinolones and rifampicins inhibit nucleic acid synthesis.
- Macrolides, aminoglycosides, and tetracyclines inhibit ribosome function.
- Trimethoprim and sulfonamides inhibit folate metabolism.

All antibiotics facilitate the growth of resistant bacteria consequent to the destruction of susceptible bacteria. Although the wide use of antimicrobial agents for veterinary and agricultural purposes has contributed to the emergence of multiresistant microorganisms,

Table 14-3 Cephalosporins

Drugs	Characteristics/Comments
First generation (eg, cefazolin, cephalexin)	Active against β-lactamase gram-positive cocci and gram-negative bacilli Usually ineffective against *Bacillus, Pseudomonas, Enterobacter,* and methicillin-resistant *Staphylococcus aureus* (MRSA) Do not cross the blood–brain barrier well
Second generation (eg, cefamandole, cefoxitin, cefaclor, cefuroxime)	Expanded coverage against gram-negative bacilli and *Haemophilus*
Third generation (eg, cefotaxime, ceftriaxone, ceftazidime)	More effective against gram-negative bacilli Less effective against gram-positive cocci (eg, staphylococci) and Enterobacteriaceae Cross blood–brain barrier, more effective for treatment of meningitis Ceftriaxone effective against Lyme disease, gonorrhea; represents the best all-purpose drug of the 3rd-generation cephalosporins
Fourth generation (eg, cefepime, cefpirome)	Good coverage against most gram-negative and gram-positive organisms and anaerobes Expensive
Fifth generation (ceftaroline)	Approved in Canada Broad spectrum Effective against MRSA

Table 14-4 New Classes of Antibiotics

Drugs	Characteristics/Comments
Streptogramins, or synergistins (eg, quinupristin-dalfopristin)	Kill bacteria rapidly; show little cross-resistance Excellent activity against staphylococci (including VISA), *Mycoplasma, Neisseria, Haemophilus, Legionella,* and *Moraxella* Offer treatment options for multidrug-resistant infections Adverse effects include gastrointestinal upset, rash, myalgias, and elevated serum alkaline phosphatase
Oxazolidines (eg, linezolid, furazolidine, eperezolid)	Effective against many multidrug-resistant bacteria Possible drug interactions due to monoamine oxidase inhibitor effect
Ketolides (eg, telithromycin)	Semisynthetic 14-membered-ring macrolides Effective against many multidrug-resistant bacteria May be hepatotoxic; exacerbate myasthenia gravis
Lipopeptides (eg, daptomycin)	Effective against gram-positive bacteria Offer treatment options for multidrug-resistant infections Reduce the nephrotoxicity of aminoglycosides when used in combination (protective effect)

the excessive use of antibiotics, especially in hospitals, has been the most significant catalyst for resistance. Bacteria resist antibiotics by inactivation of the antibiotic, decreased accumulation of the antibiotic within the microorganism, or alteration of the target site on the microbe. For example, resistance to penicillins and cephalosporins is initiated by β-lactamase enzymes that hydrolyze the β-lactam ring, thus destroying the antibiotic's effectiveness. Resistance can be mediated by chromosomal mutations or the presence of extrachromosomal DNA, also known as *plasmid resistance.* Plasmid resistance is more important from an epidemiologic point of view because it is transmissible and usually highly stable; also, it confers resistance to many different classes of antibiotics simultaneously and is often associated with other characteristics that enable a microorganism to colonize and invade a susceptible host.

Resistance-conferring plasmids have been identified in virtually all bacteria. Moreover, many bacteria contain transposons that can enter plasmids or chromosomes. Plasmids can therefore pick up chromosomal genes for resistance and transfer them to species that are not currently resistant.

Bacteria that have acquired chromosomal and plasmid-mediated resistance can neutralize or destroy antibiotics in 3 different ways (they can use one or more of these mechanisms simultaneously):

- by preventing the antibacterial agent from reaching its receptor site
- by modifying or duplicating the target enzyme so that it is insensitive to the antibacterial agent
- by synthesizing enzymes that destroy the antibacterial agent or modify the agent to alter its entry or receptor binding

Antimicrobial susceptibility testing permits a rational choice of antibiotics, although correlation of in vivo and in vitro susceptibility is not always precise. Disk-diffusion susceptibility testing has provided qualitative data about the inhibitory activity of commonly used antimicrobials against an isolated pathogen, and these data are usually sufficient. In serious infections, such as infective endocarditis, it is useful to quantify the drug concentrations that inhibit and kill the pathogen. The lowest drug concentration that prevents the growth of a defined inoculum of the isolated pathogen is the *minimal inhibitory concentration (MIC)*; the lowest concentration that kills 99.9% of an inoculum is the *minimal lethal concentration (MLC).* For bactericidal drugs, the MIC and MLC are usually similar.

The antimicrobial activity of a treated patient's serum can be estimated via measurement of serum bactericidal titers. Clinical experience suggests that intravascular infections are usually controlled when the peak serum bactericidal titer is 1.8 or greater. Bactericidal therapy is preferred for patients with immunologic compromise or life-threatening infection. Other patients may be treated effectively with either bactericidal or bacteriostatic drugs. Although synergistic combinations are useful in certain clinical situations (eg, enterococcal endocarditis, gram-negative septicemia in granulocytopenic patients), combined antimicrobial therapy should be used judiciously so that potential antagonism and toxicity can be minimized.

β-Lactam antibiotics

The β-lactam group includes the penicillins, cephalosporins, and monobactams, all of which possess a β-lactam ring that binds to specific microbial binding sites and interferes with cell-wall synthesis. The carbapenems and carbacephems are often grouped with β-lactams but have a slightly different ring structure. Most new agents have been created by side-chain manipulation of the β-lactam ring, which has improved resistance to enzymatic degradation. However, some of the newer antibiotics (such as third-generation cephalosporins) show diminished potency against gram-positive cocci, especially staphylococci.

Penicillins The first *natural penicillins,* types G and V, were degraded by the enzyme penicillinase. The *penicillinase-resistant penicillins,* such as methicillin, nafcillin, oxacillin, and cloxacillin, were developed for treating resistant *Staphylococcus* species, and except for strains of methicillin-resistant *S epidermidis,* they were effective. The next generation of penicillins included the *aminopenicillins,* ampicillin and amoxicillin, created by placing an amino group on the acyl side chain of the penicillin nucleus. This change broadened their effectiveness to include activity against *H influenzae, E coli,* and *Proteus mirabilis.* The next advance was development of the *carboxypenicillins,* carbenicillin and ticarcillin, which are active against aerobic gram-negative rods such as *P aeruginosa, Enterobacter* species, and indole-positive strains of *Proteus.* The carboxypenicillins are particularly effective for intra-abdominal infections. The fourth-generation penicillins, known as *acylureidopenicillins,* include azlocillin, mezlocillin, and piperacillin. Currently, their usefulness is in treating Enterobacteriaceae and *P aeruginosa* infections; febrile neutropenia; and infections secondary to a combination of flora found in skin, soft-tissue, intra-abdominal, and pelvic infections. However, because of the possibility of emergence of resistance, the newer penicillins are usually administered with an aminoglycoside.

Allergic reactions are the chief adverse effects encountered in using the penicillins. Among antimicrobial agents, the penicillins are the leading cause of allergy; symptoms range from mild rashes to anaphylaxis.

Cephalosporins The cephalosporins also belong to the β-lactam group of antibiotics, and cross-allergenicity may occur in 3%–5% of patients with penicillin allergies. The cephalosporins and their characteristics are outlined in Table 14-3.

The benefits of continuous intravenous infusion of β-lactam antibiotics, such as nafcillin and ceftazidime, have been demonstrated. This method of dosing provides continuous and stable therapeutic levels of the antibiotic in blood and tissue.

Polenakovik HM, Pleiman CM. Ceftaroline for methicillin-resistant *Staphylococcus aureus* bacteremia: case series and review of the literature. *Int J Antimicrob Agents.* 2013;42(5): 450–455.

Monobactams *Monobactams* are a monocyclic class of antibiotics that use only the β-lactam ring as their core structure. *Aztreonam,* the first approved monobactam antibiotic, has an excellent safety profile and good success rate in the treatment of infections caused by aerobic gram-negative bacilli, but has poor activity against gram-positive and anaerobic organisms. Aztreonam has the spectrum of an aminoglycoside antibiotic without the ototoxicity or nephrotoxicity. Aztreonam is usually combined with a semisynthetic antistaphylococcal penicillin or clindamycin in presumptive therapy of known mixed infections.

Carbapenems *Carbapenems* are a class of antibiotics with a basic ring structure similar to that of penicillins, except that a carbon atom replaces sulfur at the number 1 position. The antibacterial spectrum of the carbapenems is broader than that of any other existing antibiotic and includes *S aureus, Enterobacter* species, and *P aeruginosa,* although some resistance is emerging. Carbapenems produce a postantibiotic killing effect against some organisms, with a delay in regrowth of damaged organisms similar to that observed with aminoglycosides but not with cephalosporins or acylureidopenicillins. This quality can be particularly important for settings in which host defenses are compromised, such as granulocytopenia or sequestered foci of infection.

Imipenem-cilastatin combines a carbapenem, imipenem, with an inhibitor of renal dehydropeptidase, cilastatin. Cilastatin has no antimicrobial activity and is present solely to prevent degradation of imipenem by dehydropeptidase. As monotherapy for mixed infections, imipenem-cilastatin is an appropriate compound. Up to 50% of patients who are allergic to penicillin are also allergic to imipenem.

Meropenem, biapenem, panipenem, ertapenem, faropenem, tomopenem, and *ritipenem* are newer penems that have increased stability against degradation by dehydropeptidases. *Doripenem* is a new agent that appears to be most effective in treating carbapenem-resistant gram-negative bacilli and penicillin-resistant streptococci.

Loracarbef is an oral carbacephem, a type of antibiotic that is structurally similar to cephalosporins but possesses a broader spectrum due to higher stability against both plasmid and chromosomally mediated β-lactamases. Loracarbef provides good coverage for most gram-positive and gram-negative aerobic bacteria.

Clavulanic acid, sulbactam, and *tazobactam* are β-lactam molecules that possess little intrinsic antibacterial activity but are potent inhibitors of many plasmid-mediated class A β-lactamases. Currently, 4 combinations of β-lactam antibiotics plus β-lactamase inhibitors are available in the United States: *Augmentin* (oral amoxicillin and clavulanic acid), *Timentin* (intravenous ticarcillin and clavulanic acid), *Unasyn* (intravenous ampicillin and sulbactam), and *Zosyn* (intravenous piperacillin and tazobactam). These drugs have excellent activity against β-lactamase–producing gram-positive and gram-negative bacteria as well as many anaerobes. Recent research has illuminated new broad-spectrum inhibitors that can simultaneously inactivate several classes of β-lactamases (including classes A, C, and D) and has explored potential new cephalosporin-derived β-lactamase inactivators.

Glycopeptides

Vancomycin has regained popularity because of the emergence of methicillin-resistant staphylococci and the recognition that *C difficile* is a cause of pseudomembranous colitis. This drug has excellent activity against *Clostridium* and against most gram-positive bacteria, including methicillin-resistant staphylococci, *Corynebacterium* species, and other diphtheroids. Vancomycin has been used alone to treat serious infections caused by methicillin-resistant staphylococci.

Vancomycin-resistant enterococcal infections have recently become more common. In one study of hospitalized patients, approximately 1% carried vancomycin-resistant enterococci in their gastrointestinal tract. These infections are very difficult or impossible to treat because of multidrug resistance. In vitro studies have shown that plasmid-mediated vancomycin resistance can also be easily transferred to staphylococci. The CDC has issued recommendations regarding appropriate use of vancomycin to help counteract the emergence of bacterial drug resistance.

Teicoplanin, an investigational glycopeptide, has several advantages over vancomycin, including longer half-life, lower nephrotoxicity, and no requirement for monitoring drug levels. Teicoplanin is effective for treatment of staphylococcal infections, including endocarditis, bacteremia, osteomyelitis, and septic arthritis. Teicoplanin may be preferable to vancomycin for surgical prophylaxis because of its excellent tissue penetration, lower toxicity, and long half-life, allowing single-dose administration in several surgical procedures. The antibacterial activity of teicoplanin is similar to that of vancomycin but with increased potency, particularly against *Streptococcus* and *Enterococcus.* Teicoplanin is active against many vancomycin-resistant organisms. The new investigational glycopeptides oritavancin, telavancin, and dalbavancin and the glycolipodepsipeptide ramoplanin are highly active against vancomycin-resistant infections.

Cui L, Iwamoto A, Lian JQ, et al. Novel mechanism of antibiotic resistance originating in vancomycin-intermediate *Staphylococcus aureus. Antimicrob Agents Chemother.* 2006;50(2):428–438.

Quinolones

The introduction of a fluorine into the basic quinolone nucleus of nalidixic acid has produced compounds known as *fluoroquinolones,* which have excellent activity against gram-positive bacteria. The subsequent addition of piperazine produced compounds such as norfloxacin and ciprofloxacin, which have a broad spectrum of activity, encompassing staphylococci and most of the significant gram-negative bacilli, including *Pseudomonas.* Ciprofloxacin is available in both oral and parenteral forms and can be used to treat urinary tract infections, gonorrhea, and diarrheal diseases, as well as respiratory, skin, and bone infections. Other fluoroquinolones in the US market include ofloxacin, temafloxacin, lomefloxacin, enoxacin, levofloxacin, moxifloxacin, gemifloxacin, and besifloxacin. Fluoroquinolones awaiting FDA approval include nadifloxacin and prulifloxacin.

The newer fluoroquinolones possess even greater activity against gram-positive and gram-negative bacteria. Either moxifloxacin or levofloxacin appears to be a good treatment choice for pneumococcal infections that are resistant to penicillin and the macrolides. Oral quinolones are an alternative form of therapy to β-lactams and aminoglycosides and have allowed physicians to treat more patients outside the hospital setting. Reported adverse effects include tendon rupture (especially in elderly patients), retinal detachment, and peripheral neuropathy. Of the quinolones, moxifloxacin carries the highest risk of dysglycemia.

Zhang JZ, Ward KW. Besifloxacin, a novel fluoroquinolone antimicrobial agent, exhibits potent inhibition of pro-inflammatory cytokines in human THP-1 monocytes. *J Antimicrob Chemother.* 2008;61(1):111–116.

Macrolides

The macrolide *erythromycin* is often employed for the initial treatment of community-acquired pneumonia. This agent is effective against infections caused by pneumococci, group A streptococci, *M pneumoniae, Chlamydia,* and *Legionella.* Erythromycin is used to treat upper respiratory tract infections and sexually transmitted diseases in patients who are allergic to penicillin.

Clarithromycin and *azithromycin* are macrolide antibiotics that are chemically related to erythromycin. Both are well-tolerated alternatives to erythromycin and may offer particular advantages in treating gonococcal and chlamydial infections and in the treatment of *M avium* and other recalcitrant infections associated with AIDS and HIV infection. The treatment of MAC in an HIV-infected patient is clarithromycin and ethambutol. Prophylactic therapy with azithromycin, clarithromycin, rifabutin, or combined therapy may help prevent disseminated MAC in AIDS patients. Azithromycin is subclassified as an *azalide,* and it causes far fewer drug interactions than erythromycin. There is increasing cross-resistance among the macrolides. Telithromycin and cethromycin, newer ketolide antibiotics that belong to a new class of semisynthetic 14-membered-ring macrolides, are discussed in the section titled New Antibiotic Classes, later in this chapter.

Clindamycin has a gram-positive spectrum similar to that of erythromycin and is also active against most anaerobes, including *Bacteroides fragilis.* Except for treating anaerobic infection, clindamycin is rarely the drug of choice, although it is well absorbed orally, and parenteral formulations are available. Its major adverse effect is diarrhea, which may progress to pseudomembranous enterocolitis in some patients. Macrolides can increase an individual's risk for arrythmias, including QT interval prolongation in the case of azithromycin.

Aminoglycosides

The aminoglycoside antibiotics inhibit protein synthesis by binding to bacterial ribosomes. Gentamicin, tobramycin, amikacin, kanamycin, streptomycin, and netilmicin can be considered a group because of their similar activity, pharmacology, and toxicity. Because of poor gastrointestinal absorption, parenteral administration is necessary to produce therapeutic levels.

Aminoglycosides are used to treat serious infections caused by gram-negative bacilli, including bacteremia in immunocompromised hosts, hospital-acquired pneumonia, and peritonitis. They may be combined with penicillin to treat enterococcal endocarditis. Aminoglycosides are not effective against meningitis because they do not cross the blood–brain barrier. Aminoglycosides are not used for most gram-positive infections because the β-lactams are less toxic.

The major adverse effects of the aminoglycosides are nephrotoxicity and ototoxicity. Blood urea nitrogen, creatinine, and aminoglycoside peak and trough serum levels should be monitored, particularly in patients with known renal disease. Combined administration of a loop diuretic such as furosemide with aminoglycosides has a synergistic ototoxic effect, potentially leading to permanent loss of cochlear function. Penicillins may decrease the antimicrobial effectiveness of parenteral aminoglycosides, particularly in patients with impaired renal function.

Tetracyclines

The tetracyclines are bacteriostatic agents that reversibly inhibit ribosomal protein synthesis. Although they are active against a wide range of organisms (including *Staphylococcus, Rickettsia, Chlamydia, Nocardia,* and *Actinomyces*), resistance is widespread, especially among *S aureus* and gram-negative bacilli. The principal clinical uses of tetracyclines are in the treatment of nongonococcal urethritis, Rocky Mountain spotted fever, chronic bronchitis, and sebaceous disorders such as acne rosacea. In addition, tetracyclines are an alternative for the penicillin-allergic patient with syphilis. Tetracyclines are well absorbed when taken on an empty stomach; however, their absorption is decreased when taken with milk, antacids, calcium, or iron. Tetracyclines are distributed throughout the extracellular fluid, but cerebrospinal fluid penetration is unreliable. Adverse effects include oral or vaginal candidiasis with prolonged use, gastrointestinal upset, photosensitivity, elevation of the blood urea nitrogen level, and idiopathic intracranial hypertension. Tetracyclines can prolong the international normalized ratio (INR) in patients taking warfarin, and they should not be administered to pregnant women or to children younger than 10 years because of effects on developing bone and teeth. Lymecycline is a newer tetracycline agent available in Europe.

Miscellaneous antibacterial agents

Rifampin was originally developed as an anti-TB agent, but it is also used to treat several intractable bacterial infections. The drug is usually employed adjunctively because bacteria develop resistance to the drug when it is used as a single agent. Rifampin often demonstrates higher effectiveness in vivo than in vitro, perhaps because it penetrates directly into leukocytes and kills phagocytosed bacteria. It also penetrates well into bone and abscess cavities. Rifampin in combination with other agents is used successfully in treating *S aureus* and prosthetic valve endocarditis caused by *S epidermidis.* It is effective in eradicating the carrier state of nasal *S aureus.* The drug is also effective prophylactically against *N meningitidis* and may be useful for treating oropharyngeal carriers of *H influenzae* type b.

Another oral antibiotic with potential for treating deep-seated infections is TMP-SMX. After a single oral dose, the mean serum levels of TMP-SMX are approximately 75% of the concentration that would be achieved through the intravenous route. In addition to its excellent pharmacokinetics, TMP-SMX has an extremely broad spectrum of activity, including effectiveness against Enterobacteriaceae and some organisms that are resistant to cephalosporins. A misconception is that TMP-SMX has limited activity against gram-positive bacteria; however, most streptococci, staphylococci, and *Listeria monocytogenes* are susceptible to it. Beyond the broad-spectrum effect of TMP-SMX, the concomitant use of metronidazole creates an antibiotic combination with activity against microorganisms that surpasses that of a third-generation cephalosporin. TMP-SMX has been increasingly used in the treatment and prophylaxis of *Pneumocystis* infection and toxoplasmosis.

Chloramphenicol is a bacteriostatic agent that reversibly inhibits ribosomal protein synthesis. This drug is active against a wide variety of gram-negative and gram-positive organisms, including anaerobes. The major concern with this agent is hematopoietic toxicity, including reversible bone marrow suppression and irreversible aplasia. Aplastic anemia is an idiosyncratic late reaction to the drug and is usually fatal. Other adverse effects include hemolysis, allergy, and peripheral neuritis.

New Antibiotic Classes

Pharmacologic research has provided entirely new classes of antibiotics (see Table 14-4) that offer additional treatment options for emerging resistant bacterial strains. Most of these newer drugs are targeted against resistant strains of gram-positive bacteria. Other newer antibiotics used to treat multidrug-resistant infections include the glycylcycline antibiotic *tigecycline,* which is related to the tetracyclines; the bacteriocins *nisin* and *sakacin;* the temporins *temporin A* and *temporin L;* the DNA nanobinders; the peptide deformylase inhibitors; a folic acid antagonist, *iclaprim;* nucleoside analogues; bacteriophage endolysins, which are derived from viral phage–infected bacterial cells; and antimicrobial proteins (AMPs), natural endogenous proteins able to kill bacteria, fungi, and viruses at nanomolar concentrations.

Bailey J, Summers KM. Dalbavancin: a new lipoglycopeptide antibiotic. *Am J Health Syst Pharm.* 2008;65(7):599–610.

Doripenem (doribax)—a new parenteral carbapenem. *Med Lett Drugs Ther.* 2008;50(1278): 5–7.

Dryden MS. Novel antibiotic treatment for skin and soft tissue infection. *Curr Opin Infect Dis.* 2014;27(2):116–124.

Giannarini G, Mogorovich A, Valent F, et al. Prulifloxacin versus levofloxacin in the treatment of chronic bacterial prostatitis: a prospective, randomized, double-blind trial. *J Chemother.* 2007;19(3):304–308.

Hammerschlag MR, Sharma R. Use of cethromycin, a new ketolide, for treatment of community-acquired respiratory infections. *Expert Opin Investig Drugs.* 2008;17(3): 387–400.

Zhanel GG, Karlowsky JA, Rubinstein E, Hoban DJ. Tigecycline: a novel glycylcycline antibiotic. *Expert Rev Anti Infect Ther.* 2006;4(1):9–25.

Antifungal Agents

Imidazoles function by inhibiting fungal cytochrome P-450–dependent enzymes, thereby blocking synthesis of the fungal cell membrane. The imidazoles (fluconazole, itraconazole) offer a less toxic alternative to amphotericin B in treating cryptococcal meningitis and other invasive fungal diseases and may play a role in long-term suppression of *Cryptococcus* after remission of acute infection in severely immunocompromised patients. Ketoconazole is often less effective than the newer imidazoles and carries a higher risk of hepatotoxicity. Voriconazole, a second-generation triazole, is available in both intravenous and oral formulations. It offers a better treatment option for invasive aspergillosis and other serious fungal infections. Additional new investigational imidazoles include flutrimazole, croconazole, ravuconazole, posaconazole, sertaconazole, albaconazole, lanoconazole, bifonazole, eberconazole, and luliconazole.

Treatment of serious, deep-seated, systemic fungal infections may require the use of intravenous amphotericin B, sometimes in combination with either flucytosine or an imidazole. Lipid complex and liposome-encapsulated formulations of amphotericin B are available to reduce the drug's toxicity. Nystatin, which is structurally similar to amphotericin B, is classified as a topical antifungal agent. However, a new intravenous liposomal formulation of nystatin is currently in clinical trials for treatment of systemic fungal infections. *Terbinafine,* an allylamine oral antifungal agent, and *butenafine,* a benzylamine, are effective in controlling onychomycosis due to chronic dermatophyte infections.

Several novel antifungal agents include echinocandins, pneumocandins, and improved imidazoles. *Caspofungin, micafungin,* and *anidulafungin* are echinocandins that are approved for treatment of invasive *Candida* and *Aspergillus* infections. Other promising new drugs in preclinical development include inhibitors of fungal protein, fatty acid, lipid, and cell-wall synthesis.

Anttila VJ, Salonen J, Ylipalosaari P, Koivula I, Riikonen P, Nikoskelainen J. A retrospective nationwide case study on the use of a new antifungal agent: patients treated with caspofungin during 2001–2004 in Finland. *Clin Microbiol Infect.* 2007;13(6):606–612.

Juang P. Update on new antifungal therapy. *AACN Adv Crit Care.* 2007;18(3):253–260.

Kwon DS, Mylonakis E. Posaconazole: a new broad-spectrum antifungal agent. *Expert Opin Pharmacother.* 2007;8(8):1167–1178.

Pasqualotto AC, Denning DW. New and emerging treatments for fungal infections. *J Antimicrob Chemother.* 2008;61(Suppl 1):i19–i30.

Antiviral Agents

Acyclovir is a nucleoside analogue that is effective against HSV and VZV infections. It inhibits viral DNA replication. One phosphorylation step of acyclovir is catalyzed by the enzyme thymidine kinase. The virus-induced thymidine kinase is far more active than the host cell thymidine kinase. Therefore, acyclovir is very active against viruses within infected host cells and yet is generally well tolerated.

Acyclovir has proven effective in treating a variety of herpetic infections. Oral acyclovir effectively treats acute severe genital herpes and can be used for long-term suppression in immunocompetent patients with frequently recurring genital herpes. Intravenous acyclovir is effective against herpes simplex encephalitis. Acyclovir in doses of 500 mg/M^2 every 8 hours has been used successfully in treating herpes zoster infections in immunocompromised patients.

Oral acyclovir may be used to treat herpes zoster ophthalmicus. Doses of 800 mg 5 times daily are usually effective in reducing the incidence of ocular complications of herpes zoster ophthalmicus. However, postherpetic neuralgia is not affected by this therapy. A randomized controlled study of acyclovir and oral corticosteroids demonstrated that the latter did not help to reduce the incidence of postherpetic neuralgia when added to oral acyclovir.

Famciclovir and *valacyclovir* are currently approved in the United States for the treatment of herpes zoster and herpes simplex infections, and studies have shown that they are effective against the latter. Both of these newer drugs allow less frequent dosing intervals (every 8–12 hours, depending on the indication). *Valganciclovir* is used for the prevention and treatment of CMV infections in patients who have undergone organ transplantation or who have AIDS, and it has also been found to be effective for treating acute retinal necrosis caused by VZV.

Adefovir is a nucleoside analogue and a potent inhibitor of many viruses, such as HIV, HSV, hepatitis B, HPV, and EBV. The nucleoside analogue *brivudine* appears to have a stronger antiviral effect against VZV than does acyclovir or penciclovir. The efficacy of brivudine has been documented in several clinical trials in patients with herpesvirus-related infections, particularly in herpes zoster and herpes simplex infections.

Ganciclovir, foscarnet, and cidofovir are additional antiviral agents used for treating CMV infections, including retinitis. Amantadine and rimantadine are M2 protein inhibitors that are effective for treating influenza A and for the prophylactic treatment of contacts of infected patients. However, the rapid onset of drug resistance, ineffectiveness against influenza B, and CNS adverse effects have prevented wide acceptance of these agents. Oseltamivir is an oral neuraminidase inhibitor that initially exhibited excellent efficacy against influenza in humans, but reports in early 2009 showed a high incidence of viral resistance (up to 100%) to this agent in infections caused by influenza type A H1N1. Another neuraminidase inhibitor, zanamivir, appears to be effective for influenza, but resistance has been reported with this agent as well.

Bailey J, Summers KM. Dalbavancin: a new lipoglycopeptide antibiotic. *Am J Health Syst Pharm.* 2008;65(7):599–610.

Chacko M, Weinberg JM. Famciclovir for cutaneous herpesvirus infections: an update and review of new single-day dosing indications. *Cutis.* 2007;80(1):77–81.

Cui L, Iwamoto A, Lian JQ, et al. Novel mechanism of antibiotic resistance originating in vancomycin-intermediate *Staphylococcus aureus. Antimicrob Agents Chemother.* 2006;50(2): 428–438.

Doripenem (doribax)—a new parenteral carbapenem. *Med Lett Drugs Ther.* 2008;50(1278): 5–7.

Dryden MS. Novel antibiotic treatment for skin and soft tissue infection. *Curr Opin Infect Dis.* 2014;27(2):116–124.

Giannarini G, Mogorovich A, Valent F, et al. Prulifloxacin versus levofloxacin in the treatment of chronic bacterial prostatitis: a prospective, randomized, double-blind trial. *J Chemother.* 2007;19(3):304–308.

Hammerschlag MR, Sharma R. Use of cethromycin, a new ketolide, for treatment of community-acquired respiratory infections. *Expert Opin Investig Drugs.* 2008;17(3): 387–400.

Polenakovik HM, Pleiman CM. Ceftaroline for methicillin-resistant *Staphylococcus aureus* bacteremia: case series and review of the literature. *Int J Antimicrob Agents.* 2013;42(5): 450–455.

Superti F, Ammendolia MG, Marchetti M. New advances in anti-HSV chemotherapy. *Curr Med Chem.* 2008;15(9):900–911.

Zhanel GG, Karlowsky JA, Rubinstein E, Hoban DJ. Tigecycline: a novel glycylcycline antibiotic. *Expert Rev Anti Infect Ther.* 2006;4(1):9–25.

Zhang JZ, Ward KW. Besifloxacin, a novel fluoroquinolone antimicrobial agent, exhibits potent inhibition of pro-inflammatory cytokines in human THP-1 monocytes. *J Antimicrob Chemother.* 2008;61(1):111–116.

CHAPTER 15

Perioperative Management in Ocular Surgery

Recent Developments

- New oral anticoagulant drugs, including dabigatran, rivaroxaban, and apixaban, lack a specific antidote to reverse anticoagulant effects; empirical discontinuation before surgical intervention should be considered.
- Malignant hyperthermia susceptibility is inherited in an autosomal dominant pattern; genetic screening is available.

Introduction

While morbidity and mortality associated with ocular surgery are generally considered to be low, the perioperative management of ophthalmic surgery patients can be challenging. Often, these patients are older and have numerous medical conditions. Indeed, the ophthalmic condition requiring surgery is sometimes directly related to underlying systemic disease, such as diabetes mellitus or thyroid disease. Also, for some delicate surgical procedures there may be specific requirements about the patient's level of alertness during the operation, which would make the level of sedation particularly important. This chapter discusses some of the key issues to consider in the preoperative medical assessment and intraoperative management of the ocular surgery patient.

Preoperative Assessment

All patients require a history and physical examination as part of the preoperative assessment. However, preoperative testing in an asymptomatic patient, including electrocardiogram and routine blood tests, is not necessary. Preoperative testing is performed only when indicated; that is, the tests would have been done even if the patient were not planning surgery. The American Academy of Ophthalmology advisory opinion on the responsibilities of the ophthalmologist, Appropriate Examination and Treatment Procedures, provides general guidance on determining the appropriateness and necessity of diagnostic procedures and perioperative treatment. Although ophthalmologists may delegate the acquisition of the data required for the preoperative history and physical examination, the surgical planning and synthesis of information prior to surgery must be done by the operating ophthalmologist.

Avoiding surgical complications begins with the decision to operate. The risks and benefits of surgery, as well as any alternatives to it, are considered and the surgical plan is devised. Typically, the patient is involved in this process; informed consent is contingent on the patient's (or legal guardian's) receipt of a detailed, understandable explanation of the surgical plan. Open communication between the surgeon and the patient enhances patient education and ensures realistic expectations regarding the anesthesia depth, surgical procedure, anticipated recovery, and expected outcomes. Furthermore, a preoperative anesthesia evaluation is performed to identify any disease or disorder that might affect perioperative anesthesia care. A careful review of medication allergies, reactions to previous anesthetics, or family history of a reaction to anesthesia is critical in identifying patients at risk for malignant hyperthermia (see the section Malignant Hyperthermia later in this chapter). For a patient with an implantable cardioverter-defibrillator, the ophthalmologist should discuss the status and possible perioperative disabling of the device with the cardiologist before ocular surgery to avoid surgical complications.

The operating physician typically provides postoperative eye care. Any transfer of management should be discussed and approved, ideally before surgery, by the referring physician, the physician assuming future care, and the patient.

American Academy of Ophthalmology Ethics Committee. Appropriate Examination and Treatment Procedures. Advisory Opinion of the Code of Ethics. San Francisco: American Academy of Ophthalmology; 2007. Available at www.aao.org/about/ethics/exam_procedures.cfm. Accessed July 7, 2014.

Keay L, Lindsley K, Tielsch J, Katz J, Schein O. Routine preoperative medical testing for cataract surgery. *Cochrane Database Syst Rev.* 2009;2:CD007293.

Children and Adolescents

If surgery is planned on a child who is healthy and does not routinely take prescribed medications, no laboratory tests are necessary, even when general anesthesia is to be used. There is no evidence that abnormalities in a complete blood count affect the choice of anesthetic management for asymptomatic children. However, African American patients should be screened for sickle cell disease or trait if they have not previously been tested, because some aspects of anesthetic management will change in patients with hemoglobinopathy. Routine pregnancy testing of female patients of childbearing age, prior to anesthesia, is a complex issue and even more complex in minors, because individual states may have statutes concerning parental notification of test results. The anesthesiologist will likely discuss the need for preoperative pregnancy testing; however, consent for a pregnancy test is required.

The decision whether or not to perform elective eye surgery in children with an upper respiratory tract infection requires judgment. A child who is already ill will likely feel even worse after surgery, and the significance of a postoperative fever may be difficult to interpret. Furthermore, contaminated nasal discharge could enter the ocular area. If the child has a fever above 101°F, has purulent nasal discharge, or appears systemically ill, a bacterial lower respiratory tract infection should be considered. This circumstance argues for a delay to avoid increased risk of laryngospasm and bronchospasm with general anesthesia. However, in the absence of such findings, such as with a child who appears well except for a runny nose, many anesthesiologists elect to proceed.

Medication Use in the Preoperative Period

In general, medication regimens should not be interrupted for eye surgery. Treatment of asthma, hypertension, angina, and congestive heart failure should be continued throughout the day of surgery. However, diabetic patients require modification of glucose management (see the section Diabetes Mellitus later in this chapter). The following are guidelines, although individual practice can vary.

Antihypertensive medications should be continued until the time of surgery so that the rebound hypertension that can occur with abrupt discontinuation of antihypertensive therapy is avoided. Rebound hypertension occurs most commonly with centrally acting adrenergic agents (particularly clonidine) and with β-blockers. Oral antihypertensive medications can be taken with a sip of water the day of surgery, whether or not the patient is fasting. For patients exhibiting perioperative hypertension, more specifically, blood pressure measuring 180/110 mm Hg or higher, the benefits of delaying surgery to optimize blood pressure should be weighed against the risks of such a delay.

Holding diuretics on the day of surgery is desirable. A patient under local anesthesia may become uncomfortable from a full bladder caused by a preoperative dose of diuretic. Of greater concern is that a patient undergoing general anesthesia who continues diuretic use may become hypotensive because of intravascular volume depletion.

In patients undergoing noncardiac surgery, β-blockers have been shown to reduce mortality. The surgical procedures that carry the highest cardiac risk and the greatest benefit from the preoperative use of β-blockers are major operations in older patients, including ocular surgeries such as orbital surgery and facial surgery. Select patients with previous myocardial infarction, patients with a positive stress test result, and patients with 2 or more risk factors for coronary artery disease may also benefit from preoperative use of β-blockers. (See Chapter 3 for a complete discussion of antihypertensive medications.)

Digoxin can be withheld the day of surgery for many patients, given its long half-life. However, if a patient is receiving digoxin to control the ventricular response to atrial fibrillation, the resting heart rate must be appropriate on the morning of surgery. If the resting heart rate is more than 90 beats per minute, digoxin or another medication should be considered.

Similarly, thyroid medications, with their long half-life, can be held the day of surgery.

Anticonvulsant medications should be administered on the patient's usual schedule, because stress and particularly general anesthesia can lower the seizure threshold.

A patient who has taken systemic corticosteroids for more than a month within 3 months of surgery may require corticosteroid supplementation with hydrocortisone, depending on the type of surgical procedure. Typically, patients undergoing cataract surgery or other procedures under local anesthesia do not require such supplementation. However, for procedures involving greater surgically induced physiologic stress, patients may be administered hydrocortisone perioperatively to avoid acute adrenal insufficiency.

Nicotinic acid should be discontinued before general anesthesia because it can cause an exaggerated hypotensive response from vasodilation. It is generally taught that monoamine oxidase inhibitors should be discontinued 2–3 weeks prior to elective surgery. This is an issue best discussed with the anesthesiologist.

Use of echothiophate iodide eyedrops, which is rare today, requires that only certain muscle relaxants be administered before endotracheal intubation. Ideally, the drops should be stopped 3 weeks before elective surgery to allow recovery of the cholinesterase enzyme system. In patients who must continue echothiophate iodide, succinylcholine cannot be used during intubation, because a drug interaction involving these agents would enhance succinylcholine's effects, causing prolonged respiratory paralysis.

Although it is common to withhold aspirin before general surgical procedures, this is generally not necessary with cataract surgery. The risk of significant hemorrhage during cataract surgery is so low that the risk associated with continued anticoagulant or antiplatelet drug use is minimal. Indeed, stopping antiplatelet therapy may be associated with increased morbidity or mortality. Failure to continue aspirin and other antiplatelet therapy for 6–12 months after a coronary artery stenting procedure has been associated with increased risk of cardiac ischemia.

The management of anticoagulation in the perioperative setting must be individualized because the risk of thrombosis and the strength of the indication for anticoagulation vary greatly, as does the risk of bleeding during various surgical procedures. No single regimen satisfies all patient needs. Consultation with the patient's primary physician is advisable if anticoagulation must be stopped. Warfarin can be stopped 5 days before surgery, and if the international normalized ratio (INR) level drops below 2.0, heparin therapy with either intravenous (IV) unfractionated heparin or subcutaneous low-molecular-weight heparin can be given to maintain adequate anticoagulation until just before surgery. Intravenous heparin should be discontinued approximately 12 hours prior to surgery and restarted 24 hours after surgery. If gastrointestinal function is normal, warfarin may be restarted on the day of surgery. If anticoagulation is critical, heparin may be used until therapeutic warfarin levels have been reached.

Unlike warfarin, the new oral anticoagulant drugs, including dabigatran, rivaroxaban, and apixaban, present a unique challenge, as they lack a specific antidote to allow reversal of their anticoagulant effects. Most patients taking these agents can undergo cataract surgery without altering their anticoagulation regimen. For more invasive surgical procedures, empirical discontinuation perioperatively and/or bridging with heparin should be considered on an individual basis.

A number of over-the-counter drugs and nutritional supplements exhibit antiplatelet activity. Patients who use supplements such as vitamin E and St John's wort and nonsteroidal anti-inflammatory agents such as ibuprofen may fail to report taking these drugs because they are not "prescribed." Many nutritional supplements are not medically indicated and can be stopped before surgery.

In general, *antimicrobial prophylaxis* of bacterial endocarditis before ocular surgery is not necessary in patients with cardiac valvular disease. Guidelines for infective endocarditis prophylaxis are available from the American Heart Association (www.heart.org/HEARTORG/) and the European Society of Cardiology (www.escardio.org).

American College of Cardiology website; www.cardiosource.org.

Fleisher LA, Beckman JA, Brown KA, et al. ACC/AHA 2007 guidelines on perioperative cardiovascular evaluation and care for noncardiac surgery: a report of the American College of Cardiology/American Heart Association Task Force on Practice Guidelines. *J Am Coll Cardiol.* 2007;50(17):159–241.

Diabetes Mellitus

Oral hypoglycemic medications are usually withheld the day of surgery. These medications have a relatively long duration of action, which could lead to hypoglycemia late in the day if the patient's oral caloric intake is inadequate.

Management of blood glucose is important in avoiding central nervous system dysfunction. No single regimen works for all patients, however. Insulin-dependent patients should undergo surgery early in the day, whenever possible, to minimize disruption of their metabolic status, and their glucose levels should be monitored postoperatively. For a diet-controlled diabetic patient undergoing a brief surgical procedure, management generally involves only monitoring of the blood glucose level immediately after surgery and every 3 hours until oral intake is resumed.

For patients with relatively well-controlled insulin-requiring diabetes mellitus and reasonable glucose control (<250 mg/dL), one option is to hold all short-acting insulin and give half the usual dose of intermediate-acting or long-acting insulin the morning of the surgery. It is imperative to provide close perioperative monitoring of glucose and electrolyte levels. In patients with elevated glucose levels (≥250 mg/dL) prior to surgery, titration of dextrose 5% as part of a maintenance solution with an initial IV rate of 75 mL/hour should prevent hypoglycemia or hyperglycemia. Blood glucose should be monitored hourly and the infusion rate adjusted to maintain the glucose level at 100–200 mg/dL.

For patients who are taking insulin and undergoing procedures lasting less than 2 hours, the "no insulin, no glucose" regimen works well preoperatively on the morning of surgery. Monitoring of blood glucose levels before, during, and after surgery is important. The availability of one-touch monitoring makes such measurements very easy, even in the operating room. During the procedure, IV solutions without dextrose (lactated Ringer's or saline) are given. After the surgical procedure, and once oral intake is established, the patient should receive a portion (usually one-half or one-third) of the usual insulin dose. If a procedure lasts more than 2 hours, insulin may have to be given as an infusion of at least 4 units per hour, with monitoring of the blood glucose level every 30–60 minutes. The anesthesiologist and primary care physician should be involved in managing the blood glucose level in such patients.

Patients using an insulin pump can be easily managed during the perioperative period. The pump is left on the basal rate and, because the patient is not taking meals before surgery, the dosing used for meals is not given.

Respiratory Diseases

Patients with chronic obstructive pulmonary disease (COPD) can present distinct challenges in ophthalmic surgery. These patients may have difficulty breathing while lying flat on an operating table. They may also be prone to intraoperative and postoperative coughing, which can increase intraocular pressure. Cessation of smoking is extremely helpful for reducing intraoperative and postoperative coughing. Excessive cough suppression, however, may result in retained secretions, atelectasis, and limited air exchange. Preoperative bronchopulmonary care with chest physiotherapy can decrease susceptibility to infection and improve air exchange. In patients with COPD, general anesthesia may be preferred over local anesthesia because the anesthesiologist may have better control over tracheobronchial secretions and the cough reflex. See Chapter 7 for additional discussion.

Preoperative Fasting

Questions often arise as to how long a patient must abstain from eating and drinking before surgery. A pediatric patient who fasts for 10–12 hours preoperatively may become hypotensive as a result of dehydration. The use of clear liquids orally up to 2 hours before surgery does not lead to a higher incidence of aspiration or other gastrointestinal complications in the setting of general or local anesthesia.

The purpose of preoperative fasting is to reduce the particulate matter in the stomach and to lower the gastric fluid volume and acidity in case aspiration of stomach contents occurs. Diabetic patients, particularly those with autonomic neuropathy, are at risk for gastroparesis. Pregnant patients have a higher-than-normal risk of aspiration.

Patients with known gastroesophageal reflux disease and those with peptic ulcer disease may also have an increased risk of aspiration.

Oral administration of an H_2 blocker such as ranitidine or famotidine 2–4 hours before surgery reduces the percentage of patients with low gastric pH or high gastric volume. Metoclopramide and cisapride (restricted access in Europe; not available in the United States) also promote intestinal motility and decrease reflux; these drugs are especially useful in a nonfasting patient who requires urgent surgery. Table 15-1 lists selected perioperative medications and their uses.

Latex Allergy

According to the US Centers for Disease Control and Prevention, the prevalence of latex allergy in the general population is 1%–6% and among health care workers, 8%–12%. Health care workers and hospital employees can experience progressive sensitization to latex because of repeated occupational exposure. This sensitivity is accentuated in those with a history of atopy. Certain medical populations are also at significant risk, for example, patients with myelodysplasia or spina bifida and those who have undergone repeated urinary catheterization or frequent surgical procedures. A cross-reactivity with bananas, avocados, mangoes, and chestnuts has been demonstrated, and allergies to these foods and others have been associated with latex allergy. A history of reactivity to balloons also suggests a latex allergy.

Table 15-1 Selected Perioperative Medications and Their Uses

Use	Medications
Anti-emetic	Metoclopramide, ondansetron
Analgesic	Alfentanil, fentanyl citrate, ketorolac, morphine, sufentanil
Sedative	Diazepam, methohexital, midazolam, propofol, thiopental sodium
Histamine H_2 receptor antagonist (reduces gastric acid secretion)	Famotidine, ranitidine

Patients suspected of having latex allergy should be clearly identified, and the operating room environment made latex free. Latex is an aeroallergen and can be present in the operating room air for at least 1 hour after the use of latex gloves. Thus, whenever possible, an allergic patient should be the first case of the day.

Sussman G, Gold M. Guidelines for the management of latex allergies and safe latex use in health care facilities. Allergist website. www.acaai.org/allergist/allergies/Types/latex-allergy/Pages/latex-allergies-safe-use.aspx. Accessed September 4, 2014.

Universal Protocol

The definition of *wrong-site surgery* includes operating on the wrong site, performing the wrong procedure, or performing a procedure on the wrong person. In ophthalmology, the definition includes operating on the wrong eye or performing the wrong procedure, including implantation of a lens whose style and/or power differs from that chosen during preoperative surgical planning. Implanting a monofocal lens during cataract surgery, for example, when the plan was to implant a premium implant is considered the wrong procedure.

The Universal Protocol of the Joint Commission (www.jointcommission.org/standards_information/up.aspx) is designed to eliminate wrong-site surgery in the United States; it includes several key elements:

- agreeing on and documenting the procedure to be performed (typically done on the surgical consent form)
- marking the surgical site in the preoperative period (done by a designated member of the team, typically the surgeon)
- pausing before the beginning of surgery (time-out) to have all members of the surgical team agree that this is the correct patient and correct procedure; that the necessary equipment is present, including implants; that the patient is correctly positioned; that medical information on the patient, including x-rays, is for the correct patient; and that appropriate preoperative antibiotics, if indicated, have been given.

The requirement that 2 unique patient identifiers be confirmed by the surgical team before the initiation of surgery aims to reduce potential errors, including performing surgery on the wrong patient. The identifiers, used during a time-out, include name, date of birth, and medical record number. For the time-out to be effective, it is important that members of the surgical team feel empowered to speak up if they do not agree that all elements of the Universal Protocol have been satisfied. Wrong-site surgery is considered a sentinel event and in many states must be reported to the state board of medicine.

AAO Wrong-Site Task Force, Hoskins Center for Quality Eye Care. Patient Safety Statements. *Recommendations of American Academy of Ophthalmology Wrong-Site Task Force.* San Francisco: American Academy of Ophthalmology; 2008. Available at: http://one.aao.org/patient-safety-statement/recommendations-of-american-academy-ophthalmology-. Accessed July 8, 2014.

The Joint Commission website; www.jcrinc.com.

Intraoperative Considerations

Systemic Anesthetic Agents

The use of balanced general anesthesia, in which small amounts of several different types of medications are titrated to avoid the adverse effects of a large dose of any one type, has been effective in reducing prolonged anesthesia and prolonged recovery time. Neuromuscular blocking agents of short duration (12 minutes for mivacurium and 30 minutes for atracurium and vecuronium) administered with an infusion pump allow the anesthesiologist to fine-tune the degree of neuromuscular blockade during balanced anesthesia.

The shorter-acting narcotics such as sufentanil have potencies up to 1000 times those of morphine. These agents help provide short-term stability of hemodynamics during intensive stimulation without the cost of prolonged excessive sedation postoperatively. Using such agents immediately before intubation as part of an anesthetic induction has become nearly universal.

Management of postoperative nausea and vomiting after general anesthesia has become easier with more powerful antinausea medications such as ondansetron and metoclopramide. These drugs do not cause sedation, as droperidol does, which means the patient in a same-day surgery setting recovers more quickly.

Postoperative pain can be prophylactically treated during the procedure with IV ketorolac in a 30-mg to 60-mg dose or with small titrated doses of IV fentanyl in the range of 50–100 μg. Because of the reported gastrointestinal complications of higher doses of ketorolac, patients older than 60 years should receive a total of no more than 30 mg of IV ketorolac. Also, there is evidence that IV ketorolac, because of its pain-reducing qualities, can reduce the amount of postoperative nausea and vomiting in patients who have undergone strabismus surgery or other procedures requiring general anesthesia. There is no evidence that this particular nonsteroidal anti-inflammatory drug increases postoperative bleeding after ophthalmic surgery.

Sedation is an important part of comfortable regional or general anesthesia in a patient undergoing elective surgery. Anxiolytics such as midazolam can be given intramuscularly (1–4 mg) 30–60 minutes before the procedure or intravenously (0.5–2.0 mg) 2–3 minutes before the stimulus of the anesthetic block. Midazolam is a more appropriate sedative than diazepam for outpatient surgery because its elimination half-life is 2–4 hours; diazepam's half-life is 20–40 hours. The effects of midazolam can also be reversed with flumazenil. Careful IV titration of sedatives and narcotics is important in older patients to avoid oversedation or respiratory depression.

Alfentanil can be given intravenously in titrated doses with appropriate anesthesia monitoring. Its peak effect occurs in 1–2 minutes and lasts 10–20 minutes. Fentanyl citrate, which has a peak effect in 3–5 minutes and lasts approximately 30 minutes, is also given in titrated doses during regional or topical anesthesia. These agents are used for sedation as well as for their analgesic properties. The effects of narcotics can be reversed with the antagonist naloxone, given intravenously. The duration of naloxone reversal is 1 hour or less.

Thiopental sodium, given in increments every 30 seconds, can be used to ensure amnesia and hypnosis for regional anesthesia or local infiltration of anesthetic agents. However, too rapid or too large a dose can depress hemodynamics and respiration. Methohexital can be similarly used in increments given intravenously every 20–30 seconds.

Propofol is a drug with unique properties of rapid hypnosis and a tendency to produce bradycardia, with rapid clearance and faster recovery. It must be given through a large-bore vein or administered after a lidocaine flush of the IV line to avoid significant burning on administration. Propofol is a lipid-based medication that supports rapid bacterial growth at room temperature. Indeed, extrinsically contaminated propofol has been associated with postoperative infections, including endogenous endophthalmitis. It is therefore imperative that hospital personnel involved in the preparation, handling, and administration of this drug adhere to strict aseptic technique during its use.

Local Anesthetic Agents

Local anesthetic injection into the retrobulbar space can lead to apnea, respiratory arrest, and cranial nerve palsies on the side being injected, or even on the opposite side. Anatomical studies of the position of the retrobulbar needle in relation to the optic nerve during injection show that it is possible to inject anesthetic into the subdural space with a standard Atkinson-type needle. Cases of cranial nerve palsies associated with respiratory difficulties represent actual brainstem anesthesia from injection of the anesthetic agent into the subdural space, with subsequent diffusion into the circulating cerebrospinal fluid.

Several suggestions have been made to avoid such complications, including changing the traditional positioning of the eye during the retrobulbar anesthetic injection so that the nerve is rotated away from the track of the needle (having the patient look straight ahead, rather than up). Using less sharp, nondisposable retrobulbar needles that are less than 1¼" long also reduces the chance of perforating the optic nerve sheath. Although one series implicated the concentration of anesthetic as the cause of respiratory arrest, it is more likely that a larger volume and, therefore, a larger total dose of anesthetic was delivered to the brainstem through an inadvertent subdural injection. If apnea, respiratory arrest, or cranial neuropathies occur after a retrobulbar injection, the patient's airway must be supported with mask ventilation. Intubation and mechanical ventilation may be necessary. Apnea seldom lasts more than 30–50 minutes, but it is important that experienced medical personnel stabilize the patient's condition during this time. The peribulbar technique was devised, in part, to avoid such complications.

Respiratory distress and dysphagia can result from the Nadbath block, an injection into the stylomastoid foramen that is used to provide facial akinesia. These complications occur when the anesthetic agent is injected deeply into the area of the facial nerve as it exits the stylomastoid foramen, and the anesthetic bathes cranial nerves IX, X, and XI as they exit the jugular foramen. This leads to paralysis of these nerves, and the patient becomes dysphagic, begins to cough or has a hoarse voice, and may develop stridor or severe respiratory insufficiency. The complications tend to occur in thin persons, in whom it is easier to bury the needle deeply. Managing the respiratory distress requires suctioning the pharynx, positioning the patient on his or her side, and supplementing the patient's inspired gases with oxygen or even intubation. This complication can be avoided by use of a short hypodermic needle, advancing it only partway into the area to be injected, and injecting a small volume (<3 mL).

Anesthetic toxicity can occur when high concentrations of anesthetic agent are given. For example, if lidocaine 4% is used for a peribulbar injection, the total volume that can be safely given to a 154-lb (70-kg) patient is limited to 8 mL. A smaller patient would be able to tolerate no more than 5 mL of lidocaine 4% without risking complications of systemic toxicity, including confusion, cardiac arrhythmias, and respiratory depression.

Seizures have occurred from the intra-arterial injection of local anesthetic agent into the ophthalmic artery. Such seizures are nearly instantaneous with injection; supportive measures should include airway maintenance and blood pressure support. The seizures are of short duration.

Malignant Hyperthermia

The preoperative history can help determine whether or not a patient is at risk for *malignant hyperthermia (MH),* an autosomal dominant disorder of hypermetabolism involving the skeletal muscle. Patients determined to be at high risk for MH may require a muscle biopsy for muscle contracture evaluation or genetic testing. MH is associated with mutations in 2 genes: ryanodine receptor 1 *(RYR1),* most commonly; and calcium channel A1S *(CACNA1S).* Nevertheless, such preoperative screening is not infallible, and the surgeon and anesthesiologist should be prepared to respond to this complication. MH is a disorder of calcium binding by the sarcoplasmic reticulum of skeletal muscles. In the presence of an anesthetic triggering agent, unbound intracellular calcium increases, which stimulates muscle contracture. This increased metabolism outstrips oxygen delivery, and anaerobic metabolism develops, with the production of lactate and subsequent massive acidosis. Hyperthermia results from the hypermetabolic state.

The earliest signs of MH include tachycardia that is greater than expected for the patient's anesthetic and surgical status and elevated end-tidal carbon dioxide level, as measured by capnography. Labile blood pressure, tachypnea, sweating, muscle rigidity, blotchy discoloration of skin, cyanosis, and dark urine all signal progression of the disorder. Temperature elevation, which can reach extremely high levels, is a relatively late sign. Ultimately, respiratory and metabolic acidosis, hyperkalemia, hypercalcemia, myoglobinuria, and renal failure can occur, as can disseminated intravascular coagulation and death.

Table 15-2 Malignant Hyperthermia Protocol

1. Stop the triggering agents immediately, and conclude surgery as soon as possible.
2. Hyperventilate with 100% oxygen at high flow rates.
3. Administer:
   a. Dantrolene: 2–3 mg/kg initial bolus with increments up to 10 mg/kg total. Continue to administer dantrolene until symptoms are controlled. Occasionally, a dose greater than 10 mg/kg may be needed.
   b. Sodium bicarbonate: 1–2 mEq/kg increments guided by arterial pH and P_{CO_2}. Bicarbonate will combat hyperkalemia by driving potassium into cells.
4. Actively cool patient:
   a. If needed, administer IV iced saline (not lactated Ringer's) 15 mL/kg every 10 minutes × 3. Monitor closely.
   b. Lavage stomach, bladder, rectum, and peritoneal and thoracic cavities with iced saline.
   c. Surface cool with ice and hypothermia blanket.
5. Maintain urine output. If needed, administer mannitol 0.25 g/kg IV, furosemide 1 mg/kg IV (up to 4 doses each). Urine output greater than 2 mL/kg/h may help prevent subsequent renal failure.
6. Calcium channel blockers *should not* be given when dantrolene is administered, as hyperkalemia and myocardial depression may occur.
7. Insulin for hyperkalemia: Add 10 units of regular insulin to 50 mL of 50% glucose, and titrate to control hyperkalemia. Monitor blood glucose and potassium levels.
8. Postoperatively: Continue dantrolene 1 mg/kg IV every 6 hours × 72 hours to prevent recurrence. Lethal recurrences of MH may occur. Observe in an intensive care unit.
9. For expert medical advice and further medical evaluation, call the MHAUS MH hotline at 800-644-9737 (outside the United States: 00 +1 209-417-3722). For nonemergency professional or patient information, call 800-986-4287 or go to www.mhaus.org.

Although volatile anesthetics such as halothane, enflurane, isoflurane, and IV succinylcholine are all known to trigger MH, haloperidol, trimeprazine, and promethazine can also cause this condition. In adult strabismus surgery, to avoid the use of succinylcholine, a laryngeal mask airway can be considered if muscle relaxation is not otherwise required. The use of the laryngeal mask airway reduces the soreness and irritation of the throat that occurs after oral endotracheal intubation.

MH is treated as a medical emergency (see Table 15-2 for the treatment protocol). The Malignant Hyperthermia Association of the United States (MHAUS; www.mhaus.org) staffs a 24-hour hotline to advise medical personnel on the diagnosis and treatment of MH: 800-644-9737 (within the US) or 00 +1 209-417-3722.

Malignant hyperthermia. Genetics Home Reference website. http://ghr.nlm.nih.gov/condition/malignant-hyperthermia. Accessed August 29, 2014.

Miller RD, Eriksson LI, Fleisher LA, Wiener-Kronish JP, Cohen NH, eds. *Miller's Anesthesia.* 8th ed. Philadelphia: Elsevier/Saunders; 2014.

CHAPTER 16

Medical Emergencies and Ocular Adverse Effects of Systemic Medications

Recent Developments

- Guidelines for cardiopulmonary resuscitation changed significantly in 2010, with an emphasis on chest compressions first, followed by airway opening and rescue breathing and the immediate use of an automated external defibrillator.
- The availability of portable defibrillators in ambulances, public places, and airline jets increases the probability of survival for patients with out-of-hospital ventricular fibrillation.
- Persons with suspected ischemic stroke should be transported to a facility capable of initiating fibrinolytic therapy within 1 hour of arrival unless that facility is more than 30 minutes away by ground ambulance.

Introduction

Though only occasionally called on to manage a medical emergency, the ophthalmologist must be aware of the diagnostic and therapeutic steps necessary for proper care of a patient in acute distress. Infrequent use of these life-support techniques makes periodic review particularly important. Also, it is advisable to have a member of the office staff who is trained in basic life support. Both the American Red Cross and the American Heart Association offer courses in basic life support (BLS), advanced cardiac life support (ACLS), and pediatric advanced life support (PALS). In addition to a review of life-support techniques, it is appropriate to periodically review office procedures, medications, and the equipment needed for each category of medical emergency. Table 16-1 lists medications used in acute medical emergencies.

Cardiopulmonary Arrest

Cardiopulmonary resuscitation (CPR) is intended to rescue patients with acute circulatory failure, respiratory failure, or both. The most important determinant of short-term

Table 16-1 Medications Used in Acute Medical Emergencies

Drugs	Indications	Adverse Effects
	Arrhythmia	
Adenosine	Regular, wide or narrow complex tachycardia with a pulse	Flushing, headache, sweating, shortness of breath
Amiodarone	VF, VT	Bradycardia, hypotension
Atropine	Bradycardia with a pulse	Induced VT or supraventricular tachycardia
Dopamine	Bradycardia with a pulse (if atropine ineffective)	Ventricular arrhythmia, tachycardia
Epinephrine (1:10,000)	Asystole, PEA, VF, VT	Hypertension with excess doses
Procainamide	Stable, wide complex tachycardia with a pulse	Hypotension, bradycardia, AV block, VF
Vasopressin	Asystole, PEA, VF, VT	Cardiac arrest, arrhythmia, shock
	Shock and Anaphylaxis	
Diphenhydramine hydrochloride	Anaphylaxis and anaphylactoid reactions	Drowsiness
Epinephrine (1:1000)	Anaphylaxis	Tachycardia, hypertension
Glucose (D 50)	Insulin shock due to profound hypoglycemia	Hyperglycemia
Hydrocortisone sodium succinate	Anaphylaxis and anaphylactoid reactions	Adrenal-pituitary axis suppression
	Seizures	
Diazepam	Seizures	Sedation
Lorezapam	Seizures	Sedation

AV = atrioventricular; PEA = pulseless electrical activity; PVCs = premature ventricular contractions; VF = ventricular fibrillation; VT = ventricular tachycardia.

and long-term neurologically intact survival is the interval from onset of the arrest to restoration of effective spontaneous circulatory and respiratory function. Numerous studies have shown that early defibrillation is the most important factor influencing survival and the minimization of sequelae. The sequences included here have been developed to optimize treatment. They are useful guidelines for most patients, but they do not preclude other measures that may be indicated for individual patients. The most crucial aspects of treatment are contained in the mnemonic *CAB*—chest compressions, airway maintenance, and breathing. The most recent published CPR protocols are the 2010 American Heart Association Guidelines for cardiopulmonary resuscitation and emergency cardiovascular care; these basic CPR steps for adults, children, and infants can be found online at http://circ.ahajournals.org and www.heart.org. Also, the University of Washington maintains a free website (http://depts.washington.edu/learncpr//) with extensive resources, including text, graphics, and video demonstrations of CPR techniques.

The following are steps for CPR using CAB; they are performed with an unconscious patient (Fig 16-1):

1. Determine the level of responsiveness. Attempt to arouse the patient by tapping on his or her shoulder and shouting, "Are you all right?" Do not shake the head

or neck until this area has been evaluated for trauma. Quickly note if breathing is absent or abnormal (eg, gasping).

2. Activate the Emergency Medical Services (EMS) system if there is no patient response (in the United States, call 911 where available). Rescuers should "phone first" for unresponsive adults and give the location and nature of the emergency.

1. Call

Check the victim for unresponsiveness. If the person is not responsive and not breathing or not breathing normally, call 911 and return to the victim. In most locations the emergency dispatcher can assist you with CPR instructions.

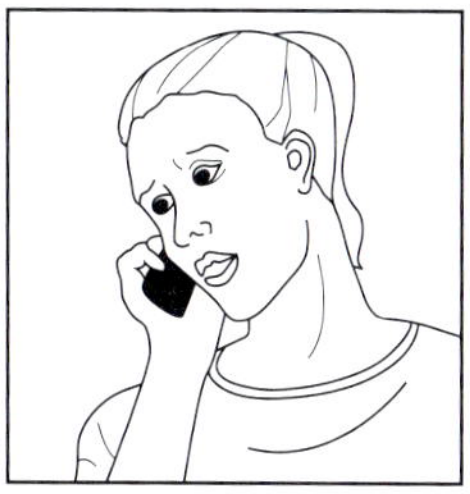

2. Pump

If the victim is still not breathing normally, coughing or moving, begin chest compressions. Push down in the center of the chest 2 inches 30 times. Pump hard and fast at the rate of at least 100/minute, faster than once per second.

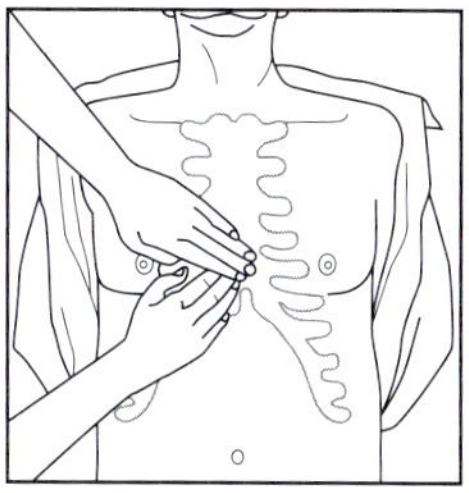

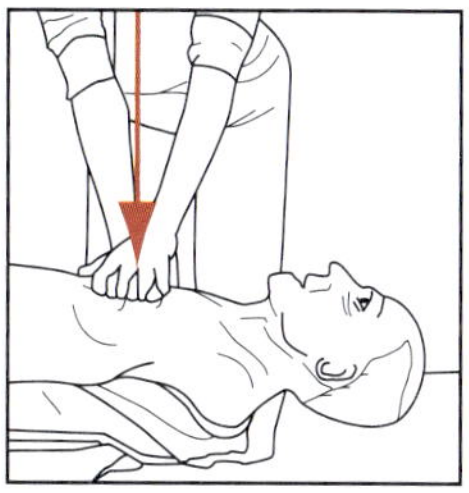

3. Blow

Tilt the head back and lift the chin. Pinch nose and cover the mouth with yours and blow until you see the chest rise. Give 2 breaths. Each breath should take 1 second.

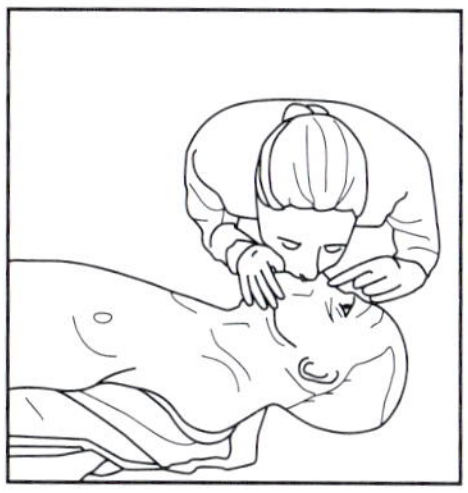

CONTINUE WITH 30 PUMPS AND 2 BREATHS UNTIL HELP ARRIVES

Note: This ratio is the same for one-person & two-person CPR. In two-person CPR the person pumping the chest stops while the other gives mouth-to-mouth breathing.

Figure 16-1 Adult cardiopulmonary resuscitation in 3 simple steps. *(Reproduced with permission from the University of Washington. Learn CPR page. University of Washington website. http://depts.washington.edu/learncpr/index.html. Accessed February 14, 2014.)*

3. Retrieve an automated external defibrillator (AED) or send someone for the AED.
4. Position the victim supine on a firm, flat surface.
5. In an unresponsive patient without respirations, initiate chest compressions. (Determination of a pulse is no longer indicated.) Place the heel of 1 hand at the midsternal region, with the bottom of the hand 1–2 finger-breadths above the xiphoid process.
6. "Push hard and push fast." The recommended cardiac compression rate is at least 100 per minute. The depth of chest compression is critical; optimal compressions are 1.5 to 2.0 inches deep for children and at least 2.0 inches deep for adults. The chest must be allowed to fully recoil between compressions.
7. Deliver 30 chest compressions.
8. As soon as the AED is available, the unit should be connected to the patient and instructions followed for assessing the heart rhythm. Interruptions to chest compressions should be minimized by having a second rescuer (eg, the person who retrieved the AED) charge and apply the AED. Resume chest compressions immediately after the shock, and continue until 30 compressions are given.
9. Open the airway. Rescue breathing (see step 10 for technique) should be performed at a rate of 10–12 ventilations per minute. Use the head-tilt, chin-lift maneuver to provide a good airway. This is done by applying firm pressure to the forehead while placing the fingers of the other hand under the chin, supporting the mandible. If a neck injury is suspected, the modified jaw thrust without head extension should be used.
10. Pinch the nose closed. Cover the patient's mouth with yours, making a tight seal, and ventilate twice with full breaths (1 second each). A 2-second pause should be observed between breaths. Visible chest rise should be seen with each breath. Resume chest compressions immediately.
11. For 1- and 2-rescuer CPR: When the victim's airway is unprotected, 30 compressions should be performed before the victim is ventilated twice. About 4 seconds should be taken for 2 ventilations, including the pause between ventilations.
12. If 2 rescuers are present, chest compression duties should be switched every 2 minutes or 5 compression/ventilation cycles.
13. Continue with compression/ventilation cycles until EMS arrives.

CPR is most effective when started immediately after cardiac arrest. If cardiac arrest has persisted for more than 10 minutes, CPR is unlikely to restore the patient's central nervous system (CNS) to prearrest status. If there is any question about the exact duration of cardiac arrest, the patient should be given the benefit of the doubt and resuscitation should be started.

The risk of disease transmission through mouth-to-mouth ventilation is very low, but a variety of face shields and masks are available for the health care professional. Masks are more effective than face shields in delivering adequate ventilation. Alternative airway devices (eg, laryngeal mask airway or esophageal/tracheal dual lumen airway device) may also be acceptable for rescuers trained in their use.

Patients with suspected stroke should be rapidly transported to a hospital capable of initiating fibrinolytic therapy within 1 hour of arrival unless that facility is more than 30 minutes away by ground ambulance. These patients merit the same priorities for dispatch as patients with acute myocardial infarction or major trauma.

The following adjuncts are helpful in CPR and are suggested components for a medical emergency tray or crash cart:

- oxygen, to enhance tissue oxygenation and to prevent or ameliorate a hypoxic state
- airways, adult and child, oral and nasal, to be used on unconscious or sedated patients
- a barrier device, such as a face shield or mask-to-mouth unit, to prevent disease transmission. Both can be used with supplemental oxygen and are especially useful if the rescuer is inexperienced in using a standard bag-valve device, which should also be included as standard equipment to help secure the airway.
- Intravenous (IV) drugs (see Table 16-1)
- IV solutions: dextrose 5% and water, D5 Ringer's lactate, normal saline
- syringes (1, 5, and 10 mL), hypodermic needles (20, 22, and 25 gauge), and venous catheters
- a suction apparatus, tourniquet, taped tongue blade, and tape
- laryngoscope and endotracheal tubes (adult and child)

If there is no 911 community emergency phone system, it is essential to have the phone number of the local paramedic emergency squad posted near all office telephones.

BLS also outlines methods for aiding persons who are choking. These methods include the Heimlich maneuver and appropriate manual techniques for removing foreign bodies from the oral pharynx. Epigastric thrusts should be attempted; up to 10–12 thrusts may be necessary. If these techniques fail to restore effective respiratory function, ventilation should be attempted. Using a finger sweep to clear a foreign body from the oral pharynx is recommended by the American Medical Association but not indicated in many modern protocols. Transtracheal ventilation by means of cricothyrotomy may be necessary if other techniques fail to clear the airway.

The American Heart Association has established guidelines and procedures for ACLS. ACLS includes intubations, defibrillation, cardioversion, pacemaker placement, administration of drugs and fluids, and communication with ambulance and hospital systems. Because of the comprehensive and changing nature of ACLS algorithms, these procedures are beyond the scope of this chapter.

Competency in pediatric emergency care may be enhanced with training in pediatric life support (PLS) and PALS. In addition, ophthalmologists should be familiar with the ophthalmic manifestations of child abuse and abusive head trauma (shaken baby syndrome). These are discussed in BCSC Section 6, *Pediatric Ophthalmology and Strabismus.*

Berg RA, Hemphill R, Abella BS, et al. Part 5: adult basic life support: 2010 American Heart Association Guidelines for Cardiopulmonary Resuscitation and Emergency Cardiovascular Care. *Circulation.* 2010;122(18 Suppl 3):S685–S705.

Syncope

Vasovagal episodes (syncope) are common, usually benign, events. These episodes occur more often in older persons and are sometimes caused by cardiac abnormalities. Because many eye patients are older, the ophthalmologist may encounter and thus should be prepared to handle this condition in the office. Syncope is defined as transient loss of consciousness and postural tone due to cerebral hypoperfusion. A syncopal episode can be triggered by a wide array of events. Often, the patient has premonitory signs and symptoms before the episode; these include lightheadedness, nausea, the feeling of temperature changes, or tinnitus. Patients with a history of cardiac problems who experience a syncopal episode have a higher risk of morbidity and mortality and should be evaluated thoroughly. A person experiencing a syncopal episode should be placed supine—preferably in a cool, quiet place—and the legs should be elevated.

Shock

Shock is a state of tissue hypoperfusion that leads to impaired cellular metabolism and—if uncorrected—progresses to multiple organ failure and death.

Classification

Shock is classified according to the 4 primary pathophysiologic mechanisms involved:

- oligemic, or hypovolemic (eg, hemorrhage, diabetic ketoacidosis, burns, or sequestration)
- cardiogenic (eg, myocardial infarction or arrhythmia)
- obstructive (eg, pericardial tamponade, pulmonary embolus, or tension pneumothorax)
- distributive, characterized by maldistribution of the vascular volume secondary to altered vasomotor tone (eg, sepsis, anaphylaxis, spinal cord insult, beriberi, or arteriovenous fistula)

The type of shock can often be determined by the history, physical examination, and appropriate diagnostic tests. Regardless of the event that precipitated the state of shock, microcirculatory failure is the common factor that eventually leads to death in advanced shock. Ventilatory failure appears to be the most significant factor in the morbidity and mortality of shock, with subsequent hypoxemia and metabolic acidosis leading to many complications.

If one rules out vasovagal syncope (by virtue of its short duration and because of knowledge of the situations that produce this condition), the basic life-support measures for the initial emergency care of the unconscious patient are similar to the measures used in treating patients with shock. The most important aspects of treatment are the CABs, the same principles used in CPR.

Failure of respiratory gas exchange is the most frequent single cause of death in patients with shock; thus, respiratory obstruction must be ruled out first. Oxygen is then given by mask; if respiratory movements are shallow, mechanical ventilation is necessary.

Respiratory obstruction can be assumed if there is stridor with respiratory movements or if cyanosis persists even when adequate ventilatory techniques have been applied. A conscious patient in distress who cannot speak and who is developing cyanosis may be choking on food or a foreign body.

Assessment

The vital signs must be monitored. The clinical syndrome is usually characterized by an altered sensorium, relative hypotension, tachycardia, tachypnea, oliguria, metabolic acidosis, weak or absent pulse, pallor, diaphoresis, and cool skin (however, the skin may be warm in septic shock). Decreased pulse pressure is often an early sign of shock, and systolic pressures of less than 90 mm Hg are often associated with vital organ hypoperfusion. Blood pressure is not always a reliable indicator of tissue perfusion, however.

Treatment

Specific guidelines for the treatment of shock, which is often quite complex, are beyond the scope of this text. General guidelines are as follows:

- The EMS system should be activated or the patient transferred to an emergency department.
- The patient should be positioned supine, with the legs elevated.
- Supplemental oxygen should be administered to enhance tissue oxygenation. Mechanical ventilation may be necessary to maintain the Po_2 at normal levels and to prevent respiratory acidosis.
- Fluid resuscitation with IV infusion of a crystalloid solution (ie, normal saline or Ringer's lactate) should be administered rapidly.
- Vasopressor drugs (norepinephrine first) may be necessary for augmentation of systemic vascular tone and/or cardiac output to help perfuse vital organs after an adequate circulating volume is established.
- Blood cultures should be drawn and antibiotic therapy initiated promptly if sepsis is suspected.
- Sodium bicarbonate, given intravenously, is indicated for correction of severe metabolic acidosis.

Experimental drugs used in the treatment of septic shock include vasopressin and polyclonal IV immunoglobulin.

Anaphylaxis

One specific cause of shock that requires immediate and specific therapy is anaphylaxis. *Anaphylaxis* is an acute allergic reaction following antigen exposure in a previously sensitized person. It is usually mediated by immunoglobulin E antibodies and involves release of chemical mediators from mast cells and basophils. *Anaphylactoid reactions,* which are more common and less severe, are the result of direct release of these chemical mediators and are triggered by nonantigenic agents. Anaphylaxis or anaphylactoid reactions may occur after exposure to pollen, drugs, foreign serum, insect stings, diagnostic agents such as iodinated contrast materials or fluorescein, vaccines, local anesthetics, and food products. The most important parameter for predicting such an attack is a history of a previous allergic reaction to any other drug or possible antigen. Unfortunately, a history of known sensitivity may not always be elicited. Studies indicate that there has been an increase in anaphylaxis in recent years.

Anaphylaxis is particularly important to the ophthalmologist, in view of the increasing number of surgical procedures and fluorescein angiograms being performed in the office setting. It is estimated that allergic reactions to fluorescein (including urticaria) occur in up to 1% of all angiograms. In one survey, the overall risk of a severe reaction was 1 in 1900 patients, including a risk of respiratory compromise in 1 in 3800 subjects. If diaphoresis, apprehension, pallor, a rapid and weak pulse, or any combination thereof develops in a patient after administration of a drug, the patient should be considered to have an allergic reaction until proven otherwise. The diagnosis is certain if there is associated generalized itching, urticaria, angioedema of the skin, dyspnea, wheezing, or arrhythmia. This process may lead rapidly to loss of consciousness, shock, cardiac arrest, coma, or death.

Once an acute allergic reaction is suspected, prompt treatment is indicated:

- Oxygen should be administered to patients in respiratory distress.
- Epinephrine (0.3 mL of 1:1000 solution) injected intramuscularly in a limb opposite to the antigenic agent exposure site is usually effective to maintain circulation and blood pressure.
- IV volume expansion may be necessary to restore and maintain tissue perfusion. Methylprednisolone should be administered for serious or prolonged reactions. When given early, corticosteroids help control possible long-term sequelae.
- Antihistamines are helpful in slowing or halting the ongoing allergic response but are of limited value in acute anaphylaxis.
- Tracheotomy or cricothyrotomy is indicated when laryngeal edema is unresponsive to the previous methods or when oral intubation cannot be performed.
- All patients with anaphylaxis or anaphylactoid reactions should be observed for at least 6 hours.

In cases of mild allergic reactions, the physician can give 25–50 mg of diphenhydramine hydrochloride orally or intramuscularly and observe the patient closely to determine whether further treatment is necessary. Pretreating high-risk patients with an antihistamine, corticosteroids, or both prior to fluorescein angiography may reduce the risk of an allergic reaction. In all cases of anaphylaxis, supportive treatment should be maintained until the emergency medical team arrives.

For patients with a known history of anaphylaxis, personal emergency kits containing epinephrine are available and can be used until medical help arrives. The kits are designed to allow self-treatment by the patient or administration by a family member or an informed bystander. One commercially available allergy kit contains a syringe and needle preloaded with 0.6 mL of 1:1000 epinephrine. The physician who prescribes this kit must give detailed instructions concerning the use of the device. Epinephrine auto-injectors are also available. Each contains a spring-loaded automatic injector, which does not permit graduated doses to be given but automatically injects 0.3 mg of epinephrine (0.15 mg in the pediatric version) when the device is triggered by pressure on the thigh. The epinephrine ampules contained in these self-treatment kits have a limited shelf life and should be replaced when the expiration date is reached or if the solution becomes discolored. Any person given epinephrine requires 4–6 hours of observation to ensure that there is no rebound effect. Novel treatments for allergic reactions include sublingual immunotherapy, in which the patient is exposed to the offending antigen via the gastrointestinal system to improve tolerance.

Dellinger RP, Levy MM, Rhodes A, et al. Surviving Sepsis Campaign: international guidelines for management of severe sepsis and septic shock, 2012. *Intensive Care Med.* 2013;39(2):165–228.

Jones AE, Puskarich MA. The Surviving Sepsis Campaign guidelines 2012: update for emergency physicians. *Ann Emerg Med.* 2014;63(1):35–47.

Seizures and Status Epilepticus

A *seizure* is a paroxysmal episode of abnormal electrical activity in the brain, resulting in involuntary transient neurologic, motor activity, behavioral, or autonomic dysfunction. Typically, seizures are divided into 2 major categories, partial and generalized. Although seizures can present with many different clinical manifestations, most fit into the subcategories of simple partial, complex partial, or generalized tonic–clonic. See Chapter 11 for detailed discussion of these categories.

Status epilepticus is defined as a prolonged seizure (30 minutes or longer) or as multiple seizures without intervening periods of normal consciousness. Status epilepticus, like seizures, may have a local onset with secondary generalization or may be generalized from onset. This condition often occurs concomitantly with hyperthermia, acidosis, hypoxia, tachycardia, hypercapnia, and mydriasis and, if persistent, may be associated with irreversible brain injury. Status epilepticus that is completely stopped within 2 hours usually has relatively minor morbidity compared with episodes lasting longer than 2 hours.

Major causes of seizures and status epilepticus include

- drug withdrawal, such as from anticonvulsants, benzodiazepines, barbiturates, or alcohol
- metabolic abnormalities, such as hypoglycemia, hyponatremia, hypocalcemia, or hypomagnesemia
- conditions that affect the CNS, such as infection, trauma, stroke, hypoxia, ischemia, or sleep deprivation
- toxic levels of various drugs

Emergency *medical* management of seizures is best left to physicians who perform this routinely. However, there are some general considerations in the treatment of seizures that the clinician should be aware of. The first consideration is now maintenance of circulation. Airway maintenance, which used to be the first consideration, is the second consideration. Maintenance of circulation becomes particularly important if the seizure progresses to status epilepticus.

In management, it is important not only to stop the seizure activity but also to identify and treat the underlying cause when possible. Additional steps are to note the time of seizure onset, monitor and maintain an airway, and monitor vital signs. Activation of the emergency response (911) team is indicated in all cases of acute seizure onset. In the setting of an ophthalmology office, it may be appropriate to check blood glucose levels, as many seizure patients have diabetes mellitus.

Refractory cases of status epilepticus have responded successfully to repeated electroconvulsive therapy sessions, IV sedatives such as ketamine or propofol, surgical ablation and stimulation procedures, and topiramate and levetiracetam.

Riviello JJ Jr, Claassen J, LaRoche SM, et al. Treatment of status epilepticus: an international survey of experts. *Neurocrit Care.* 2013;18(2):193–200.

Toxic Reactions to Local Anesthetic Agents and Other Drugs

Toxic overdose can cause acute distress and unconsciousness. Clinicians should be prepared to respond to this emergency whenever a patient is undergoing a procedure that requires local anesthesia. Table 16-2 lists commonly used local anesthetics with their maximum safe dose.

Reactions following administration of local anesthetics are almost always toxic and only rarely allergic. A high blood level of local anesthetic can be produced by the following: too large a dose, unusually rapid absorption (including inadvertent administration directly into a vein), and unusually slow detoxification or elimination (especially in liver disease). Though rare, hypersensitivity (ie, decreased patient tolerance) and idiosyncratic reactions to local anesthetic agents may occur, as with any drug. True allergic or anaphylactic reactions are also uncommon but may occur, particularly with agents belonging to the amino ester class (eg, tetracaine).

Toxic reactions cause overstimulation of the CNS, which may lead to excitability, restlessness, apprehension, disorientation, tremors, and convulsions (cerebral cortex effects), as well as nausea and vomiting (medulla effects). Cardiac effects initially include tachycardia and hypertension. Ultimately, depression of the CNS and the cardiovascular system occurs, which may result in drowsiness or coma (cerebral cortex effects), as well as in irregular respirations, sighing, dyspnea, and respiratory arrest (medulla effects). Cardiac effects of CNS depression are bradycardia and hypotension.

Table 16-2 Maximum Recommended Local Anesthetic Doses

Agent	Commercially Available Concentrations (%) 1% = 10 mg/mL	Plain Solutions, mg	Epinephrine-Containing Solutions, mg
Chloroprocaine	1.0, 2.0, 3.0	800	1000
Lidocaine	0.5, 1.0, 1.5, 2.0, 4.0, 5.0	300	500
Mepivacaine	1.0, 1.5, 2.0	300	225
Bupivacaine	0.25, 0.5, 0.75	175	225
Tetracaine	1.0	100	100

Injected local anesthetic can have a direct toxic effect on muscle tissue. In the case of peribulbar or retrobulbar injections, this can result in muscle weakness, which in some patients is followed by muscle contracture. Extraocular motility can be affected, resulting in diplopia (usually hypertropia) that may require surgical revision. Hyaluronidase may be partially protective by allowing more rapid diffusion of the anesthetic agent following injection.

Increased metabolic activity of the CNS and poor ventilation can lead to cerebral hypoxia. Treatment consists of oxygenation, supportive airway care, and titrated IV administration of midazolam, which is used to suppress cortical stimulation.

Other emergency procedures that must be applied in cases of toxic overdose include suctioning if vomiting occurs, and using a taped tongue blade if convulsions develop. If shock develops, the appropriate drugs can be administered by IV infusion.

The addition of *epinephrine* to the local anesthetic can also cause adverse reactions. Reactions to epinephrine can produce symptoms similar to those of early CNS overstimulation by local anesthetic, such as anxiety, restlessness, tremor, hypertension, and tachycardia. Unlike local anesthetic toxicity, however, epinephrine overdose does not produce convulsions or bradycardia as the toxic reaction proceeds. Oxygen is useful in the treatment of epinephrine overdoses.

The administration of retrobulbar *bupivacaine* has been associated with respiratory arrest. This reaction may be caused by intra-arterial injection of the local anesthetic, with retrograde flow to the cerebral circulation. It can also result from puncture of the dural sheath of the optic nerve during retrobulbar block, with diffusion of the local anesthetic along the subdural space in the midbrain. A large prospective study comparing retrobulbar injection of 0.75% bupivacaine plus 2.0% lidocaine to 0.75% bupivacaine plus 4.0% lidocaine found that patients receiving 4.0% lidocaine mixed with bupivacaine had an almost 9 times greater risk of respiratory arrest than patients receiving 2.0% lidocaine mixed with bupivacaine.

The use of IV *edrophonium chloride* in the diagnosis of myasthenia gravis can have toxic adverse effects. The signs and symptoms result from cholinergic stimulation and may include nausea, vomiting, diarrhea, sweating, increased bronchial and salivary secretions, muscle fasciculations and weakness, and bradycardia. Some of these signs may be transient and self-limited because of the very short half-life of IV edrophonium. However, whenever the test is to be performed, a syringe containing 0.5 mg of atropine sulfate must be immediately available. (Some physicians routinely pretreat with atropine all patients undergoing such testing.)

If signs of excess cholinergic stimulation occur, 0.5 mg of atropine sulfate should be administered intravenously. This dose may be repeated every 3–10 minutes if necessary. The total dose of atropine necessary to counteract the toxic effects is seldom more than 2 mg. If toxic signs progress, the treatment described earlier for toxic overdose may be necessary.

Guo S, Wagner R, Gewirtz M, et al. Diplopia and strabismus following ocular surgeries. *Surv Ophthalmol.* 2010;55(4):335–358.

Moorthy SS, Zaffer R, Rodriguez S, Ksiazek S, Yee RD. Apnea and seizures following retrobulbar local anesthetic injection. *J Clin Anesth.* 2003;15(4):267–270.

Ocular Adverse Effects of Systemic Medications

Because of the development of medical specialties and the proliferation of specific therapeutic agents, patients frequently have multiple simultaneous drug regimens. Often, no single physician is aware of all the drugs the patient is taking. The clinical problem is compounded by several factors. The physician may not be familiar with drugs used outside his or her specialty. In addition, the patient may have a drug interaction that affects a bodily system not usually monitored by the specialist. Finally, the patient might not associate a symptom with a particular drug that has been used, if that symptom is not related to the system for which the drug was given. The advent of electronic medical records has helped physicians deal with the multiple drug regimens but has not eliminated the problem.

The effects of some systemic drugs are widely known. For example, the commonly prescribed erectile dysfunction agent sildenafil has been noted to block photoreceptor signals, causing electroretinographic changes, visual disturbances (including changes in color perception), and increased light sensitivity. The spectrum of systemic side effects of commonly used ophthalmic drugs is covered extensively elsewhere in this series (see BCSC Section 9, *Intraocular Inflammation and Uveitis,* and Section 10, *Glaucoma*). The ocular adverse effects of several commonly prescribed systemic medications are presented in Table 16-3. Drug interactions are always a concern in patients who use multiple topical and systemic medications.

The ophthalmologist can minimize adverse effects from multiple-drug therapy by doing the following:

- Maintain a high level of suspicion for drug interactions.
- Question the patient closely about other drug therapy and general symptoms.
- Encourage all patients to carry a card listing the drugs they use.
- Keep in close communication with the patient's primary care physician.
- Consult with a clinical pharmacologist or internist whenever a question of drug interaction arises.
- Utilize resources provided through electronic medical records. For example, some electronic medical record systems link to pharmacy records.

Unrecognized adverse effects of topical or systemic medications should be reported to the National Registry of Drug-Induced Ocular Side Effects at

Casey Eye Institute - National Registry of Drug-Induced Ocular Side Effects
OHSU Foundation
Mailstop 45
PO Box 4000
Portland, OR 97208-9852
Fax: 503-494-4286

Members of the American Academy of Ophthalmology (AAO) can access this database free of charge at www.eyedrugregistry.com. This website also provides an AAO annual

Table 16-3 Potential Ocular Adverse Effects of Popular Drugs

Drug	Adverse Effects
Antibiotics	
Cefaclor	Mild inflammation of ocular surface (rare); eyelid problems; nystagmus; visual hallucinations
Cefuroxime axetil	Mild inflammation of ocular surface (rare)
Ciprofloxacin	Eyelid problems; exacerbation of myasthenia; visual sensations; retinal detachment
Moxifloxacin (oral)	Iris transillumination; sphincter paralysis, retinal detachment
Rifampin	Conjunctival hyperemia; exudative conjunctivitis; increased lacrimation
Tetracycline, doxycycline, minocycline	Papilledema secondary to IIH; transient myopia; blue-gray, dark blue, or brownish pigmentation of the sclera; hyperpigmentation of eyelids or conjunctiva; diplopia
Antidepressants/anxiolytics	
Alprazolam	Diplopia; decreased or blurred vision; decreased accommodation; abnormal extraocular muscle movements; allergic conjunctivitis
Fluoxetine	Blurred vision; photophobia; mydriasis; dry eye; conjunctivitis; diplopia
Imipramine	Decreased vision; decreased accommodation; slight mydriasis; photosensitivity
Antiepileptics	
Topiramate	Conjunctivitis; abnormal accommodation; photophobia; strabismus; mydriasis; anterior uveitis; acute myopia; anterior chamber shallowing; secondary angle-closure glaucoma (bilateral); visual field defects; suprachoroidal effusions
Analgesics, anti-inflammatory drugs	
Aspirin	Transient blurred vision; transient myopia; hypersensitivity reactions
Ibuprofen	Blurred vision; decreased vision; diplopia; photosensitivity; dry eyes; decrease in color vision; optic or retrobulbar neuritis
Hydroxychloroquine	Retinopathy (bull's-eye maculopathy), with decreased vision and color perception
Naproxen	Decreased vision; changes in color vision; optic or retrobulbar neuritis; papilledema secondary to IIH; photosensitivity; corneal opacities
Disease-modifying agents	
Bisphosphonates	Anterior uveitis; conjunctivitis; scleritis; blurred vision
Interferon	Cotton-wool spots
Isotretinoin	Corneal opacities; night blindness; decreased color vision; sicca syndrome; papilledema
Asthma, allergy drugs	
Antihistamines	Decreased vision; may induce or aggravate dry eye; pupillary changes; decreased accommodation; blurred vision; decreased mucoid or lacrimal secretions; diplopia
Corticosteroids	Decreased vision; posterior subcapsular cataracts; increased intraocular pressure

(Continued)

Table 16-3 *(continued)*

Drug	Adverse Effects
Cardiovascular drugs	
Amiodarone	Photophobia; blurred vision; corneal deposits; anterior subcapsular lens opacities; optic neuropathy
β-Blockers	Decreased vision; dry eye syndrome; visual hallucinations; decreased intraocular pressure; decreased lacrimation
Selective α_{1a} antagonists	Intraoperative floppy iris syndrome (IFIS), with a sluggish hypotonic iris, miosis, iris prolapse
Calcium channel blockers	Decreased or blurred vision; periorbital edema; ocular irritation (general)
Captopril, enalapril	Angioedema of the eye and orbit; conjunctivitis; decreased vision
Digitalis glycosides	Decreased vision; color vision defects; glare phenomenon; flickering vision
Diuretics (thiazide-type)	Decreased vision; myopia; color vision abnormalities; retinal edema
Flecainide	Blurred vision; decreased vision; decreased accommodation; abnormal visual sensations; decreased depth perception; nystagmus
Warfarin	Retinal hemorrhages in susceptible persons; hyphema; allergic reactions; conjunctivitis; lacrimation; decreased vision
Drugs used in the treatment of impotence	
Sildenafil Tadalafil	Possible retinal vascular occlusions; decreased color perception; conjunctivitis; photophobia
Hormones, hormone-related drugs	
Clomiphene	Visual sensations; decreased vision; mydriasis; visual field constriction; photophobia; diplopia
Danazol	Decreased vision; diplopia; papilledema secondary to IIH; visual field defects
Estradiol	Decreased vision; retinal vascular disorders; papilledema secondary to IIH; fluctuations of corneal curvature and corneal steepening; color vision abnormalities
Leuprolide	Blurred vision; papilledema secondary to IIH; retinal hemorrhage and branch vein occlusion; eye pain; eyelid edema
Oral contraceptives	Decreased vision; retinal vascular disorders; papilledema secondary to IIH; color vision abnormalities
Tamoxifen	Decreased vision; corneal deposits; retinal edema or hemorrhage; papilledema; retinopathy; decreased color vision; optic neuritis or neuropathy

IIH = idiopathic intracranial hypertension.

meeting syllabus, entitled "Drug-Related Adverse Effects of Clinical Importance to the Ophthalmologist."

Fraunfelder FT, Fraunfelder FW, Chambers WA. *Clinical Ocular Toxicology: Drug-Induced Ocular Side Effects.* Philadelphia: Elsevier/Saunders; 2008.

The authors would like to thank Courtland Keteyian, MD, for his contribution to this chapter.

Basic Texts

General Medicine

Advanced Cardiovascular Life Support Provider Manual. Dallas: American Heart Association; 2011.

Bonow RO, Mann DL, Zipes DP, Libby P, eds. *Braunwald's Heart Disease: A Textbook of Cardiovascular Medicine.* 9th ed. Philadelphia: Elsevier/Saunders; 2012.

Bope ET, Kellerman RD, eds. *Conn's Current Therapy 2014.* Philadelphia: Elsevier/Saunders; 2013.

Cush JJ, Kavanaugh AF, Stein CM. *Rheumatology: Diagnosis and Therapeutics.* 2nd ed. Philadelphia: Lippincott Williams & Wilkins; 2004.

DeVita VT Jr, Lawrence TS, Rosenberg SA, DePinho RA, Weinberg RA, eds. *DeVita, Hellman, and Rosenberg's Cancer: Principles and Practice of Oncology.* 9th ed. Philadelphia: Lippincott Williams & Wilkins; 2011.

Firestein GS, Budd RC, Gabriel SE, McInnes IB, O'Dell JR, eds. *Kelley's Textbook of Rheumatology.* 9th ed. Philadelphia: Elsevier/Saunders; 2013.

Godara H, Hirbe A, Nassif M, Otepka H, Rosenstock A, eds. *The Washington Manual of Medical Therapeutics.* 34th ed. Philadelphia: Lippincott Williams & Wilkins; 2013.

Goetz CG, ed. *Textbook of Clinical Neurology.* 3rd ed. Philadelphia: Elsevier/Saunders; 2007.

Goldman L, Schafer AI, eds. *Goldman's Cecil Medicine.* 24th ed. Philadelphia: Elsevier/Saunders; 2012.

Ham RJ, Sloane PD, Warshaw GA, Potter JF, Flaherty E, eds. *Ham's Primary Care Geriatrics.* 6th ed. Philadelphia: Elsevier/Saunders; 2014.

Longo DL, Fauci AS, Kasper DL, Hauser SL, Jameson JL, Loscalzo J, eds. *Harrison's Principles of Internal Medicine.* 18th ed. New York: McGraw-Hill; 2012.

Mandell GL, Bennett JE, Dolin R, eds. *Mandell, Douglas, and Bennett's Principles and Practice of Infectious Diseases.* 7th ed. Philadelphia: Elsevier/Churchill Livingstone; 2010.

McGill JB, Henderson KE, Clutter WE, Baranski TJ, eds. *The Washington Manual Endocrinology Subspecialty Consult.* 3rd ed. Philadelphia: Lippincott Williams & Wilkins; 2012.

Melmed S, Polonsky KS, Larsen PR, Kronenberg HM, eds. *Williams Textbook of Endocrinology.* 12th ed. Philadelphia: Elsevier/Saunders; 2011.

Miller RD, Eriksson LI, Fleisher LA, Wiener-Kronish JP, Young WL, eds. *Miller's Anesthesia.* 7th ed. Philadelphia: Elsevier/Churchill Livingstone; 2009.

Moore DP, Jefferson JW. *Handbook of Medical Psychiatry.* 2nd ed. Philadelphia: Elsevier/Mosby; 2004.

Papadakis M, McPhee SJ, eds. *Current Medical Diagnosis and Treatment 2014.* 53rd ed. New York: McGraw-Hill; 2013.

Porter RS, Kaplan JL, eds. *The Merck Manual of Diagnosis and Therapy.* 19th ed. Whitehouse Station, New Jersey: Merck Sharp & Dohme Corp; 2011.
Ropper AH, Samuels MA, Klein JP, eds. *Adams and Victor's Principles of Neurology.* 10th ed. New York: McGraw-Hill; 2014.
Volberding PA, Sande MA, Lange J, Greene WC, Gallant JE, eds. *Global HIV/AIDS Medicine.* Philadelphia: Elsevier/Saunders; 2008.

Related Academy Materials

The Academy is dedicated to providing a wealth of high-quality clinical education resources for ophthalmologists.

Print Publications and Electronic Products

For a complete listing of Academy products related to topics covered in this BCSC Section, visit our online store at http://store.aao.org/clinical-education/topic/comprehensive-ophthalmology.html. Or call Customer Service at 866.561.8558 (toll free, US only) or +1 415.561.8540, Monday through Friday, between 8:00 AM and 5:00 PM (PST).

Online Resources

Visit the Ophthalmic News and Education (ONE®) Network at www.aao.org/clinical-education to find relevant videos, online courses, journal articles, practice guidelines, self-assessment quizzes, images and more. The ONE Network is a free Academy-member benefit.

Access free, trusted articles and content with the Academy's collaborative online encyclopedia, EyeWiki, at www.aao.org/eyewiki.

Requesting Continuing Medical Education Credit

The American Academy of Ophthalmology is accredited by the Accreditation Council for Continuing Medical Education to provide continuing medical education for physicians.

The American Academy of Ophthalmology designates this enduring material for a maximum of 10 *AMA PRA Category 1 Credits*™. Physicians should claim only the credit commensurate with the extent of their participation in the activity.

The American Medical Association requires that all learners participating in activities involving enduring materials complete a formal assessment before claiming continuing medical education (CME) credit. To assess your achievement in this activity and ensure that a specified level of knowledge has been reached, a posttest for this Section of the Basic and Clinical Science Course is provided online. A minimum score of 80% must be obtained to pass the test and claim CME credit.

To take the posttest and request CME credit online:

1. Go to www.aao.org/cme-central and log in.
2. Click on "Claim CME Credit and View My CME Transcript" and then "Report AAO Credits."
3. Select the appropriate Academy activity. You will be directed to the posttest.
4. Once you have passed the test with a score of 80% or higher, you will be directed to your transcript. *If you are not an Academy member, you will be able to print out a certificate of participation once you have passed the test.*

CME expiration date: June 1, 2018. *AMA PRA Category 1 Credits*™ may be claimed only once between June 1, 2015, and the expiration date.

For assistance, contact the Academy's Customer Service department at 866-561-8558 (US only) or +1 415-561-8540 between 8:00 AM and 5:00 PM (PST), Monday through Friday, or send an e-mail to customer_service@aao.org.

Study Questions

Please note that these questions are not part of your CME reporting process. They are provided here for your own educational use and identification of any professional practice gaps. The required CME posttest is available online (see "Requesting CME Credit"). Following the questions are a blank answer sheet and answers with discussions. Although a concerted effort has been made to avoid ambiguity and redundancy in these questions, the authors recognize that differences of opinion may occur regarding the "best" answer. The discussions are provided to demonstrate the rationale used to derive the answer. They may also be helpful in confirming that your approach to the problem was correct or, if necessary, in fixing the principle in your memory. The Section 1 faculty thanks the Self-Assessment Committee for reviewing these self-assessment questions.

1. A power calculation is performed before a clinical study for what purpose?
   a. to determine the chance of changing clinical practice with a proven hypothesis
   b. to determine the sample size required to evaluate a predicted difference in outcome
   c. to determine the statistical significance of measured differences in outcome
   d. to determine the proper study design to test the hypothesis

2. An organizational framework to improve clinical quality should include which component?
   a. identifying the team member who is limiting quality
   b. understanding the process of care
   c. determining whether the outcomes of care are being measured
   d. providing one-time feedback to the group of interest

3. Which of the following studies demonstrated reduced complications with intensive glycemic control in patients with type 2 diabetes mellitus?
   a. Diabetes Prevention Program
   b. United Kingdom Prospective Diabetes Study (UKPDS)
   c. Diabetes Control and Complications Trial (DCCT)
   d. Action to Control Cardiovascular Risk in Diabetes (ACCORD)

4. What combination of laboratory tests is recommended in screening for thyroid dysfunction?
   a. TSH alone
   b. TSH, free T_3
   c. TSH, free T_4
   d. TSH, T_4

5. What recommendation do the Eighth Joint National Committee (JNC 8) guidelines provide for the treatment of hypertension in the general population aged 60 years or older?
   a. goal of <120 mm Hg for systolic blood pressure (SBP) and ≤80 mm Hg for diastolic BP (DBP)
   b. goal of <150 mm Hg for SBP and/or <90 mm Hg for DBP
   c. goal of <140 mm Hg for SBP and ≤90 mm Hg for DBP
   d. goal of <160 mm Hg for SBP and/or ≤80 mm Hg for DBP

6. Prophylactic implantable cardioverter-defibrillators are indicated treatment for which of the following patient groups?
   a. patients with chronic atrial fibrillation
   b. patients who have survived an episode of hemodynamically unstable ventricular tachycardia
   c. patients not expected to survive more than 6 months regardless of treatment
   d. patients without inducible ventricular arrhythmias on electrophysiologic testing

7. What finding would meet one of the stated criteria for the diagnosis of metabolic syndrome?
   a. male with a fasting glucose level of 99 mg/dL
   b. female with a high-density-lipoprotein (HDL) level of 53 mg/dL
   c. male with blood pressure of 128/82 mm Hg
   d. female with a waist circumference of 36 in

8. The risk of myopathy from the use of simvastatin is increased if the patient is also taking which medication?
   a. metoprolol
   b. aspirin
   c. gemfibrozil
   d. clopidogrel

9. A 55-year-old male patient in the emergency department has crushing chest pain and elevated levels of serum cardiac-specific troponins; the electrocardiogram shows ST-segment depression. Which diagnosis is the most likely?
   a. unstable angina
   b. non–ST-segment elevation myocardial infarction (NSTEMI)
   c. ST-segment elevation MI (STEMI)
   d. costochondritis

10. The patient discussed in the previous question undergoes reperfusion therapy with placement of a drug-eluting stent. What additional medical therapy is recommended?
    a. aspirin as the sole anticoagulant
    b. avoidance of metoprolol
    c. use of captopril or lisinopril
    d. continued cigarette smoking

11. What is the only antiplatelet agent that has been shown to be effective in early treatment of ischemic stroke?
    a. heparin
    b. clopidogrel
    c. aspirin
    d. dipyridamole

12. What is an example of a restrictive lung disease?
    a. cystic fibrosis
    b. idiopathic pulmonary fibrosis
    c. chronic bronchitis
    d. emphysema

13. What is a common β_2-agonist used in the treatment of asthma?
    a. ipratropium bromide
    b. theophylline
    c. cromolyn sodium
    d. salmeterol

14. What condition is associated with obstructive sleep apnea syndrome?
    a. Fuchs dystrophy
    b. nonarteritic anterior ischemic optic neuropathy
    c. entropion
    d. idiopathic central serous chorioretinopathy

15. What is the best screening test for paroxysmal nocturnal hemoglobinuria?
    a. Ham test
    b. serum haptoglobin
    c. flow cytometry
    d. sucrose hemolysis test

16. What is the most common inherited bleeding disorder?
    a. hemophilia A
    b. hemophilia B
    c. von Willebrand disease
    d. Osler-Weber-Rendu disease

17. What immunosuppressant medication should be considered as a last option in a 15-year-old female with diabetes mellitus and bilateral, vision-threatening HLA-B27-associated panuveitis?
    a. methotrexate
    b. infliximab
    c. corticosteroids
    d. cyclophosphamide

18. What is the most common type of thrombosis associated with antiphospholipid syndrome?
    a. deep venous thrombosis
    b. superficial thrombophlebitis
    c. pulmonary embolism
    d. renal vein thrombosis

19. What is a potential adverse effect of anticytokine drugs such as etanercept and infliximab?
    a. disc edema
    b. angle-closure glaucoma
    c. optic neuropathy
    d. increased risk of diabetes mellitus

20. An ophthalmologist suspects that an older patient who presents with hyphema has been abused. What is the first step in the care of this patient?
    a. Call the patient's primary care physician about the suspected abuse.
    b. Treat the suspected eye injury and address the nature of the injury on a follow-up examination, after obtaining further information from the family.
    c. Advise the caregiver to watch the patient for unstable balance and possible falls.
    d. Complete a written report promptly, document suspicious injuries, and report any suspicions to the appropriate authorities.

21. What are the possible features of a major depressive disorder in an elderly patient?
    a. temporal headache and jaw claudication
    b. unexplained bruises, black eyes, and fractures
    c. unexplained vision loss and loss of interest or pleasure in activities
    d. significant weight gain and night sweats

22. What are some of the hallmarks of schizophrenia?
    a. hallucinations, delusions, disorganized thinking
    b. persistent low mood and slowed thought processes
    c. elevated mood sufficiently severe to cause impairment in functioning
    d. disorientation or memory loss caused by any disease, drug, or trauma directly affecting the central nervous system

23. What are the features of a somatoform disorder?
    a. symptoms suggesting physical illness or injury with concurrent physical findings
    b. symptoms within the person's willful and purposeful control
    c. symptoms including a preoccupation with fear of having a serious disease
    d. symptoms concurrent with other psychiatric symptoms, such as hallucinations

24. According to the 2013 American Cancer Society guidelines, what is an acceptable option in screening for colorectal cancer in a 52-year-old patient?
    a. single fecal occult blood card completed in the physician's office
    b. CT colonography every 5 years
    c. colonoscopy every 15–20 years
    d. Barium swallow

25. According to the US Preventive Services Task Force, yearly prostate-specific antigen testing to screen for prostate cancer should be performed in which group of individuals listed below?
    a. all 30-year-old men
    b. all 55-year-old men
    c. 60-year-old men with a positive family history of prostate cancer
    d. 60-year-old men, with no discussion of risks and benefits

26. What is the most radiosensitive structure in the eye?
    a. retina
    b. optic nerve
    c. lens
    d. cornea

27. What was the first angiogenesis inhibitor approved for treatment of cancer in the United States?
    a. ranibizumab
    b. bevacizumab
    c. aflibercept
    d. pegaptanib

28. What is the standard antiviral treatment of cytomegalovirus (CMV) retinitis?
    a. ganciclovir implant
    b. valganciclovir and intravitreal ganciclovir or foscarnet
    c. nonsteroidal anti-inflammatory drugs (NSAIDs)
    d. oral acyclovir

29. Achilles tendon rupture is a potential adverse effect of what medication?
    a. azithromycin
    b. rifampin
    c. fluconazole
    d. ciprofloxacin

30. What is the appropriate treatment for ocular syphilis?
    a. moxifloxacin
    b. intramuscular injection of penicillin G
    c. intravenous penicillin G
    d. dapsone

31. The Universal Protocol of the Joint Commission focuses on what patient-safety recommendation?
    a. utilizing 2 patient identifiers
    b. employing proper hand hygiene
    c. using appropriate perioperative antibiotics
    d. avoiding wrong-site, wrong-procedure surgery

32. The risk of chronic obstructive pulmonary disease (COPD) is most effectively reduced with what intervention?
    a. weight loss
    b. exercise
    c. reduction of respiratory infections by hand washing
    d. smoking cessation

33. What is the most frequent cause of death of patients with shock?
    a. arrhythmia
    b. hypertension
    c. hypervolemia
    d. respiratory failure

Answer Sheet for Section 1 Study Questions

Question	Answer	Question	Answer
1	a b c d	18	a b c d
2	a b c d	19	a b c d
3	a b c d	20	a b c d
4	a b c d	21	a b c d
5	a b c d	22	a b c d
6	a b c d	23	a b c d
7	a b c d	24	a b c d
8	a b c d	25	a b c d
9	a b c d	26	a b c d
10	a b c d	27	a b c d
11	a b c d	28	a b c d
12	a b c d	29	a b c d
13	a b c d	30	a b c d
14	a b c d	31	a b c d
15	a b c d	32	a b c d
16	a b c d	33	a b c d
17	a b c d		

Answers

1. **b.** Before a clinical study is conducted, a power analysis is performed to measure the probability that the study will correctly reject the null hypothesis when it is false. Before conduction of a clinical study, a power calculation is used to determine the sample size required for studying a predicted difference in outcome. It can also be used to predict a minimum difference measurement in outcome based on a given sample size.
2. **b.** Many factors affect the quality of patient care. A determination of whether the outcomes of care are being measured should be part of the planning process, not the organizational framework. An organizational framework to improve clinical quality should provide continual, not one-time, feedback.
3. **b.** The United Kingdom Prospective Diabetes Study (UKPDS) showed that intensive glycemic control in type 2 diabetes reduced rates of retinopathy, nephropathy, and neuropathy. Similarly, the Diabetes Control and Complications Trial (DCCT) showed reduced complication rates in type 1 diabetes under strict glycemic control. The Action to Control Cardiovascular Risk in Diabetes (ACCORD) study raised concerns regarding intensive glucose control in patients with type 2 diabetes, given the increased risk of cardiovascular mortality suggested by the study results. The Diabetes Prevention Program demonstrated that moderate walking could reduce the risk of progression from impaired glucose tolerance to type 2 diabetes.
4. **c.** The American Thyroid Association recommends the combination of TSH and free T_4 in screening for thyroid dysfunction. The combination of free T_4 and sensitive TSH assays has a sensitivity of 99.5% and a specificity of 98.0%.
5. **b.** For the general population aged 60 years and older, JNC 8 guidelines recommend that the systolic blood pressure target be less than 150 mm Hg and/or the diastolic blood pressure less than 90 mm Hg.
6. **b.** If a patient is not expected to survive at least 1 year with good functional status, an implantable cardioverter-defibrillator (ICD) is not recommended under current American College of Cardiology/American Heart Association (ACC/AHA) guidelines. Survival and functional status are improved with an ICD in the setting of previous cardiac arrest, hemodynamically unstable ventricular tachycardia, or inducible ventricular arrhythmias on electrophysiologic testing. ICDs are not indicated for chronic atrial fibrillation.
7. **d.** Patients with the metabolic syndrome have 3 or more of the following: a decreased high-density-lipoprotein cholesterol (HDL-C) level (<40 mg/dL for men, <50 mg/dL for women), increased abdominal obesity (United States: >40-in waist circumference for men, >35 in for women), elevated triglyceride level (≥150 mg/dL), hypertension (blood pressure >130/85 mm Hg), and an elevated fasting glucose level (≥100 mg/dL). An elevated HDL-C level is generally a protective factor, reducing the risk of cardiovascular events.
8. **c.** Gemfibrozil, amiodarone, and some calcium channel blockers increase the risk of myopathy when taken in conjunction with simvastatin. Other fibric acid agents such as fenofibrate may be safely used in combination with a statin drug. Aspirin and β-blockers do not increase the risk of myopathy.

9. **b.** In non–ST-segment elevation myocardial infarction (NSTEMI), the electrocardiogram (ECG) typically shows ST-segment depression; in ST-segment elevation MI (STEMI) the ECG most often shows ST-segment elevation. A patient with costochondritis would not have the ECG or serum troponin findings, and elevated troponin levels would not occur in unstable angina.
10. **c.** An angiotensin-converting enzyme (ACE) inhibitor such as captopril or lisinopril is part of the medical regimen after myocardial infarction. Whenever possible, aspirin should be used in combination with a second antiplatelet agent for at least 1 year after placement of a drug-eluting stent. β-Blockers are recommended following an MI, and cigarette smoking should be avoided.
11. **c.** Although aspirin, clopidogrel, and aspirin/extended-release dipyridamole combination are acceptable drug choices for secondary stroke prevention, aspirin is the only antiplatelet agent that is effective in early treatment of ischemic stroke. Heparin and related agents are not effective in reduction of mortality or recurrent stroke in patients with cardioembolic or noncardioembolic stroke. In fact, these agents are associated with higher mortality and worse outcome.
12. **b.** Idiopathic pulmonary fibrosis is a restrictive lung disease. Cystic fibrosis, chronic bronchitis, and emphysema are obstructive lung diseases.
13. **d.** Salmeterol is a common long-acting β_2-agonist used in the treatment of asthma. Ipratropium bromide is an anticholinergic agent, theophylline is a xanthine derivative, and cromolyn sodium is a mast-cell stabilizer.
14. **b.** Nonarteritic anterior ischemic optic neuropathy (NAION) can be associated with obstructive sleep apnea syndrome. There is no proven association between obstructive sleep apnea syndrome and Fuchs dystrophy, entropion, or idiopathic central serous chorioretinopathy.
15. **c.** In the past, paroxysmal nocturnal hemoglobinuria (PNH) was diagnosed by indirect tests involving complement-mediated lysis of the PNH red blood cells. Currently, the best screening test is flow cytometry, which has largely replaced the classic sucrose hemolysis test and the Ham test.
16. **c.** Von Willebrand disease (vWD) is the most common inherited bleeding disorder: low levels of von Willebrand factor (vWF) are found in 1% of the population. vWD is an autosomal dominant disorder; mild disease is codominant, and more severe disease is recessive. Many women with vWF have significant menorrhagia, endometriosis, and postpartum hemorrhage. Hemophilia A and hemophilia B are X-linked disorders.
17. **d.** Corticosteroids are often used in the acute setting for patients with severe uveitis. Patients who are diabetic require close monitoring of blood glucose levels to prevent hyperglycemic episodes. Methotrexate and infliximab are frequently used, often in combination, to treat uveitis in the pediatric population. Cyclophosphamide is a potent immunosuppressive drug that, given its potential to cause sterility, is reserved for recalcitrant disease.
18. **a.** Deep venous thrombosis occurs in one-third of patients with antiphospholipid syndrome. In addition, arterial thrombosis, superficial thrombophlebitis, and pulmonary embolism can be seen.
19. **c.** Etanercept and infliximab have been associated with demyelinating disease and optic neuritis. The antiepileptic medication topiramate has been associated with acute angle-closure glaucoma. The newer atypical antipsychotic agents, such as olanzapine and clo-

zapine, may be associated with initiating or worsening diabetes mellitus. Cyclosporine has been associated with disc edema.

20. **d.** Complete a written report promptly, document any suspicious injuries, and report your suspicions to the appropriate authorities. The ophthalmologist may be the first physician to see an older patient who has been abused or neglected. The signs may be subtle, and early recognition is key. In the United States, the prevalence of elder maltreatment has been reported as 7.6%–10.0% of study participants and is estimated to affect 11.4% of adults older than 60 years.
21. **c.** Depressed mood, unexplained vision loss, and loss of interest or pleasure in activities can all be signs of a major depressive disorder in elderly persons. The ophthalmologist may conclude that further evaluation by the primary care physician is necessary. Unexplained bruises, black eyes, or fractures may be signs of elder abuse.
22. **a.** The hallmarks of schizophrenia include hallucinations, delusions, disorganized thinking, and "negative" symptoms such as emotional and cognitive blunting and social and occupational dysfunction. Motor disturbances range from uncontrolled, aimless activity to catatonic stupor, in which the patient may be immobile, mute, and unresponsive yet fully conscious. Repetitive, purposeless mannerisms and an inability to complete goal-directed tasks are also common. Patients may have other mental health conditions, such as depression or anxiety disorders, but these are not essential features of the disease.
23. **c.** Somatoform disorders are mental conditions characterized by symptoms suggesting physical illness or injury in the absence of physical findings or a known physiologic mechanism to account for the symptoms. The symptoms are considered to be outside the patient's voluntary control.
24. **b.** CT colonography every 5 years is an acceptable option in colorectal cancer screening. Three fecal occult blood cards completed at home and submitted are acceptable, as is a double-contrast barium enema or a colonoscopy at least every 10 years.
25. **c.** The risks and benefits of the prostate-specific antigen (PSA) test, as well as the risks associated with treatment, should be discussed with all men aged 50 years and older. Because of the risk of overdiagnosis and overtreatment, many medical societies now suggest yearly PSA testing only in high-risk patients, such as those with a strong family history.
26. **c.** The lens is the most radiosensitive structure in the eye, followed by the cornea, retina, and optic nerve.
27. **b.** Bevacizumab was approved by the US Food and Drug Administration for the treatment of colorectal cancer in 2004, and aflibercept was approved for the treatment of colorectal cancer in 2012. Ranibizumab and pegaptanib are not FDA-approved cancer treatments.
28. **b.** The current standard-of-care treatment of cytomegalovirus retinitis is valganciclovir and intravitreal ganciclovir or foscarnet. The ganciclovir implant is no longer in use, oral acyclovir is ineffective, and nonsteroidal anti-inflammatory drugs (NSAIDs) possess no antiviral properties.
29. **d.** Ciprofloxacin is a fluoroquinolone antibiotic that has been associated with Achilles tendon rupture, especially in elderly patients. Azithromycin carries a risk of QT interval prolongation, and rifampin can cause hepatotoxicity. Fluconazole is generally well tolerated.
30. **c.** The treatment for ocular syphilis is the same as that for neurosyphilis, which requires the use of intravenous penicillin G. The treatment of CNS-sparing syphilis is intramuscular

injection of penicillin G. Moxifloxacin and dapsone are not suitable alternatives to penicillin for the treatment of syphilis.

31. **d.** The Universal Protocol of the Joint Commission was created to address the continuing occurrence of wrong-site, wrong-procedure, and wrong-person surgery.
32. **d.** Smoking cessation is the single most effective intervention to reduce the risk of chronic obstructive pulmonary disease or slow its progression. Ophthalmologists should not underestimate the impact of discussing with their patients the harmful effects of smoking.
33. **d.** Failure of respiratory gas exchange is the most frequent single cause of death in patients with shock, so respiratory obstruction must be ruled out first. Oxygen is then given by mask; if respiratory movements are shallow, mechanical ventilation is necessary. Respiratory obstruction can be assumed if there is stridor with respiratory movements or if cyanosis persists even when adequate ventilatory techniques have been applied. A conscious patient in distress who cannot speak and who is developing cyanosis may be choking on food or a foreign body; the Heimlich maneuver has been shown to be an effective means of treatment.

Index

(*f* = figure; *t* = table)